Fundamentals of Medical
BACTERIOLOGY
and MYCOLOGY
for Students of Medicine
and Related Sciences

Fundamentals of Medical
BACTERIOLOGY
and MYCOLOGY
for Students of Medicine
and Related Sciences

QUENTIN N. MYRVIK, Ph.D.
Professor and Chairman
Department of Microbiology
The Bowman Gray School of Medicine
Wake Forest University
Winston-Salem, North Carolina

NANCY N. PEARSALL, Ph.D.
Assistant Professor of Microbiology
Department of Microbiology
University of Washington School of
  Medicine
Seattle, Washington

RUSSELL S. WEISER, Ph.D.
Professor of Immunology
Department of Microbiology
University of Washington School of
  Medicine
Seattle, Washington

LEA & FEBIGER 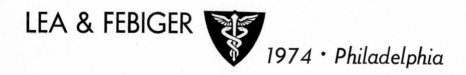 *1974 • Philadelphia*

Cover photograph: Electron micrograph of *Mycobacterium leprae* (negative stain: uranyl acetate $\times$ 200,000) showing a surface network of peptido-glycolipid filaments unique to bacteria of the genus *Mycobacterium*. This material is of singular biological interest since it is evidently the essential active constituent of tubercle bacilli that endows them with their strong adjuvanticity and their remarkable capacity to induce delayed hypersensitivity to associated protein antigens. (J. Gordon and R. G. White. Clin. and Exp. Immunol. *9*:539, 1971.)

Library of Congress Cataloging in Publication Data

Myrvik, Quentin N.   1921-
    Fundamentals of bacteriology and mycology.

    1. Bacteriology, Medical. 2. Medical mycology. I Pearsall, Nancy N., joint author. II. Weiser, Russell S., 1906-   joint author. III. Title. [DNLM: 1. Bacteriology. 2. Mycology. QW4 M998f 1974]
QR46.M97   616.01   74-2293
ISBN 0-8121-0423-4

Published in Great Britain by Henry Kimpton Publishers, London

PRINTED IN THE UNITED STATES OF AMERICA

Contributors:

Chapter 2

Dr. Stephen H. Richardson,
Professor of Microbiology,
Bowman Gray School of Medicine,
Winston-Salem, N.C.

Chapters 3 and 4

Dr. Henry Drexler,
Associate Professor of Microbiology,
Bowman Gray School of Medicine,
Winston-Salem, N.C.

Preface

THE tremendous additions to knowledge that continue to be made in the medical and allied sciences have placed an almost overwhelming burden on the students in these fields. This in turn has resulted in revolutionary changes in curricula involving revisions in both the subject matter taught and teaching methods. Faced with the dilemma of "so much to be taught and so little time to teach it" medical educators in particular have searched their souls (as has always been true of educators) in an effort to devise suitable curricula and improve teaching methods. This has resulted in "core curricula," "independent study," "integrated courses," "dropping of laboratory courses," "elective curricula," "pathway curricula," "no lecture-mechanical device teaching," and so on. Philosophies differ markedly, the pendulum is swinging and medical education is still in a state of great turmoil. It is hazardous, indeed, to speculate about what the medical student should know and be taught in order to best serve the public's medical needs. This makes it essentially impossible to develop texts that will satisfy the majority of instructors in any discipline in the medical sciences.

In designing this textbook, the second of three covering the areas of immunology and medical microbiology, we have adhered to the core concept with the goal of compiling a text having the attributes of being concise, up to date, instructive, and hopefully highly readable, challenging and stimulating. We realize that it is extremely difficult to achieve all of these objectives but we have tried to attain our goals in so far as possible. We believe that the three separate volumes, rather than one, augment our endeavor. Also these small texts are easily carried and used, are amenable to timely and frequent revisions, and, if so desired, only one or two may be used.

It has been our plan to emphasize basic principles and the why and wherefore. To challenge the reader we have occasionally engaged in prediction and philosophy. We have taken the view that the medical student profits most from texts in medical microbiology in which the greatest emphasis is placed on the fundamentals that determine the natural history of disease with special attention to mechanisms of pathogenesis and host resistance, especially at the cellular, biochemical and molecular levels; knowledge in these areas has the greatest predictive value with respect to the course and outcome of disease and best serves as the guide to diagnosis, therapy and research.

Medical perspectives have been stressed because we feel strongly that knowledge of the natural history and ravages of infectious diseases uninfluenced by the intervention of public health or medical practitioners is a highly important part of medical education. It is only with adequate perspectives that the medical student can fully understand an infectious disease and appreciate its potential hazards in the event of neglect or breakdown in sanitation or medical services or the mutational emergence of a new pathogen. The adage that "he who ignores history lives dangerously" is as true of infectious disease as any other area of human relations.

A special comment about omission of material on intermediary metabolism is in order. Since, in most medical schools, material on intermediary metabolism applicable to microbes is usually covered in biochemistry or in integrated courses in cell biology, it is given little attention in this text.

In the interest of brevity, we have chosen to present in some detail the most important pathogens of the various genera as models while giving brief attention to related pathogens of lesser importance.

As an introduction to the literature, selected references are presented at the end of each chapter. They consist of reviews and historical and recent references and are intended to provide the student with the opportunity of pursuing the subject in depth.

This text is not designed to meet the needs of advanced students in medical bacteriology and mycology or to serve as a reference book. It is primarily intended to serve students of medicine and related biological sciences. We sincerely hope that it will be of value to many who study in these fields.

Winston-Salem, North Carolina   QUENTIN N. MYRVIK
                                                       NANCY N. PEARSALL
Seattle, Washington   RUSSELL S. WEISER

Contents

Chapter 1

The Impact of Microbiology on the Health of Man

Among the major afflictions of man—famine, pestilence and war—the greatest progress has been made in controlling pestilence; in terms of lives saved, measures for controlling infectious diseases stand as the most important achievements in the history of medicine. Even more remarkable is the fact that essentially all of these achievements have been accomplished within the last century. No longer do pandemics of infectious diseases sweep continents with great destruction of life, such as occurred when the black plague crossed Europe in the early 14th century killing one-fourth or more of the population; no longer do chronic diseases such as syphilis and tuberculosis ravage populations on a worldwide basis, as in Koch's time in the 1880s when one of every three died of tuberculosis by middle age and no longer are certain acute infections, such as streptococcal meningitis, invariably fatal.

The great progress made in the control of infectious diseases stemmed from the discovery of bacteria by Anton van Leeuwenhoek in 1683—a man of great talent but modest means, whose hobby was microscopy. Leeuwenhoek presented the first reliable evidence of the existence of bacteria. He was a self-trained expert at lens grinding, and among the hundreds of single-lens microscopes he built many were superior to any others of his time, having effective resolution powers up to 300×. Although secretive about his techniques, which probably included some form of dark-field illumination, his scientific reports were voluminous and comprised some 200 letters to the Royal Society of London written over a period of many years. He examined essentially every conceivable object that struck his fancy from the hairs on a louse to the "beasties" or "animalcules" (small animals) in scrapings from his teeth. His discourses on the shapes and movements of various bacteria of the mouth were remarkably accurate; he described them as varying greatly in their movements, as being a million times smaller than the eye of a louse, and as being more numerous in a man's mouth than "all of the men in the kingdom." The only reward of his hobby was the reward of discovery; but what a reward it must have been, for he spent essentially every spare moment at his microscopes dur-

1

ing many years extending from 1660 until nearly the time of his death at the age of 91 years in 1723. He was elected to membership in the Royal Society of London, to which he bequeathed many of his microscopes, the remainder, some 247, being sold at auction for 61 pounds.

The germ theory of disease was proposed centuries before Leeuwenhoek's time (Varro, 116-26 B.C.; Columella, 60 B.C.) and was most clearly conceived by the illustrious poet-physician Gerolamo Fracastoro in 1546, who expressed the view that infection is transmitted by the tiniest of particles (*seminaria*) that we cannot perceive with our senses, *particulae minimae et insensibilis*. He envisioned infectious agents to be specific living organisms capable of multiplying and spreading within the body. Despite the fact that the germ theory was well documented in Fracastoro's book *De Contagione et Contagiosis Morbis* in 1547, the discovery of bacteria by Leeuwenhoek did not promptly spark the idea that these "animalcules" could be the causative agents of infectious disease. Instead microbiology languished for almost two centuries as a purely descriptive and abstract science literally awaiting the perfection of the compound microscope and the development of pure culture techniques. Other investigators had only limited success in confirming Leeuwenhoek's observations. It is unfortunate that he was so secretive about his "darkfield technique," for had he made it known to others, progress in bacteriology might have been greatly advanced. It is quite possible that with his technique the anthrax bacillus could have been detected in the blood of infected animals, a feat which was not accomplished until some two centuries later by Davaine with the aid of the compound microscope. Like all sciences, the history of microbiology is largely the history of breakthroughs in methodology and instrumentation; the perfection of the compound microscope was one such breakthrough.

For more than a century after Leeuwenhoek's time the attention of bacteriologists was focused principally on the theory of spontaneous generation of life. The world of "animalcules" remained the last stronghold for the proponents of spontaneous generation despite strong opposing evidence provided by the classical experiments of Spallanzani (1776) and Schwann (1836) on the preservative effects of heat treatment on organic materials. The much-investigated but unsettled question of spontaneous generation absorbed the early attentions of Louis Pasteur, whose experiments culminated in the famous concluding remarks of his Sorbonne lecture of 1864 in which he stated that his sterile medium did not become contaminated "because I have kept it sheltered from the only living thing that man does not know how to produce; from the germs which float in the air, from Life, for Life is a germ and a germ is Life. Never will the doctrine of spontaneous generation recover from the mortal blow of this simple experiment."

Although Pasteur is regarded as the father of experimental and theoretical microbiology, he was also a practical man intent on science serving mankind. He was an unusually vigorous, perceptive, and imaginative investigator, a chemist by training and a superb experimentalist. By well-designed and painstaking experiments he avoided the pitfalls which plagued most investigators of his day and thus was able to solve problem after problem rapidly. He settled the dispute about the role of yeast in alcoholic fermentation and established that different fermentations were carried out by different and specific microbes, each demanding particular cultural conditions for its growth and activities. He introduced autoclaving to destroy heat-resistant forms (spores) and devised liquid media for growing cultures. He was also the first to employ synthetic media and to discover microbes that could live without air (anaerobes). Pasteur's interests were unusually wide and ranged from "diseases of beer and wine" to diseases of plants, animals, and man. Through his work on pebrine of silkworms, anthrax of sheep, and spoilage of wine he came to be regarded as the savior of the silk, sheep, and wine industries of France. In view of his training, it is not surprising that his interests remained focused throughout his life on the biochemical activities of microbes and that he regarded animal diseases literally to represent fermentations in the animal body.

About 1880 Pasteur directed his attentions to antimicrobial immunity. Among his many contributions one of the most important was his discovery of the enduring principle that mutant strains of pathogens of attenuated virulence can be isolated and that they commonly make the best vaccines. In recognition of his successful development of rabies vaccine in 1885, many research institutes named in his honor were established throughout the world, the largest of which is the Institut Pasteur in Paris.

Another giant in the early history of microbiology was Robert Koch, a country doctor who abandoned the practice of medicine for a research career in an effort to gain new insight into the causes and nature of infectious diseases. His motivation for changing to a research career stemmed from his feeling of helplessness in dealing with human infections and is reflected in his statement "mothers come to me crying—asking me to save their babies, but what can I do?—grope, fumble, reassure them, when I know there is no hope. How can I cure diphtheria when I do not even know what causes it, when even the wisest doctor in Germany does not know." Koch's wife bought her husband a microscope so that he could test the dictates enunciated by Henle, his former professor, for determining the causative agents of infectious diseases. Koch soon grew the anthrax bacillus in pure culture, thus erasing any doubt that the organism was the sole cause of anthrax (1876). Six years and some 271 experiments later Koch reported his epoch-making discovery of the tubercle bacillus, the cause of tuberculosis.

Koch was a careful and tireless investigator who planned experiments with great ingenuity and carried them out with precision and skill. His

TABLE 1-1

Some Important Milestones in the Development of Medical Microbiology

Approximate Date	Principal Contributor(s)	Contribution(s)
1546	Fracastoro	Clearly enunciated the germ theory of disease, including modes of transmission and the development of specific acquired immunity.
1683	Leeuwenhoek	Gave the first accurate account of the visualization of yeasts and bacteria.
1798	Jenner	Introduced vaccination against smallpox with cowpox virus.
1835	Bassi	Showed that "animalcules" cause a transmissible fungal disease (muscardine) of silk worms.
1836-1837	Cagniard-Latour; Schwann	Clearly established that microbes (yeasts) are biochemically active (alcoholic fermentation).
1839	Schönlein	Showed that certain skin diseases are due to fungi.
1843-1847	Holmes; Semmelweis	Showed that physicians and attendants often transmit infectious disease from one patient to another and demonstrated the effectiveness of control procedures.
1849	Snow	Proved that cholera is waterborne and set forth the epidemiological principles of infectious diseases.
1850-1872	Davaine	First to observe bacteria clearly in tissues (blood) during infection (anthrax) and demonstrated increased virulence with animal passage.
1861-1885	Pasteur	Demonstrated that different kinds of bacteria have distinct biological activities and cultural needs. Demonstrated that some microbes can grow without oxygen. Disproved the theory of spontaneous generation. Introduced sterilization by steam under pressure. Proved the value of attenuated vaccines.
1870	Hansen	Observed *Mycobacterium leprae* in the tissues of lepers; this was the first time that bacteria were seen in human lesions.
1871	Weigert	Introduced successful methods for staining bacteria with aniline dyes.
1872	Cohn	Established the basis of systematic classification of bacteria.
1876-1883	Koch*	Observed the sporulation cycle of *Bacillus anthracis* and conclusively proved it to be the specific cause of anthrax. Introduced pure culture methods using solid media and perfected methods for staining bacteria. Discovered the tubercle bacillus and described delayed hypersensitivity to tuberculin. Set forth criteria for ascertaining the causative agents of infectious diseases (Koch's postulates).

TABLE 1-1 *(Continued)*
Some Important Milestones in the Development of Medical Microbiology

Approximate Date	Principal Contributor(s)	Contribution(s)
1878	Tyndall	Proved conclusively that microbes are associated with dust particles in air and that they consist of thermolabile (vegetative) and thermostable (spore) forms.
1878	Lister	Introduced the practice of antiseptic surgery; obtained the first pure cultures of bacteria by an *in vitro* method, extinction dilution.
1880-1883	Ogston	Established that wound suppuration is commonly caused by cocci of two types, cocci in clusters and cocci in chains; introduced the concept that systemic infection can arise by spread from localized infection.
1884	Chamberland	Introduced the bacterial filter; perfected the autoclave.
1884	Gram	Developed the Gram stain.
1884	Metchnikoff*	Introduced the concept that antimicrobial immunity is "cellular" and results from the activities of phagocytes.
1884-1886	Salmon and Theobald Smith	Introduced the use of killed vaccines.
1889	Roux and Yersin	Proved that bacterial toxin can account for the pathogenicity of an organism; e.g., *Corynebacterium diphtheriae*.
1890	H. Buchner	First to clearly enunciate the theory of humoral immunity.
1890	von Behring* and Kitasato	Discovered Abs (tetanus and diphtheria antitoxins).
1894	Pfeiffer	Described specific bacteriolysis by immune serum *in vitro* and *in vivo* (Pfeiffer phenomenon).
1894	Denys and Havet	Established that immune serum and phagocytes can act conjointly in antibacterial defense.
1895-1901	Bordet*	Conclusively established that specific Ab and "alexine" (later termed "complement") can lyse certain bacteria and mammalian cells and, with Gengou, developed the complement fixation test.
1896	Durham and Gruber	Provided the first clear and systematic description of specific bacterial agglutination.
1896	Widal	Introduced specific serodiagnosis of infectious diseases with his "Widal test" for typhoid fever.

TABLE 1-1 *(Continued)*
Some Important Milestones in the Development of Medical Microbiology

Approximate Date	Principal Contributor(s)	Contribution(s)
1896-1909	Ehrlich*	Introduced methods for standardizing toxins and antitoxins. Introduced the procedure of acid-fast staining. Set forth a theory of Ab production. Introduced chemotherapy (arsenicals for syphilis).
1897	E. Buchner*	Discovered the role of yeast zymase in alcoholic fermentation.
1897	Kraus	Developed the precipitin test for measuring the reaction of Abs with soluble Ags.
1898	Nocard, Roux, and associates	Discovered *Mycoplasma mycoides* (the cause of pleuropneumonia of cattle) the first of the Mycoplasma described.
1898	Beijerinck	Discovered filterable viruses (tobacco mosaic virus).
1903	Wright and Douglas	Discovered specific opsonization.
1905-1908	von Pirquet	Advanced the concept that allergy plays a major role in determining the lesions, symptoms, and course of infectious diseases.
1909	Ricketts	Discovered *Rickettsia rickettsii* (the cause of Rocky Mountain spotted fever) the first of the Rickettsiaceae described.
1913	Schick	Introduced the diphtheria toxin skin test (Schick test) for measuring immunity to diphtheria.
1915-1917	Twort; d'Herelle	Discovered bacteriophage.
1921-1925	Zinnser and associates	Provided evidence supporting the concept advanced earlier by von Behring that antimicrobial immunity and delayed hypersensitivity "are parallel and perhaps causally related phenomena."
1923	Ramon	Introduced the principle of converting toxin to a nontoxic immunizing agent, toxoid.
1922-1928	Fleming*	Discovered the bacteriolytic agent lysozyme. Discovered penicillin, the first antibiotic later used successfully for antibacterial chemotherapy.
1930-1937	Dienes and Schoenheit; Dienes and Edsall	Described the capacity of tubercle bacilli to direct the immune response of associated Ags toward the development of delayed hypersensitivity. First to recognize wall-less bacteria (formerly called L forms by Klieneberger-Nobel, 1935).

TABLE 1-1 *(Continued)*
Some Important Milestones in the Development of Medical Microbiology

Approximate Date	Principal Contributor(s)	Contribution(s)
1935	Boivin and Mesrobeanu	Discovered the endotoxins of gram-negative bacteria.
1935	Domagk*	Discovered Prontosil, the precursor of sulfanilamide, and ushered in the modern era of chemotherapy.
1934-1941	Ruska; Marton	Developed the electron microscope.
1937	Freund	Developed Freund's adjuvant mixture, a tubercle bacillus-water-in-oil mixture which enhances Ab production and "directs" the immune response toward the development of delayed hypersensitivity and cellular immunity.
1940	Florey*, Chain*, and colleagues	Purified penicillin and developed procedures for its production and use as a chemotherapeutic agent.
1942-1945	Landsteiner* and Chase; Chase	Accomplished passive transfer of delayed type hypersensitivity with lymphoid cells.
1944	S. A. Waksman* and associates	Discovered streptomycin, the first antibiotic effective against tuberculosis.
1944	Avery, MacLeod, and McCarty	Discovered genetic transformation of bacteria by DNA.
1952	Bruton	Presented the first example of an hereditary immunologic deficiency disease, sex-linked agammaglobulinemia.
1951-1953	Freeman; Groman	Discovered lysogenic conversion of bacteria by bacteriophage (toxin production by *C. diphtheriae*).
1952	Westphal and associates	Purified and determined the structure of endotoxin.
1957	Germuth and associates; Dixon and associates	Demonstrated that soluble Ag-Ab complexes can cause allergic injury.
1959	Watanabe	Discovered episomal transfer of multiple antibiotic resistance in bacteria.
1960	Shepard	Produced the first experimental infection with *M. leprae*, using the mouse footpad.
1962	Mackaness and associates	Demonstrated that lymphocytes are initiator cells and that macrophages are effector cells in specific antimicrobial cellular immunity.
1969	H. Muller-Eberhard	Made major contributions toward an understanding of the complexity and functions of the complement system.

*Recipients of Nobel Prize.

staining and improved pure culture methods permitted precise studies on the cultural characteristics of bacteria and conclusive establishment of organisms as the specific causative agents of disease according to his famous postulates (see Chapter 9). His agar plating technique for isolating pure cultures is routine to this day. As the result of epidemiological studies on waterborne disease, he proposed the use of sand filtration for purifying water supplies, a practice still in common use. Koch's pure cultural technique was so successful that the causative agents of most of the common bacterial diseases of man were discovered within the next two decades.

Since both Pasteur and Koch were men of great compassion, it is no surprise that they were attracted to the study of infectious disease, the greatest medical problem of their day.

With the recent development of techniques for purifying and handling macromolecules a new and promising area of research in medical microbiology has opened, the molecular aspects of pathogenesis of infectious diseases.

Space does not permit a detailed recounting of the many contributions that have played important roles in the development of medical microbiology. However, a limited list of key advances is presented in Table 1-1.

References

Avery, O. T., MacLeod, C. M., and McCarty, M.: Induction of transformation by a deoxyribonucleic acid fraction isolated from pneumococcus type. III. J. Exp. Med. *79*:137, 1944.

Bruton, O. C.: Agammaglobulinemia. Pediatrics *9*:722, 1952.

Chase, M. W.: The cellular transfer of cutaneous hypersensitivity to tuberculin. Proc. Soc. Exp. Biol. Med. *59*:134, 1945.

Dienes, L., and Schöenheit, E. W.: Certain characteristics of the infectious processes in connection with the influence exerted on the immunity response. J. Immunol. *19*:41, 1930.

Dienes, L., and Edsall, G.: Observations on the L-organisms of Klieneberger. Proc. Soc. Exp. Biol. Med. *36*:740, 1937.

Dixon, F. J.: Characterization of the antibody response. J. Cellular Comp. Physiol. *50*:27, 1957.

Dixon, F. J.: The role of antigen-antibody complexes in disease. The Harvey Lectures Series 58, 1962-63.

Fleming, A.: On a remarkable bacteriolytic element found in tissues and secretions. Proc. Roy. Soc. Ser. B *93*:306, 1922.

Fleming, A.: On the antibacterial action of cultures of a penicillium, with special reference to their use in the isolation of *B. influenzae*. Brit. J. Exp. Pathol. *10*:226, 1929.

Freeman, V. J.: Studies on the virulence of bacteriophage-infected strains of *Corynebacterium diphtheriae*. J. Bacteriol. *61*:675, 1951.

Freund, J., and McDermott, K.: Sensitization to horse serum by means of adjuvants. Proc. Soc. Exp. Biol. Med. *49*:548, 1942.

Florey, H. W., Chain, E., Heatley, N. G., Jennings, M. A., Sanders, A. G., Abraham, E. P., and Florey, M. E.: *Antibiotics*. Vol. I and II. London: Oxford Univ. Press, 1949.

Germuth, F. G., and McKinnon, G. E.: Studies on the biological properties of antigen-antibody complexes. Bull. Johns Hopkins Hosp. *101*:13, 1957.

Groman, N. B.: Evidence for the induced nature of the change from nontoxigenicity to toxigenicity in *Corynebacterium diphtheriae* as a result of exposure to specific bacteriophage. J. Bacteriol. *66*:184, 1953.

Landsteiner, K., and Chase, M. W.: Experiments on transfer of cutaneous sensitivity to simple compounds. Proc. Soc. Exp. Biol. Med. *49*:688. 1942.

von Luderitz, O., and Westphal, O.: Uber die chromatographie auf rundfiltern. Zeit. fur Natursforsch. G. *76*:136, 1952.

Mackaness, G. B.: The immunology of antituberculous immunity. Amer. Rev. Resp. Dis. *97*: 337, 1968.

Marton, L.: La microscopie electronique des objets biologiques. Bull. Acad. Roy. Belg. Cl. Sci. *20*:439, 1934.

Marton, L.: The electron microscope. J. Bacteriol. *41*:397, 1941.

Muller-Eberhard, H. J.: Complement. Ann. Rev. Biochem. *38*:389, 1969.

Nocard, E., Roux, E. R., Borrel, M., Salimbeni and Dujardin-Beaumetz: Le microbe de la peripneumonie. Ann. Inst. Pasteur *12*:240, 1898.

Von Pirquet, C.: Allergy. München Med. Wschr. *30*:1457, 1906.

Ricketts, H. T.: A microorganism which apparently has a specific relationship to Rocky Mountain spotted fever. J.A.M.A. *52*:379, 1909.

Ruska, E.: Uber fortschritte im bau und in der leistung des magnetischen elektronenmikroskops. (Aus dem Hochspannunginstitut Neubabelsberg der Technischen Hochschule Berlin). Z. Physik. *87*:580, 1934.

Shepard, C. C.: The experimental disease that follows the injection of human leprosy bacilli into footpads of mice. J. Exp. Med. *112*:445, 1960.

Watanabe, T.: Infective heredity of multiple drug resistance in bacteria. Bacteriol. Rev. *27*:87, 1963.

Watanabe, T., and Fukasawa, T.: "Resistance transfer factor," an episome in *Enterobacteriaceae*. Biochem. Biophys. Res. Comm. *3*:660, 1960.

Zinnser, H., and Mueller, J. H.: On the nature of bacterial allergies. J. Exp. Med. *41*:159, 1925.

Chapter 2

Biology of Bacteria

In this chapter special consideration will be given to the relationships between structure and function of pathogenic bacteria with particular emphasis on those properties which characterize them as pathogens. Of the thousands of microbes which have been described during the past 100 years relatively few cause serious health problems for man. Among the remaining microorganisms many play major roles in man's total environment by acting as essential cogs in the nitrogen, carbon, and sulfur cycles as well as serving as an integral part of the food web upon which all biological systems depend. Bacteria and fungi are employed extensively in food production and processing and in manufacturing; ironically in recent years microbes have served as the major source of the antibiotics whose effects have so markedly improved infectious disease management in the last 25 years.

Since the advent of biochemical genetics in the early 1940s, microorganisms, especially bacterial viruses, have provided valuable model systems for studying molecular genetics. For example, the great value of using bacterial cells as models for metabolic studies, regulatory functions, and virus-host interactions, is commonly accepted. Much of the information being accumulated with cultured mammalian cells is being obtained from studies similar to those which have used the common intestinal inhabitant *Escherichia coli.*

A. Common Characteristics of Bacteria

Organisms whose dimensions are 0.01 mm or less generally fall within the province of microbiology. However, most microbes have dimensions in the range of micrometers or nanometers. Except to draw parallels relative to specific structures or to point out differences in chemical composition, the present discussion will be largely limited to the bacteria with emphasis on those attributes which determine pathogenicity and the capacity of the host to resist infection.

Pathogenic bacteria are remarkably well suited to survive, grow, and replicate within the host. Being extremely small (about the size of the average-sized organelle in host cells), they are capable of unusually high growth rates. For example, a single cell of *E. coli* growing under ideal circumstances can reproduce itself in 20 minutes. This rapid rate of multiplication is attainable because in a cell of such small size the required nutrients and growth factors can diffuse with great speed to reach all sites within the cell, including the sites of macromolecular synthesis; consequently, the biosynthetic activities of bacterial cells are more efficient than those of cells of larger dimensions. A practical consequence of this rapid diffusion and high metabolic rate is that inhibitory substances, such as antibiotics, can enter extracellular bacteria more readily than neighboring host cells.

The unique biosynthetic prowess of bacteria can be at one and the same time an asset and a liability to them. For example, the ability of *Diplococcus pneumoniae* to produce specific polysaccharide capsules protects it from phagocytosis, whereas the unique composition and reactions involved in the synthesis of its cell wall have permitted man to develop antibiotics which can specifically inhibit cell-wall synthesis without harming host cells.

The bacteria and blue-green algae are *procaryotes*, whereas all other cells are *eucaryotes*. Eucaryotic cells are distinguished from procaryotic cells mainly on the basis of the complexity of their internal structure. They contain membrane-bound organelles such as nuclei and mitochondria and undergo true mitotic division. Procaryotic cells have a relatively simple internal structure with no comparable cytoplasmic organelles. Mitochondrial functions in procaryotic cells are localized in the cytoplasmic membrane while the remainder of the metabolic processes are structurally analogous to those found in eucaryotic cells.

The concept of the *procaryotic cell* as an entity distinct from the eucaryotic cell was relatively slow in its evolution. This was pimarily due to the limitations of the ordinary light microscope for studying bacteria. If bacteria are suspended in a drop of aqueous liquid for observation, very little can be learned with the light microscope other than rough approximations of their size, shape, and whether they are motile. This is because the cytoplasm of the average bacterial cell contains approximately 80% water and therefore differs little in refractive index from the surrounding medium. The other basic problem is that the maximum resolving power of the light microscope is limited to about 200 nm, which is approximately one-half the diameter of some of the smaller bacteria.

Introduction of routine staining procedures, such as the Gram stain and negative stain, and the development of pure culture techniques were major steps for defining bacteria in terms of size and shape. The Gram stain became the basis for differentiating bacteria into two large groups, the gram-positive and gram-negative bacteria. As will be pointed out in a later section in this chapter (4d), these tinctorial properties are only superficial manifestations of complex differences between the cell walls of these two major groups of bacteria.

B. Bacterial Morphology

The introduction and subsequent widespread use of the electron microscope in the late 1940s wrought a revolution in the study of bacterial ultrastructure. The electron microscope has a resolving power of 1 nm or less, which permits primary magnifications at least 300 times greater than the light microscope. The newest electron microscopes used in conjunction with subsequent photographic enlargement are capable of attaining magnifications of about one million thus allowing visualization of protein molecules.

The breakthrough in resolving the fine structure of bacteria came in the early 1950s with the development of thin-sectioning procedures capable of yielding sections of a thickness of 20 nm or less. Using these techniques it was possible to determine the fine structure of the bacterial cell for the first time. The usual internal organelles found in eucaryotic cells,

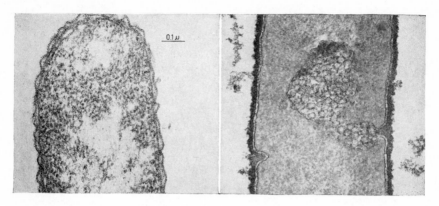

Figure 2-1. Thin-section electron micrographs of representative bacteria. (A) *Escherichia coli* (gram-negative); note the multilayered cell envelope. (B) *Bacillus subtilis* (gram-positive); the thick amorphous cell wall is adjacent to the cytoplasmic membrane. The vesicular invagination of the membrane is a mesosome. (Reprinted with permission from Bacteriol. Rev. *29*:299, 1965.)

such as a membrane-limited nucleus, mitochondria, and distinct endoplasmic reticulum are not evident in bacteria.

Electron micrographs of typical bacterial cells are presented in Figure 2-1. The most prominent structure of the gram-positive cell *Bacillus subtilis* is its amorphous cell wall. In contrast, the gram-negative bacterium *E. coli* has a more complex cell wall which is multilayered and exhibits elements of substructure. Immediately interior to the cell wall of both cells is a distinct cytoplasmic membrane with the trilaminar appearance typical of biological membranes. The cytoplasmic membrane of the gram-positive cell is invaginated and folded on itself within the cytoplasm to form a complex system of vesicles. These structures, called *mesosomes*, are commonly seen in gram-positive bacteria but are seldom observed in gram-negative species. The center of each cell is filled with lightly stained material which, on close inspection, can be seen to consist of a tightly packed bundle of intertwined fibers. This is the nuclear apparatus of the cell, and the fibers are double-stranded DNA. In rapidly growing cells more than one nucleus is often visible due to lack of synchrony between DNA replication and cell division.

A typical procaryotic cell which has been engulfed by a eurcaryotic cell, an alveolar macrophage, is shown in Figure 2-2. The relative degree of internal organization and the comparative sizes of the two types of cells are readily apparent.

1. Flagella

Some bacteria are motile; motility is due to long flexible appendages called *flagella*, which may originate from (1) one or both ends of the cell

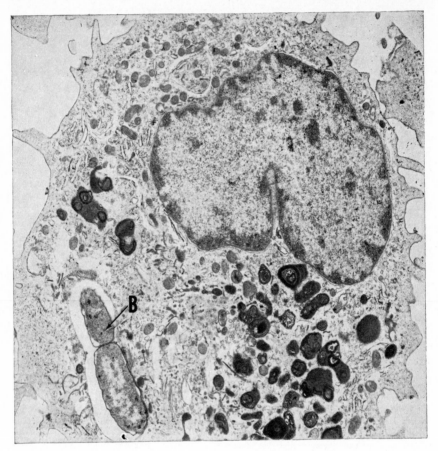

Figure 2-2. A dividing bacterium (B) engulfed by an alveolar macrophage. Compare the relatively simple internal structure and size of the bacteria with that of the surrounding organelles.

as a single element or as tufts or (2) at points around the entire cell surface (Fig. 2-3). Flagellation of the former type is referred to as *polar*; the latter as *peritrichous*. The presence and arrangement of flagella have been useful in taxonomy.

Flagella range from 3 to 10 μm in length and between 10 and 20 nm in diameter. Since the diameter is well below the resolving power of the light microscope, they cannot be seen with this instrument except by employing special stains which deposit a heavy precipitate around the flagella to increase their diameter. In some of the larger bacteria, flagella can be observed directly on living organisms by using a darkfield microscope. Much conjecture concerning the basic structure of flagella was ended when electron micrographs showed that they are composed of subunits arrayed in a

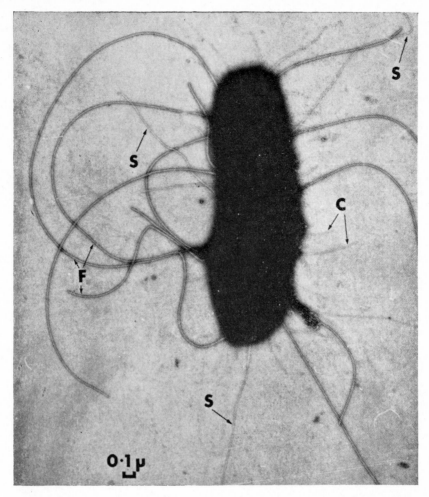

Figure 2-3. *Escherichia coli* showing sexual pili (S), common pili (C), and flagella (F). (Reprinted with permission from Bacteriol. Rev. *32*:55, 1968.)

triple helix. In contrast, the flagella of eucaryotic organisms consist of two central fibers surrounded by nine identical fibers. The flagella of eucaryotic organisms terminate in a basal body lying immediately beneath the cytoplasmic membrane; the basal body controls flagellar movement. However, no true basal bodies have been identified in bacteria, although disc-shaped and hooked structures have been seen at the base of some isolated flagella. These structures appear to be buried in the cell membrane and are thought to be in direct contact with the cytoplasm.

When flagellated bacteria are agitated at high speed in a blender their flagella are sheared off. The relatively large bacterial cells and the small

flagella can then be separated by differential centrifugation. Purified flagella exposed to low pH become amorphous, elements of which reaggre-
gate to form the original rod-shaped structures when the pH is raised.
Physiochemical studies of amorphous flagellins show that they are myosin-
like proteins with molecular weights of approximately 35,000. Although
bacteria may lose their flagella, they can readily regenerate these structures.

Flagellar proteins of different species of bacteria are antigenically specific. Agglutination tests involving serologically distinct flagellar and cell-wall
Ags of certain groups of bacteria, such as the salmonellae, have been useful
in laboratory diagnosis and for epidemiological studies.

The precise ways in which motility of bacteria may influence the induction or the course of disease are not known. However, the attribute of
motility may assist some organisms in penetrating integuments and spreading within the body.

2. Pili

Other surface appendages called *pili* or *fimbrae* are present on some
bacteria. They are short, stiff, spike-like structures 2 to 5 μm in length and
5 to 30 nm in diameter (Fig. 2-3). Pili are considerably shorter than
flagella. They occur on a number of gram-negative bacteria but have not
been observed on gram-positive organisms.

Pili are below the resolving power of the light microscope and stains
have not been devised which allow visualization. Piliation appears to be an
unstable genetic character since piliated bacteria readily lose their ability
to form pili. Presumptive evidence of the presence of pili can often be
obtained indirectly since piliated cells tend to be "sticky" and adhere to
each other, as well as to glass surfaces and red blood cells. Pili are composed of antigenically specific proteins (pilin) and can be detected using
specific antisera developed with purified pili or antisera against whole or-
gansims which are made specific by absorption with nonpiliated mutants.

The fine structure of pili is best observed in shadowed EM preparations
as shown in Figure 2-3. They are tubular structures made of spherical subunits arranged in the form of a helix with an inside diameter of 2 to 3 nm.
Purified pilins have been prepared; the subunits of these proteins have a
molecular weight of about 17,000 and contain abnormally large amounts
of neutral amino acids which impart a hydrophobic character to the pili.
Pili removed by mechanical means are rapidly regenerated.

Two basic groups of pili have been described: the first group appears to
function as "hold-fasts." The second group, commonly referred to as
"sexual pili," are involved in the transmission of extrachromosomal genetic factors between cells. These two groups of pili can be differentiated
from each other on the basis of their relative size and number (Fig. 2-3).
The common or hold-fast pili are smaller and more numerous than the
sexual pili. The hold-fast pili are usually found on pathogenic enteric or-

ganisms, such as members of the genera *Shigella* and *Salmonella,* and on urogenital tract pathogens, such as *Neisseria gonorrhoeae* and members of the genera *Proteus* and *Pseudomonas.* There is evidence that being able to stick to surfaces is an advantage to the organism in terms of pathogenesis (Chapters 13 and 20) and may be an important determinant of specific tissue localization. The fact that pili are usually found on bacteria that cause infections involving the gut and the urogenital tract is compatible with this concept.

The sexual pili are much larger than hold-fast pili and usually do not exceed two per cell. The best-studied example of sexual pili is the *F pilus* (Chapter 4), which is associated only with male bacteria and which plays a role in conjugation. Formation of the F pilus is genetically controlled by a small piece of extrachromosomal transmissible DNA called the *F factor* and is often repressed in cells in which the factor has become stabilized. Although the exact role played by F pili in conjugation is unknown, it is probable that they facilitate the passage of chromosomal components to female cells since their inside dimensions are sufficient to accommodate the passage of double-stranded DNA molecules. There are special phages which are specific for male bacteria because the sex pilus possesses surface receptors specific for the phage; apparently the phage nucleic acid injected into the pilus by the phage passes through the pilus into the male cell.

Another important function of sexual pili involves the passage of extrachromosomal genetic material, such as resistance transfer factors (RTF), which have been shown to permit the simultaneous transfer of resistance to as many as eight antibiotics. In this case the transfer of genetic factors which determine resistance to the antibiotics is accompanied by transfer of the genetic trait governing pilus production. By this mechanism an entire population of bacteria can be genetically converted to antibiotic resistance within a few hours. The rapidity of the acquisition of multiple resistance to antibiotics by this mechanism is in sharp contrast to the chance event of antibiotic resistance resulting from a single-step mutation.

It is obvious that sexual pili provide a unique system for acquiring new genetic traits which are critical for survival in adverse environments. There is little doubt that other genetic traits will be described that are transmitted by these mechanisms.

3. Capsules

Many bacteria (pathogens and nonpathogens) continuously secrete a loosely attached slime layer or capsule which covers the surface of the cell. In the case of free-living microbes, capsules appear to be nonessential to an organism's normal functions and can be removed without apparent harm to the organisms. Likewise encapsulated pathogens propagated in the laboratory can lose their capsules on serial culture suggesting that in this case the capsule is advantageous only when the organism faces the *in vivo* environment.

Capsules are amorphous substances and do not exhibit any structure *per se*. They are most easily seen when the microbes are mixed with very fine colloidal suspensions, such as India ink or nigrosin, and spread in a thin layer on a microscope slide. This procedure is called *negative staining* since the capsules show up as clear halos separating the lightly stained cells from the black background.

Capsules provide a means for distinguishing serotypes of certain microbes. For example, when specific anticapsular Ab is mixed with the corresponding capsulated cells, the capsules swell.

a. Chemical Composition of Capsules. Most capsules are polysaccharides made up of a few sugars such as rhamnose or mannose plus sugar derivatives such as glucosamine, glucuronic acid, and so forth. Often the linkages between the individual sugars are unique; it is these odd conformations plus the sequences of the repeating sugar units that confers immunological specificity on capsular materials. Not all capsules are polysaccharides (Table 2-1), the most notable example being *Bacillus anthracis,* which causes anthrax. The capsule on this pathogen is composed of polyglutamic acid, but the amino acid is in the unnatural D-form as opposed to the L-form normally found in proteins. Other capsules contain small amounts of protein, lipid, and even nucleic acid in addition to polysaccharides.

The enzymes responsible for capsule formation are located in the cell membrane. As with the formation of other cell surface components, the usual sequence is nucleotide activation of individual sugar units followed

TABLE 2-1

Chemical Composition of the Capsules of Representative Pathogenic Bacteria

Organism	Nature of Capsule	Chemical Subunits
Bacillus anthracis	Polypeptide	D-glutamic acid
Neisseria meningitidis	Polysaccharide	Sialic acid, hexosamines
Haemophilus influenzae	Polysaccharide	Polysugarphosphates
Diplococcus pneumoniae	Polysaccharides	
	Type II	Rhamnose, glucose, glucuronic acid
	Type XIV	Galactose, glucose, N-acetylglucosamine
Streptococcus spp.	Hyaluronic acid	N-acetylglucosamine, glucuronic acid
Salmonella typhi	Polysaccharide	N-acetyl-D-galactos-aminuronic acid
Other gram-negative species	Lipopolysaccharide	Lipid, protein, polysaccharide

by transport through the membranes via a lipid carrier; finally polymerization occurs, and the polymer extends through the cell wall with accumulation on the surface. In most cases there is no evidence of covalent bonding between the completed capsule and other cell-wall components. As an example of this loose attachment during the course of pneumococcal pneumonia, large quantities of the capsular polysaccharide accumulate in the blood stream.

b. Function of Capsules. The major function of capsules *in vivo* is to protect the microbes from phagocytosis. Among the encapsulated pathogens virulence is lost or decreased whenever mutation to the noncapsulated form occurs.

In many instances the presence or absence of capsules on bacteria is reflected in the gross appearance of the colonies they form. Capsulated strains generally form smooth colonies with a moist consistency and regular edges. Noncapsulated strains form rough colonies having a dry consistency and irregular edges. Loss of the capsule results in cells with a hydrophobic surface which causes cell clumping.

4. Cell Wall

When whole bacteria are examined with the electron microscope, two ultrastructural patterns emerge. No fine structure is usually seen in gram-positive bacteria except that the capsule or surface slime layer, if present, appears as an uneven halo around the cell. In contrast, most gram-negative bacteria are covered with pseudopod-like protuberances which give the surface a medusa-head appearance (Fig. 2-4).

By combining the techniques of thin sectioning and freeze-etching, distinct patterns of cell-wall structure for gram-positive and gram-negative bacteria become evident. The gram-positive cells have a single layer of complex mucopeptide (peptidoglycan or murein) 20 to 80 nm in thickness which directly overlays the cytoplasmic membrane (see Fig. 2-1).

In contrast, gram-negative bacteria usually have cell walls consisting of one dense layer 2 to 3 nm thick and as many as 3 additional distinct layers giving a total thickness of 15 to 30 nm (Fig. 2-4). The outer trilaminar membrane is composed of lipoprotein with the major portion of the protein being one species of structural protein. Beneath this outer layer is a thin layer of murein separated from the cytoplasmic membrane by a *periplasmic space* known to contain enzymes involved in cell-wall synthesis and in the degradation of macromolecules. Gram-negative cell walls have been fractionated into at least 3 different components, each derived from a distinct layer.

a. Chemical Composition of Murein. Purified gram-positive cell walls are composed primarily of the amino sugars N-acetylglucosamine and N-acetylmuramic acid (muramic acid). The latter is N-acetylglucosamine with an O-linked lactic acid residue on the number 3 carbon. Muramic acid is a unique component of procaryotic cell walls and serves to distinguish procaryotic from eucaryotic cells.

The murein of both gram-negative and gram-positive cells contains D-glutamic acid, D- and L-alanine, L-lysine, glycine and a unique diamino acid, diaminopimelic acid. Different bacteria vary in the relative amounts

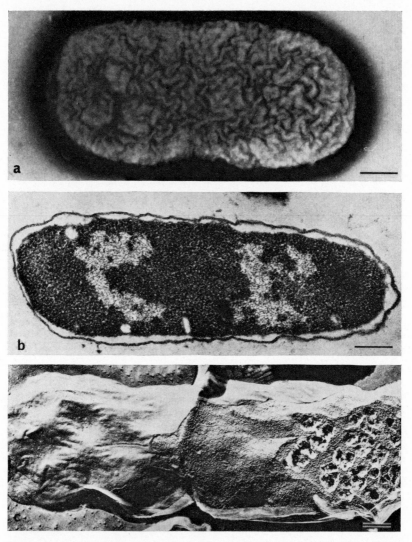

Figure 2-4. Comparison of *Escherichia coli* from logarithmically growing cultures after: (A) negative staining in silicotungstate; (B) fixation in osmium tetroxide, dehydration, embedding, and ultrathin sectioning (wall and membrane have separated); (C) freeze-etching. The intact cell surface is seen at right. The bar represents 250 nm in all micrographs. (Reprinted with permission from J. Bacteriol. *101*:304, 1970.)

of these cell-wall amino acids, but all organisms analyzed so far exhibit a similar pattern.

Murein can be considered to be a single giant macromolecule because its subunits are all covalently linked to one another. The backbone of this macromolecule is made up of alternating units of muramic acid and N-acetylglucosamine in a β 1-4 linkage (Fig. 2-5). Each muramic acid is in turn linked through a peptide bond on its lactic acid substituent to a tetra- or pentapeptide composed of alternating D and L isomers of the

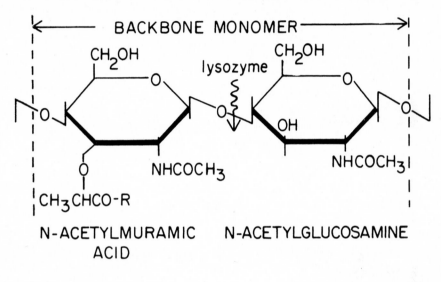

N-ACETYLMURAMIC ACID   N-ACETYLGLUCOSAMINE

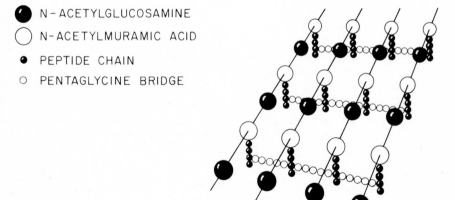

● N–ACETYLGLUCOSAMINE
○ N–ACETYLMURAMIC ACID
● PEPTIDE CHAIN
○ PENTAGLYCINE BRIDGE

Figure 2-5. (Top) Chemical configuration of the backbone unit of murein. Note the lysozyme-sensitive linkage. (Bottom) Three-dimensional view of a small segment of murein from a typical gram-positive cell. The straight lines represent lysozyme-sensitive sites.

amino acids mentioned in the preceding paragraph. Alternation of the amino acid isomers confers additional rigidity on the molecule. In gram-positive bacteria these peptides are linked to the identical peptides on adjacent sugar backbones by tetra- or pentapeptides, glycine, or by another peptide having the same sequence as that linked to the muramic acid.

In the murein layer of gram-negative bacteria the only bridges between adjacent chains are through the peptides on the muramic acid. This results in a considerably thinner layer; apparently the murein of gram-negative cells is only one molecule in thickness.

Although there is considerable variation in the amino acid composition, it appears that the murein layers of all bacteria have the same basic structure. The biosynthetic pathways employed by bacteria for the synthesis of murein involve (1) nucleotide activation and synthesis of peptides on the muramyl residue; (2) transfer to the lipid carrier, modification of the amino acid side chains, and transport through the membrane; (3) attachment to the growing murein mesh followed by cross-linking (see Figure 6-6 for the generalized pathways involved).

Each of these synthetic phases is unique biochemically and is not duplicated elsewhere in nature. Murein and its synthesis have provided a unique biochemical target that has proven vulnerable to antibacterial substances that can specifically inhibit cell-well synthesis without any harmful effect on host cells. In addition, lysozyme, an enzyme found in tears, saliva, and body fluids, specifically disrupts the β 1-4 linkages in the sugar backbone of the wall and ultimately causes the affected bacteria to lyse (Fig. 2-5). Lysozyme is particularly effective against gram-positive bacteria possessing cell walls containing as much as 50% murein. Gram-negative cells, whose murein layer lies beneath other cell-wall components, require special treatment with chelating agents or at an alkaline pH (which exposes the murein layer) before lysozyme has an effect. When susceptible gram-positive cells are treated with lysozyme, their entire murein layer eventually dissolves leaving naked *protoplasts** bounded only by the cytoplasmic membrane. Under normal osmotic conditions the high osmotic pressure inside the protoplast (5 to 20 atmospheres) causes the naked protoplast to burst. If the osmotic pressure of the medium is increased to equal intracellular pressure by adding sucrose (an osmotic stabilizer), the spherical protoplasts can survive and carry out most of their normal cellular functions except division. Protoplasts are unable to divide, presumably because they have no residual template or murein to which the newly synthesized monomeric units can attach themselves to form the cell wall, a structure which is evidently necessary for membrane septation.

* By convention gram-positive cells yield protoplasts, whereas the analogous structures derived from gram-negative cells are called "spheroplasts." This is because the latter contain residues of cell-wall material, and some are capable of reversion to rod forms when the inducing agent is removed.

b. L-forms and Mycoplasma. Occasionally when bacteria are repeatedly subcultured in the presence of a spheroplast inducer and an osmotic stabilizer, mutants arise which are unable to revert to the parental, osmotically stable form because of a defect in cell-wall synthesis. This same phenomenon may occur during the course of an active infection which can result in the emergence of permanent fragile organisms designated as *L-forms*. These L-forms have been derived from a wide variety of pathogens. Since they lack a complete cell wall, they are resistant to penicillin and its derivatives. These organisms have been alleged to be important in a number of disease states, such as rheumatoid arthritis and nongonococcal urethritis, but definite proof of their etiological role in these diseases is lacking.

A closely related group of microorganisms of the genus *Mycoplasma* has also received much attention in recent years. Organisms of this group which includes the human pathogen, *M. pneumoniae,* and some members of the normal flora are nearly identical to L-forms in size and pleomorphism. It has been hypothesized that mycoplasmas were originally derived from bacteria in the same way that L-forms are induced; however, no mycoplasma has ever been observed to revert to a bacterial form, a "mutation" which is a relatively common event among L-forms. In addition, recent studies employing DNA analysis and hybridization have not shown that mycoplasmas are related to bacteria.

c. Other Cell-wall Components of Gram-positive Bacteria. Apart from their major constituent murein, gram-positive cell walls contain another peculiar class of compounds, lacking in gram-negative walls, called teichoic acids. These polymers are composed of polyglycerol or polyribitol phosphate. As isolated, they are often covalently linked to D-alanine, N-acetylglucosamine, glucuronic acid, or glucose, making it appear that they play a structural role as additional cross-links in the murein complex.

Gram-positive cell walls of some bacteria may contain polysaccharides and small amounts of protein. In some instances these additional wall components can be detected immunologically and used to differentiate between closely related organisms.

d. The Gram-negative Cell Wall. As pointed out earlier (Fig. 2-4), the composition of the gram-negative cell wall is more complex than its gram-positive counterpart. Eighty per cent of the dry weight of these structures is composed of lipid, protein, and polysaccharide. The high lipid and relatively low murein content of these bacteria is evidently the basis of their reaction to the Gram stain. When a film (smear) of either gram-positive or gram-negative bacteria is stained with the Gram stain, crystal violet is first applied followed by an iodine solution. The crystal violet-iodine complex which forms in the cell can be readily extracted with alcohol (decolorization step) from gram-negative bacteria but not from gram-positive bacteria. Accordingly, when these respective smears are counterstained with the red dye safranin, gram-negative bacteria are stained red but gram-positive bacteria remain purple because of the excess dye-iodine complex remaining.

Since the cell walls of gram-negative bacteria have a high lipid-murein ratio, the alcohol extracts the lipid moieties which allows the dye-iodine complexes to solubilize and rapidly leach out and in effect decolorize the gram-negative cells. In contrast, the cell walls in gram-positive bacteria are composed, for the most part, of murein with little or no lipid; as a consequence, alcohol penetrates the cells poorly because the murein is alcohol insoluble. Accordingly, the solubilization of the dye-complex is retarded and the intact gram-positive cells retain most of the crystal violet-iodine complex and appear purple on the smear. Because of the high lipid content of their cell walls, certain bacteria, such as *Mycobacterium tuberculosis*, fail to take the Gram stain but can be differentiated from other organisms by the acid-fast stain (see Chapter 29).

Endotoxin and lipopolysaccharide. When isolated cell walls of gram-negative bacteria are treated with lipid solvents, such as aqueous phenol or ether, 70 to 80% of their wall material is solubilized. Analysis of the solubilized material shows that it contains a complex lipid, polysaccharide, and sometimes protein. This lipopolysaccharide (LPS) which is also released naturally when gram-negative cells lyse, is called *endotoxin*. For purposes of orientation, a schematic view showing the location of LPS in a gram-negative cell envelope (cytoplasmic membrane and cell wall) is shown in Figure 2-6.

Electron microscopy and chemical analysis of mutants that are unable to synthesize all or part of their LPS complex show that the LPS complex has the general structure illustrated in Figure 2-7. Buried in the outermost lipoprotein layer of the cell wall is a complex lipid structure designated *Lipid A.* Attached to this is a *core polysaccharide* containing 5 sugars including 2-keto-3-deoxyoctonic acid (KDO), which is found only in the core region. Linked to the polysaccharide moiety of the core region are long strands of polysaccharide made up of repeating sequences of tetra- or pentasaccharides.

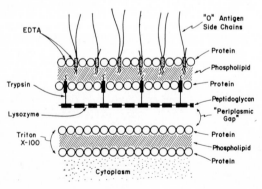

Figure 2-6. Simplified model of the cell envelope of *E. coli*. Components of the envelope are listed on the right; probable sites of attack of various disruptive agents are indicated on the left. Endotoxin is composed of the moieties exterior to the peptidoglycan layer. (Reprinted with permission from J. Bacteriol. *108*:553, 1971.)

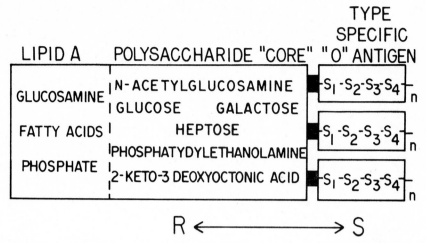

Figure 2-7. Diagrammatic representation of the lipopolysaccharide complex of gram-negative cell walls. The Lipid A and "core" composition of all gram-negative bacteria is similar. Type specificity resides in the kinds and sequences of sugars S_1-S_4 in the side chain.

These sequences confer type specificity on the somatic antigen and permit fine distinctions between bacteria which are otherwise phenotypically identical. When freshly isolated gram-negative pathogens are cultivated in the laboratory, they often undergo a smooth to rough (S → R) colony mutation analogous to that accompanying capsule loss of gram-positive organisms. When this occurs the R-mutants become deficient in their ability to synthesize the type-specific polysaccharide side chains and there is a concomitant loss of virulence. No mutants deficient in Lipid A or core polysaccharide synthesis have been isolated, suggesting that these components are essential to the maintenance of cell-wall integrity.

Analysis of R-mutants shows that most gram-negative bacteria have an essentially identical Lipid A and core polysaccharide composition. The Lipid A plus the core polysaccharide with or without the "O" specific side chains is considered to be the toxic portion of "endotoxin"; the specific polysaccharide and the protein make up the antigenic moieties (Fig. 2-7).

Biosynthesis of LPS bears a remarkable similarity to the synthesis of murein (Fig. 6-6). The individual sugar components are attached to nucleotides, transferred to lipid carriers, and then added to the Lipid A-core "backbone" as a single unit. Each individual sugar in the repeating sequence of the specific polysaccharide chain is activated by a different nucleotide, greatly increasing the specificity of the enzyme pathways involved in the synthesis of the chain.

e. **Functions of the Cell Wall.** The major function of the bacterial cell wall is to protect the protoplast against the effects of hypotonic environments. The internal osmotic pressure of bacteria is usually much greater than the surrounding environment. The strength of the wall is sufficient to prevent swelling and lysis of the microorganisms under all but the most unfavorable circumstances.

The cell wall often serves as a protective barrier against host defenses. For example, cell-wall components such as D-amino acids, muramic acid, teichoic acid, and unique sugars such as colitose and abequose are broken down very slowly if at all by the host.

5. The Protoplasmic Membrane

The appearance of the protoplasmic membrane is similar to that of any other cytoplasmic membrane having the familiar trilaminar structure approximately 8 nm thick (Fig. 2-1). Except for the mycoplasmas, bacterial membranes contain no sterols and are thus relatively fragile when compared to the membranes of eucaryotic cells. Bacteria lack the capacity to synthesize complex sterols and even mycoplasmas rely on preformed sterols.

a. Chemical Composition of Membranes. In addition to lacking sterols, bacterial membranes are generally less complex chemically than those of eucaryotic cells. They are composed of approximately equal amounts of lipid and protein, most of the lipid being phospholipid. The predominant phospholipids are phosphatidyl ethanolamine and phosphatidyl serine with small amounts of cardiolipin present in some species.

b. Functions of Bacterial Protoplasmic Membranes. One of the major functions of bacterial protoplasmic membranes is to maintain a constant environment within the interior of the cell. This is accomplished by an elaborate set of transport mechanisms located in or on the membrane. Charged molecules and nonpolar compounds larger than glycerol are largely excluded from the cytoplasm, and only very low concentrations of such materials can enter by passive diffusion. In order to achieve osmotic balance and a concentrated "pool" of nutrients inside the cell, ions such as H^+, Na^+, K^+, SO_4^{2-}, and PO_4^{3-} are actively transported through the membrane by specific receptor proteins which obey kinetics much like those of enzymes. Other loci for amino acids and sugars are also present and are often referred to as *permeases*. These active transport processes are energy dependent, temperature dependent, flow against concentration gradients, and are inhibited by metabolic poisons such as cyanide and dinitrophenol. These concentration mechanisms allow bacteria to survive in a wide diversity of environments, most of which contain only minute amounts of the nutrients required for normal bacterial function.

Another major function of the membrane is to supply the cell with energy. All of the electron transport and oxidative phosphorylation functions associated with mitochondria in eucaryotic cells are found in the cytoplasmic membrane of bacteria. Contrary to the relatively stable chemical composition of mitochondria, the electron transport systems of bacteria undergo wide fluctuations in their composition depending on the oxygen tension of the surrounding environment. *Mesosomes,* which are invaginations of the bacterial membrane, appear to have exceptionally high oxidation/reduction capacities and may represent the equivalents of the mitochondria of eucaryotic cells.

The lipid carriers and terminal enzymes responsible for cell-wall and lipopolysaccharide synthesis are also associated with cytoplasmic membranes. These enzymes are located on the outer aspects of the membrane where the final polymerization steps in fashioning the growing cell wall take place. They are thus readily accessible to the inhibitory effects of cell-wall-directed antibiotics such as penicillin and cycloserine. A number of degradative enzymes such as nucleases, amylases, and phosphatases are also loosely attached to the outer surface of the membrane. Because these enzymes are released from bacteria by gentle means in the absence of demonstrable lysis, they are referred to as *periplasmic enzymes* and are generally thought to initiate the breakdown of complex macromolecules into assimilable subunits which can be recycled to serve as a source of nutrients for the microorganisms.

The cell membrane also plays a role in DNA replication. Serial thin sections of dividing bacteria often show one or more sites where DNA is apparently attached to the growing membrane (Fig. 2-8). As the cell enlarges, the replicating DNA is pulled apart and is finally separated into two equal bundles. The membrane then begins to invaginate midway between the segregated nuclei. The attached cell wall grows inward until septation of the membrane and wall occurs to complete the division cycle. It is believed that the point of DNA attachment is also the site of DNA replication and that DNA duplication of this site signals the beginning of the complex events involved in cell division.

Because of its essential role in maintaining various normal bacterial functions in the face of marked osmotic differences, the membrane is indirectly vulnerable to agents which weaken or destroy the cell wall. Most of the known bactericidal antibiotics and host defense mechanisms act in some manner to weaken the cell wall, expose the membrane, and bring about lysis of the unprotected protoplast.

6. The Cytoplasm

The most conspicuous structures inside microorganisms are the ribosomes (Fig. 2-1). These are tightly packed spherical particles 15 to 20 nm in diameter. Although they are not aligned in an organized fashion on an intracellular reticular membrane, clusters of ribosomes called *polysomes* occur which are much more efficient for protein synthesis than single particles.

Ribosomes are composed of 40% protein and 60% RNA. Intact procaryotic ribosomes have a sedimentation coefficient of 70S and can be separated into 50S and 30S subunits when the Mg^{2+} concentration of the suspension medium is reduced. These ribosomes are slightly smaller than those of eucaryotic cells which are 80S particles composed of 60S and 40S subunits.

Ribosomes function as a surface on which the messenger RNA combines with the appropriate transfer RNA to link activated amino acids through peptide bonds into polypeptides and proteins. Because the maximum rate of protein synthesis of each ribosome or polysome is limited, the number

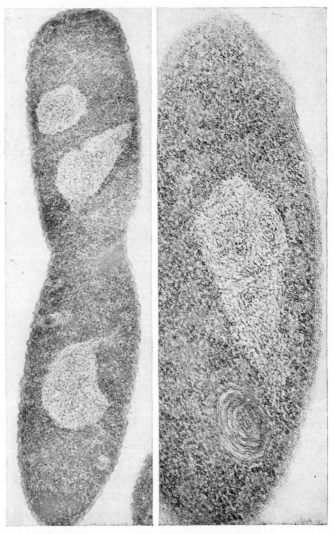

Figure 2-8. Thin sections of dividing bacteria. Note the attachment of the DNA to the cytoplasmic membrane and the connection of the mesosome to the dividing nuclear apparatus. (Reproduced with permission from Bacteriol. Rev. *32*:39, 1968.)

of ribosomes in a cell is, as a general rule, directly related to the growth rate.

A unique feature of 70S ribosomes, which are also found in eucaryotic cell organelles such as mitochondria and chloroplasts, is that they have specific binding sites for certain antibiotics such as streptomycin and chloramphenicol. When bound, the antibiotics cause the ribosomes to become disengaged from the messenger RNA or cause premature release of incomplete polypeptides thus inhibiting protein synthesis. At high concentrations these antibiotics are toxic to mammalian cells as well as to bacteria. This is presumably due to their inhibitory effect on mitochondrial protein synthesis.

7. Endospores

Members of the genera *Bacillus* and *Clostridium* are characterized by their ability to form endospores. Endospores are extremely resistant to heating and drying and are the principal reason why the autoclave is employed in sterilization of culture media and other heat-stable materials. Although many spores are resistant to boiling for 30 minutes, the standard autoclave temperature of 121°C for 20 minutes is lethal for all known endospores provided each spore is subjected to the maximum temperature for the full time period.

Endospores do not stain by Gram's method and consequently appear as empty spaces; in wet mounts they appear as refractile granules. These properties are a reflection of their relative impermeability to ordinary solvents and solutes and of the density of their interior components. Thin sections of endospores (Fig. 2-9) reveal an extremely thick exosporium surrounding several layers of compact cytoplasmic material, a few ribosomes, and a tightly packed fibrillar nuclear region.

The chemical composition of endospores resembles that of vegetative cells except that no free water is present. There is also a relatively high concentration of the calcium salt of dipicolinic acid which is not detectable in vegetative cells. This compound makes up the bulk of the exosporium and apparently contributes to its heat resistance.

The formation of endospores represents an important survival mechanism. When cells are subjected to a variety of adverse environmental changes such as desiccation or nutritional deprivation, each forms a single spore. The free spores, which are released from the sporulating cell, are essentially metabolically inert and may remain dormant indefinitely. In many instances, however, the spore will germinate and eventually give rise to a single vegetative cell identical to the organism from which it was derived. Since one cell produces one spore which in turn produces one vegetative cell, endospore formation can only be considered to be part of a specialized life cycle and not a replicative mechanism. Most sporing organisms are saprophytes whose normal habitat is soil rich in organic matter.

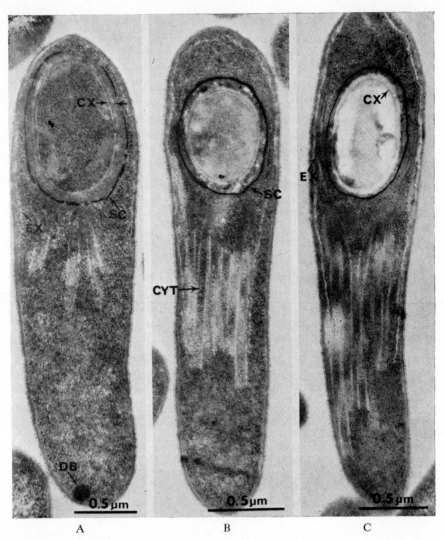

A   B   C

Figure 2-9. (A) Section through an immature spore showing the deposition of coat material (SC) between the appendages and their site of origin. Note the presence of an electron-dense body (DB), increased cortical development (CX, between the arrows), and the presence of an immature exosporium (EX). (B) Section through a developing spore with a completed spore coat (SC); the appendages are no longer contiguous with their origin. Note the presence of cytoplasmic material (CYT) within the appendage tubules. (C) Longitudinal section through a mature spore within the sporangium illustrating that some of the appendages reach almost the entire length of the sporangium. The spore possesses a well-developed cortex (CX, between the arrows) and a laminated exosporium (EX). (Reproduced with permission from J. Bacteriol. *106*:269, 1971.)

8. The Nuclear Apparatus

As pointed out earlier, the existence of a bacterial nuclear apparatus was in doubt until observations were made with the electron microscope. The apparatus as currently envisioned is a tightly packed bundle of double-stranded DNA containing approximately 5 million base pairs. The strands are in the form of a closed circle 1000 to 2000 μm long (Fig. 2-8).

Apparently the nuclear apparatus is held loosely in place by the viscosity of the cytoplasm and ionic interactions with the polyamines, spermine and spermidine. This physical state is consistent with rapid replication of procaryotic DNA which would require free intracellular diffusion of nucleotides, phosphate, and other elements involved in its synthesis.

The function of the nuclear apparatus in bacteria is essentially the same as that of any other living organism. In bacteria, however, the problems of maintaining a stable phenotype are complicated by changes imposed on the microorganisms by a constantly changing environment. To offset the problems presented by a changing environment, bacteria have evolved an elaborate set of control mechanisms which allow immediate expression or repression of a wide variety of phenotypic characteristics. These mechanisms, which will be discussed in Chapter 4, together with the more permanent alterations due to mutation followed by selection are the basis upon which the virulence and pathogenicity of infectious microbes rests.

9. Miscellaneous Cytoplasmic Inclusions

Because of their rapid metabolic rate, most bacteria do not accumulate appreciable quantities of intracellular storage products. Under conditions of nitrogen deprivation small amounts of glycogen, granulose, or the unique bacterial lipid, poly-beta-hydroxy-butyric acid, may appear in the cytoplasm. Volutin, a polymetaphosphate complex, can often be seen in *Corynebacterium* species when they are stained with methylene blue. The complexes, commonly called *metachromatic granules,* are characteristic of this genus and are sometimes used as an aid in identifying some pathogens in clinical specimens.

C. Bacterial Growth and Replication

When bacteria are inoculated into a fresh medium, their growth proceeds through a series of characteristic phases the semilog plot of which is called a *growth curve* (Fig. 2-10). Usually the organisms undergo an initial *lag phase* in cell division because the cells must readjust their phenotype to the new environment by turning on or turning off various functions such as utilization of a specific sugar, amino acids, proteins, or fats as sources of nutrients. These readjustments are mediated by the regulatory systems mentioned earlier and, in general, result in a coordinated system of enzymes and functions that are most economical for the microorganism.

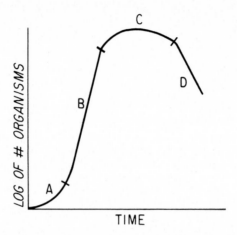

Figure 2-10. A typical growth curve for a bacterial population. Because of the large numbers of cells produced the counts are generally expressed as Log$_{10}$ of the actual number. A, lag phase; B, exponential phase; C, stationary phase; D, decline phase.

After this adjustment phase the organisms begin to enlarge during the latter part of the lag phase and then begin to divide exponentially; this represents the initiation of the phase of most rapid multiplication, the *exponential phase*. Later, as the environment becomes unfavorable the multiplication rate gradually declines until ultimately the *stationary phase* is reached, during which the multiplication rate is equal to the death rate; subsequent to this the *decline phase* occurs, during which death exceeds multiplication. The maximum rates of multiplication attainable by different bacteria vary markedly. For example, *Vibrio cholerae* under ideal circumstances has a generation time of approximately 20 minutes, whereas *M. tuberculosis* can divide only once every 14 hours under optimal conditions. However, the generation times *in vivo* are usually longer than in optimal *in vitro* environments due primarily to the forces of host defense and nutritional limitations. Compared with the maximum growth rate of mammalian cells (generation time about 8 hr), the growth rate of most bacteria is nothing short of phenomenal. The great speed of bacterial growth, which is largely a function of the exponential nature of their multiplication, is a difficult but important concept for the beginning student to grasp. For example, if a culture of *E. coli* could be provided with optimal conditions for growth, a single cell would give rise to a cell mass 4000 times that of the earth within 2 days.

Bacteria do not sustain exponential growth indefinitely because of nutritional limitations and/or the accumulation of toxic metabolites. Even under ideal conditions the maximum total populations attainable seldom exceed 10^{10} per ml.

Cell division of bacteria ordinarily takes place through a process of transverse binary fission. The details of this process have already been described in the section dealing with nuclear replication (Fig. 2-8).

The basic aspects of cell division have recently been explored using Ab specific for cell walls and which has been conjugated with a fluorescent dye to permit visualization of the growing cell wall. After the cells have been treated with the labeled Ab, they are allowed to grow; the points of growth show up as dark areas of increasing size. As shown in Figure 2-11, cocci and rods exhibit quite different patterns of growth. The cocci enlarge and develop a narrow equatorial band which produces a constriction resulting in separation of the two cells; rod-shaped organisms elongate as the result of random or dispersed growth until septation and division take place.

Following division the cells may or may not separate; consequently either single cells or aggregates of cells result, the nature of which varies and is a characteristic of the species. For example, most of the enteric gram-negative rods occur singly, whereas the gram-positive cocci tend to remain attached to one another. Among the gram-positive cocci the pattern of cell aggregation varies, depending on the order of division in different planes. Whereas staphylococci divided randomly in three planes to form grape-like clusters, pneumococci and streptococci divide in a single plane which results in aggregates of two or more cells arranged linearly. In the case of *Corynebacterium diphtheriae* a "snapping motion" commonly follows sep-

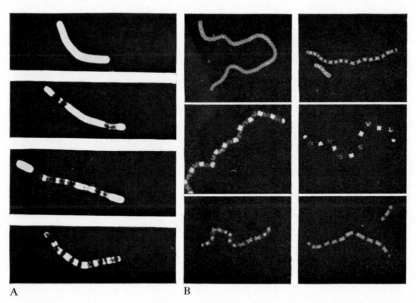

A   B

Figure 2-11. Growth of bacteria after initial labeling with fluorescent Ab specific for cell-wall components. The dark areas represent new wall growth, the brightly stained portions old wall. (A) *Bacillus cereus*; (B) *Streptococcus pyogenes*. (Reprinted with permission from Bacteriol. Rev. *29*:326, 1965.)

tation causing the cells to line up in parallel fashion or to form patterns resembling Chinese letters. These species characteristics are often reflected in the morphology of colonies growing on artificial media. For example, organisms which lyse when they reach the stationary phase of growth yield colonies with depressed centers composed of dead cells and elevated margins composed of actively growing cells. Organisms that display "snapping" post-fission movements tend to form wrinkled, "heaped-up" colonies.

D. Bacterial Nutrition and Metabolism

For the most part bacteria carry out the same biosynthetic processes that occur in other cells. All bacteria possess a glycolytic pathway, some form of a tricarboxylic acid cycle, and, with the exception of obligate anaerobes, an electron transport mechanism geared to generate ATP via oxidative phosphorylation. *The major difference between bacteria and eucaryotic cells is that bacteria have a greater capacity to adapt to new environments by undergoing phenotypic changes.* For example, *E. coli* in its normal habitat in the colon proliferates anaerobically by fermenting amino acids and sugars but can grow equally well aerobically in a simple salts solution with glucose as the only organic constituent. The genetic potential and regulatory changes which allow this marked diversity of life styles will be discussed in Chapter 4.

Many bacteria, including pathogens, can be cultivated *in vitro* on media composed of meat or plant digests plus an extract of yeast. For more fastidious pathogens, such as *Diplococcus pneumoniae*, human or animal blood may be added. In general the more parasitic an organism becomes, the more fastidious it becomes with respect to its nutritional requirements. Presumably as organisms have adapted to a parasitic existence, they have gradually lost much of their biosynthetic capacity through mutation and selection. Under conditions of obligate parasitism many of their complex nutritional requirements are supplied by the host, consequently the enzymes and genes concerned with such nutritional requirements are no longer needed by the bacterial cell and are not retained in the course of their evolution.

Knowledge of the nutritional peculiarities of microorganisms can be used for designing culture media which will prevent or inhibit the growth of unwanted bacteria and/or permit differentiation between pathogens and nonpathogens. For instance, some *selective media* used to isolate enteric pathogens contain relatively high concentrations of citrate which inhibits the growth of *E. coli* but is harmless for species of *Salmonella* and *Shigella*. This allows the clinical microbiologist to isolate the etiologic agent which may be present in relatively low numbers from fecal specimens containing huge numbers of normal flora coliforms. The addition of lactose plus certain indicators provides a mechanism for monitoring changes in the color of colonies that ferment lactose; thus lactose-fermenting pathogens can be differentiated from nonpathogens that do not ferment lactose (*differential medium*). Judicious employment of differential and selective media can markedly simplify isolation and identification of pathogens from clinical specimens.

E. Pure Cultures

To identify a microbe with certainty, it is usually necessary to isolate the organism in pure culture. This is readily accomplished by depositing a small amount of a specimen at the margin of a Petri plate containing an appropriate solid agar growth medium. The specimen is then mechanically dispersed over the surface of the medium by "streaking" with a sterile wire loop. By dragging bacteria away from the initial inoculation site they are in effect diluted out until some of the cells are deposited singly along the line of streaking. Since most motile bacteria are unable to move about on the relatively dry medium surface, the dividing bacteria accumulate and form visible colonies, many of which are the progeny of but a single organism. Such colonies represent a pure culture; other colonies may also represent pure cultures providing they arise from organisms of a single kind even if more than one cell is initially present. The latter is referred to as a colony-forming unit (CFU). Since it is not always possible to be certain that a colony arose from a single cell or more than one cell of the same type, it is common practice to select isolated colonies and repeat the streaking procedure to ensure that the culture isolate is pure.

Once a pure culture has been isolated, a panel of tests is applied to identify the unknown isolate. Because only a limited number of tests may be required to identify a given species of microbe, standard keys are usually consulted since they include outlines of tests needed for identification as well as systematic procedures. Tests commonly employed by the diagnostic medical microbiologist to identify various pathogens include (1) Gram stain reaction, (2) cell morphology and presence or absence of a capsule, (3) cell grouping, (4) motility and arrangement of flagella, (5) ability to ferment certain sugars, (6) utilization of certain amino acids as a sole source of carbon, (7) tests for distinctive end products of metabolism, (8) identification of unique indicator enzymes, (9) susceptibility to environmental conditions including oxygen tension and specific inhibitors of growth, (10) serologic tests for specific Ags, (11) animal pathogenicity, and (12) phage typing.

F. Bacterial Classification

Taxonomic schema are very important communication systems which biologists continually struggle to improve. Microbiologists have developed

TABLE 2-2
Family and Genus of Medically Important Bacteria

Family	Genus	Gram Reaction* and Identifying Features	Oxygen Requirement
Pseudomonadaceae	Pseudomonas	Straight, G–, motile rods	Aerobic
Spirillaceae	Vibrio	Curved, G–, motile rods	Facultative
Enterobacteriaceae	Salmonella Shigella Proteus Escherichia	Straight, G– rods; motile and nonmotile	Facultative
Brucellaceae	Yersinia Bordetella Brucella Haemophilus	Small, G– coccobacilli; some show polar staining	Facultative
Bacteroidaceae	Bacteroides	Straight, G– rods	Anaerobic
Neisseriaceae	Neisseria	G– cocci in pairs	Microaerophilic
Lactobacillaceae	Diplococcus Streptococcus	G+ cocci in pairs and chains	Microaerophilic
Micrococcaceae	Staphylococcus	G+ cocci in irregular clusters	Facultative
Bacillaceae	Bacillus Clostridium	G+ rods; form spores	Aerobic Anaerobic
Corynebacteriaceae	Corynebacterium	G+, pleomorphic rods with granules	Aerobic
Mycobacteriaceae	Mycobacterium	G+, acid-fast, irregular rods	Aerobic
Actinomycetaceae	Actinomyces	G+, fungus-like rods	Anaerobic
	Nocardia	G+, acid-fast, fragmented rods	Aerobic
Treponemataceae	Borrelia	G—, flexible loose spirals;	Aerobic
	Treponema Leptospira	Flexible tight spirals; silver stain	Anaerobic Aerobic
Mycoplasmataceae	Mycoplasma	G—, pleomorphic, cell wall-less	Facultative
Rickettsiaceae	Rickettsia	G—, small coccobacilli; obligate intra-cellular parasites	Facultative

*G+ = gram-positive; G— = gram-negative.

taxonomic schema similar to those employed for multicellular organisms by which bacteria and fungi are placed into orders, classes, families, genera, and species. The principle behind the system is that the more closely related two organisms are, the greater the number of features they should have in common. Since all of the traits used are phenotypic and since not all traits are given equal weight, the system is strictly artificial. However, this means of identifying bacteria is of great practical value to the clinical microbiologist because he can label an isolate possessing a given set of characteristics by name and thus communicate his findings to physicians and other microbiologists by this simple expedient.

In Table 2-2, most of the medically important genera of bacteria are grouped according to some of their primary characteristics such as the Gram stain reaction, shape, cell arrangement, visible diagnostic morphological features, and oxygen requirements. In many instances it is possible to assign an isolate to a genus with no additional information. However, differentiation of a species within a genus requires additional tests.

G. Quantification of Bacteria

It is common practice to determine the number of viable bacteria present in a sample of urine from a patient suspected of having a urinary tract infection because if it exceeds 10^5 per ml of urine the patient is probably infected. The principle used for determining the number of viable bacteria in a specimen is based on diluting the specimen and plating aliquots on the surface of a suitable agar medium. The specimen must be diluted to a point where the colonies which grow on the surface are dispersed sufficiently so that they can be counted. The number of colonies is a reflection of the number of live bacteria (per ml) in the original urine specimen or more accurately the number of CFU per ml since clumping often occurs.

Other applications in which bacterial enumeration techniques are used include analyses of water, milk, ice cream, and other food products.

H. Bacterial Attributes of Special Medical Importance

The pathogenicity of bacteria rests on their ability to enter the host and to multiply and injure tissues by whatever virulence factors they are genetically capable of expressing. These include secretory products as well as structural components. For example, encapsulated organisms and smooth gram-negative organisms possess an enhanced resistance to phagocytosis. In the case of the pathogens that can colonize the intestinal and urogenital tracts, hold-fast pili assist in establishing an infection and sexual pili permit the rapid transfer of resistance to antimicrobial drugs. The chemical composition of the cell surfaces of all pathogens prevents, to a certain extent, their destruction by host defense mechanisms. Indeed some bacteria can even multiply within phagocytes. In the host, as well as in nature, bacteria are remarkably well suited to adapt to constantly changing environments which accounts for the constant challenge microbes present to the human host and to the microbiologist.

References

Davis, B. D., Dulbecco, R., Eisen, H. N., Ginsberg, H. S., and Wood, W.B.: *Microbiology*. New York: Harper & Row, 1968.

Gunsalus, I. C., and Stanier, R. Y., eds.: *The Bacteria: A Treatise on Structure and Function*. New York: Academic Press, 1960.

Mandelstam, J., and McQuillen, K.: *Biochemistry of Bacterial Growth*. Oxford: Blackwell Scientific Publishers, 1968.

Rogers, H. J.: Bacterial growth and the cell envelope. Bacteriol. Rev. *34*:194, 1970.

Rothfield, L., and Romeo, D.: Role of lipids in the biosynthesis of bacterial cell envelope. Bacteriol. Rev. *35*:14, 1971.

Smith, H., and Pearce, J. H., eds.: *Microbial Pathogenicity in Man and Animals*. London: Cambridge University Press, 1972.

Stanier, R., Doudoroff, M., and Adelberg, E.: *The Microbial World*. 3rd ed. Englewood Cliffs, N.J.: Prentice-Hall, 1970.

Symposium on the fine structure and replication of bacteria and their parts. Bacteriol. Rev. *29*:277, 1965.

Bacterial Viruses

Virtually all types of living cells are subject to invasion by viruses, and bacteria are no exception. The viruses that infect bacteria are called *bacteriophages*, or simply *phages*. Because bacteria can be easily cultured and grow rapidly, studies on phage replication and infection are more readily accomplished than similar studies using animal viruses. Studies on bacteriophages have been of great importance in microbiology, genetics, and molecular biology. Medical microbiology, for example, has profited from phage studies in the following ways: First, the mechanisms of replication of phages and viruses that infect animals are similar. Second, phages (like all viruses) are highly specific with regard to the cells they can infect; therefore it is possible to use the infection pattern with a panel of known phages to identify bacterial strains. This procedure, known as *phage typing*, has been useful in epidemiologic studies concerned with tracing the spread of infection due to specific strains of bacteria. Finally, certain kinds of phage can infect bacterial cells and direct the production of potent bacterial exotoxins that are responsible for diseases such as diphtheria, scarlet fever, and botulism.

Many phages have been discovered. One which offers a useful model to illustrate the mechanisms of phage infection will be considered here; namely, a phage called *lambda* (λ) which attacks *Escherichia coli*.

The morphology of phage λ is shown in Figure 3-1. Although the morphology of λ and many other phages seems to be more complex than the morphology of most animal viruses, there are certain similarities between viruses of the two groups. Like all viruses, the λ particle consists essentially of a piece of nucleic acid surrounded by a protein coat (*capsid*). The complete virus particle is called a *virion*. When outside the cell, the mature λ

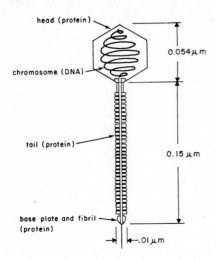

head (protein)

0.054 μm

chromosome (DNA)

tail (protein)

0.15 μm

base plate and fibril
(protein)

←.01 μm

Figure 3-1. Bacteriophage λ. (Adapted from *The Bacteriophage Lambda*. Ed. by A. D. Hershey. Cold Spring Harbor, N.Y.: Cold Spring Harbor Laboratory, 1971.)

virion is inert. However, when the phage nucleic acid reaches the cytoplasm, it is capable of diverting cellular metabolism toward production of virus particles.

When phage λ encounters an appropriate host cell, the base plate of the phage's "tail" attaches to a specific site (*receptor*) on the bacterial surface. Once *specific attachment* has occurred, the viral DNA is injected into the cell, a process called *penetration*, leaving the protein capsid outside. Thus, the phage tail functions as an organelle to facilitate specific adsorption to cells and as a tube to deliver the phage DNA into the bacterial cell through its thick cell wall.

There are two distinct types of life cycles which phage λ can undergo (Fig. 3-2).

A. The Vegetative (Lytic) Life Cycle

About 45 minutes after the λ chromosome has entered the host cell, the cell lyses and releases approximately 200 mature virus particles. The interval between penetration and host cell lysis is called the *latent period*. Much of what the virus needs in order to complete its vegetative life cycle is coded for by the phage chromosome itself. Therefore, the latent period has provided an excellent opportunity for studying gene expression. Extensive genetic mapping and study of the functions of λ have demonstrated that its chromosome is highly organized, the genes determining related functions being grouped into adjacent clusters (Fig. 3-3).

The chromosome of phage λ is a linear molecule of double-stranded DNA, about 1% as long as the host *E. coli* chromosome. Soon after infection, the λ chromosome forms a circle and serves as a template for the

synthesis of messenger ribonucleic acid (mRNA). The functions shown in
the center and lower part of the map in Figure 3-3 are expressed first.
Finally, the functions in the upper arm of the map are expressed. Although
synthesis of both phage nucleic acid and protein is substantial throughout
the latent period, no mature phage particles appear during the first half of
this period. This early part of the latent period, during which no mature
virions are present, is called the *eclipse period*. During the second half of
the latent period which is designated the *maturation period*, mature virus
particles are assembled and are released by cell lysis at the end of the
latent period.

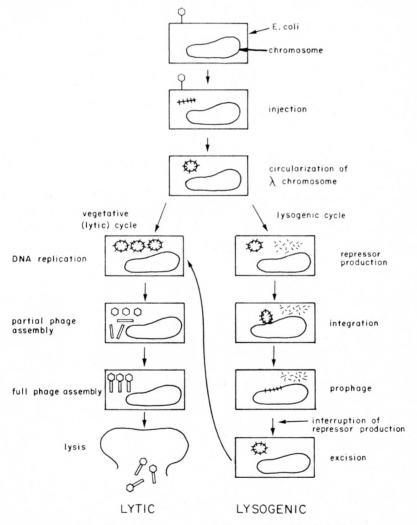

Figure 3-2. The lytic and lysogenic life cycles of bacteriophage λ.

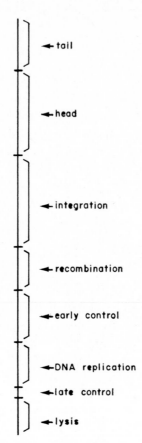

Figure 3-3. The genetic map of bacteriophage λ. Genes which control related functions are grouped together on the chromosome of λ. Therefore each of the bracketed regions represents a cluster of genes.

The mechanisms by which the expression of λ genes are controlled as well as the act of gene expression itself have been well characterized. Although some areas are still not well understood, it is appropriate to recount certain important events which occur during the eclipse phase. The steps involved are:

a. Genes specifying the proteins which are involved in the control of transcription are expressed first.

b. Following this, products needed for recombination and integration are synthesized, as well as products needed for DNA replication; copies of the virus chromosome are then synthesized.

c. A product is synthesized which is needed for efficient expression of the genes involved in lysis as well as in head and tail construction; the head and tail proteins then begin to accumulate.

d. Heads and tails begin to form which, together with DNA, are subsequently assembled into mature virus particles. Assembly of the first mature virion signals the end of the eclipse period and the beginning of the maturation period.

During the maturation period, synthesis of many virus components continues, while at the same time the final assembly of components into mature virus particles leads to the accumulation of infectious virions in the cytoplasm of the cell. The formation of mature virus takes place in an assembly-line fashion and is notably different from the multiplication of bacteria which occurs as the result of binary fission. As a terminal event, the accumulation of a phage-induced lysozyme causes lysis of the cell wall and release of the phage particles.

B. The Lysogenic Life Cycle

For reasons which are not entirely clear, some λ chromosomes are only partially expressed and then become integrated into the bacterial chromosome, a process known as *lysogenization*. Although lysogeny has been intensively studied, some aspects of the phenomenon remain obscure. A phage chromosome which is destined to become integrated expresses itself only partially, by producing a protein that specifically catalyzes integration (via recombination at specific bacterial and phage sites). Preliminary to integration another protein is synthesized, a repressor, that eventually represses the production of all mRNA of the phage except that which specifies the repressor molecule itself. The integrated λ chromosome is called a *prophage*. The DNA of the prophage is replicated along with the bacterial chromosome; however, except for the production of repressor, the prophage is a silent partner in the phage-bacterium association.

A notable finding is that the presence of prophage repressor in the lysogenic cell renders the cell "immune" to superinfection with phage λ since the repressor blocks the production of mRNA by any newly introduced λ chromosome.

The stability of prophage in a culture is illustrated by the observation that certain lysogenic strains of bacteria have been maintained by serial transfers for over 20 years. Nevertheless, the prophage is potentially lethal to the cell that carries it. In about one of every 10^5 cells the synthesis of repressor is interrupted and, as a result, λ genes are expressed; the prophage is excised from the chromosome of the organism, and λ genes initiate the lytic (vegetative) cycle leading to the production of mature λ particles and lysis of the host cell. Release of λ phage particles into the culture medium of a lysogenic strain is of no consequence to the remaining lysogenic cells in the culture since they are immune to superinfection with infectious λ particles.

The probability of a switch from the prophage state to the vegetative state can be increased by treating lysogenic cells with certain chemical and physical agents which mediate a process known as *induction*. For example, appropriate exposure of *E. coli* (λ) (i.e., *E. coli* lysogenic for bacteriophage λ) to ultraviolet (UV) irradiation leads to induction of the prophage in nearly every cell in the population and, after a period of time, there is a massive release of phage from the induced cells.

Other interesting phenomena associated with bacterial viruses (not necessarily λ) will be discussed since some of them also occur among the animal viruses.

C.   Phenotypic Mixing

The assembly-line manner of production of mature virions can lead to unusual types of virus particles in which components of similar, but genetically distinct, viruses are combined. One example involves the so-called *host range mutant* (Fig. 3-4). The cell-wall sites which serve as specific attachment receptors for the sites on the tip of the phage tail sometimes change due to mutation so that they no longer permit the adsorption of the particular phage. The phage, in turn, can sometimes undergo mutation involving one of the subunits of its base plate concerned with cell attachment so that the phage can attach to both mutant and wild-type (nonmutant) host cells. For example, phage A might be capable of adsorbing to and growing on bacterial strain a but not strain b. In contrast, phage B (a mutant of phage A) might be capable of attaching to and injecting its DNA into both strain a and strain b.

Now suppose that a cell of strain a simultaneously becomes infected with phage A and phage B. Except for one mutation (presumably caused by the alteration of a single base pair), these two phage strains are identical. As shown in Figure 3-4, during the assembly of progeny virus particles, a tail made by virus A could become attached to a head containing the DNA of virus B or vice versa. This means that a phage can be formed possessing the genotype of phage A but the phenotype of phage B or vice versa. Be-

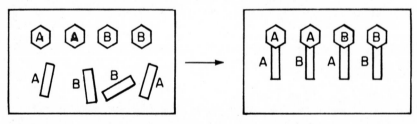

Figure 3-4. Phenotypic mixing. The assembly-line production of complete bacteriophage from component parts can lead to phenotypically mixed particles; for example, tails specified by the genes of phage A can be connected to a head containing a B-type chromosome and vice versa. Phages A and B must be related for phenotypic mixing to occur.

cause of these events, it is possible to infect cells of type b with the DNA of phage type A. As would be expected, the chromosome of phage type A will direct the production of only type A phage regardless of what kind of tail was associated with the original chromosome.

The mutation of phage A to phage B also illustrates a mechanism by which phages can vary so as to attack a wide range of hosts. In the particular model cited, the B phage would be referred to as a *host range mutant* of phage A.

D. Viral Exclusion

There are very few individual bacterial cells which can simultaneously support the replication of two unrelated phages. The reasons for this undoubtedly differ widely from one situation to another. Competition for essential constituents such as ribosomes, enzymes, and nucleotides is probably an important contributing factor in many cases of viral exclusion. Some bacteriophages, such as the coliphage T4, can exclude the growth of almost all unrelated viruses because T4 makes nucleases which destroy most heterologous DNA molecules.

E. Multiplicity Reactivation

Exposure of phage particles to harmful agents such as low doses of UV irradiation often causes a precipitous drop in viral infectivity. However, the members of a population of noninfectious irradiated phages often can cooperate to produce an infection. It is presumed that the cooperating phage particles have been damaged in different parts of their chromosomes; however, as the result of genetic recombination of undamaged genes, the cooperating chromosomes give rise to undamaged viruses.

F. Cross Reactivation

A phenomenon similar to multiplicity reactivation is cross reactivation, a circumstance in which an undamaged virus serves to repair a damaged virus. Cross reactivation can occur between heterologous as well as between homologous viruses; evidently it results from complementation of the damaged genes by complementary genes of the undamaged phage as well as through genetic recombination.

References

Hayes, W.: *The Genetics of Bacteria and Their Viruses.* 2nd ed. New York: John Wiley and Sons, 1968.

Hershey, A. D., ed.: *The Bacteriophage Lambda.* Cold Spring Harbor, N.Y.: Cold Spring Harbor Laboratory, 1971.

Stent, G. S.: *Molecular Biology of Bacterial Viruses.* San Francisco: W. H. Freeman and Company, 1963.

Stent, G. S.: *Molecular Genetics.* San Francisco: W. H. Freeman and Company, 1971.

Bacterial Genetics

Microbes are notorious for their potential variability. In fact, genetic changes in infecting organisms often occur during the course of infection. This does not obtain because the mechanisms of genetic change among bacteria are basically different from those that occur in higher organisms; instead, the unusually short generation time of bacteria leads to a more rapid selection of those organisms in a population which are best equipped to survive a given environment.

It is assumed that the student has at least a cursory knowledge of the structure of deoxyribonucleic acid (DNA), the role of DNA in heredity, and the way in which mutations occur. The purpose of this chapter is to enable the student to build a framework of knowledge which will be of practical value in clinical medicine. Four aspects of microbial genetics are considered: (1) bacteria as genetic entities; (2) the exchange of genetic information between bacteria; (3) control of genetic expression, and (4) microbial genetics in medicine.

A. Bacteria as Genetic Entities

Like all forms of life, bacteria are able to transmit their characteristics to their progeny, and the progeny in turn are able to convert this information (genetic potential or *genotype*) into products (genetic expression or *phenotype*). With respect to microbial genetics, the most-studied species is *Escherichia coli*. From corollary studies with organisms related to *E. coli,* such as *Salmonella* species as well as with members of the unrelated genus *Bacillus,* it has become apparent that much of the information obtained with *E. coli* has general application.

The chromosome of *E. coli* is about 1000 μm long and contains approximately 3×10^6 base pairs. Since an average gene contains 1000 base pairs, *E. coli* has approximately 3000 genes. To date, about 300 of these genes have been characterized and located on the chromosome; this has permitted detailed studies on mutation, expression, and heredity.

Mutation is defined as a heritable change in the genome which does not result from the incorporation of genetic material from another organism. It is well recognized that mutations occur at a relatively constant rate in all dividing cells. Certain agents (*mutagens*) are able to accelerate mutation by mechanisms known to cause natural or spontaneous mutation. The way in which a cell responds to a given mutagen is not always simple or predictable. Mutagens commonly cause mutations by inducing pairing errors of various sorts between the nitrogenous bases of DNA during its replication. Such errors may result from either chemical or physical damage to DNA by the mutagen or a variety of other causes. It is notable that many of the cells present in a population of 10^8 *E. coli* will have experienced a mutagenic event. In fact it is probable that a large population of *E. coli* contains at least one mutant for every gene possessed by the cells. As a consequence of evolution, microbes have undergone mutation and selection for perhaps millions of years; this has resulted in a large number of species that specifically fit their own particular ecological niches. Therefore, most mutants derived from wild-type *E. coli* have a reduced ability to survive in nature! Accordingly, most mutants are usually at a selective disadvantage if they must compete in the natural habitat of the wild-type species. When the natural habitat is altered, mutants may have greater ability to survive than the wild-type strain.

For example, if a large population of *E. coli* is exposed to appropriate concentrations of the antibiotic streptomycin, the chances are good that before adding the drug at least one organism in the initial population would have experienced a random mutation yielding streptomycin resistance. Consequently all of the wild-type streptomycin-sensitive cells should soon be killed, and incubation of the streptomycin-containing culture should lead to the growth of streptomycin-resistant mutants and give rise to a culture of streptomycin-resistant *E. coli*. This illustrates the important evolutionary principle that ability to undergo random mutation endows each microbial species with a remarkable degree of flexibility for meeting unfavorable alterations in the environment.

Once DNA has undergone a mutational change, there is a certain time lapse before the new mutant phenotype is expressed (*phenotypic lag*). This time lapse may occur because the product of the formerly unmutated gene must be depleted before the new phenotypic change is expressed. A lapse may also occur because many bacterial cells have two copies of the chromosome, only one of which is mutated. When the cell divides, only one of the daughter cells obtains the mutant copy.

It is important to remember that mutation occurs spontaneously and randomly; because of the short generation time of bacteria, a bacterial mutant can often be selected in an altered environment preferentially favorable to it and dominate a population within a day or two.

It is also noteworthy that phenotypic changes occur in bacteria which are not the direct result of a mutation or genetic exchange but instead involve a complex system of gene control. At any given moment, a large number of the genes of an organism are not expressed, and it is only in the face of specific stimuli (*inducers*) that certain genes are expressed. The altered response of an organism by specific stimuli is called *adaptation* or *induction* and is discussed in Section C of this chapter. It occurs much more rapidly than selection of a mutant; in general, all members of a population may become fully induced within a matter of a few hours. In this regard, pathogenic organisms can undergo adaptive change in response to host factors during the course of infection. Such change is not the result of mutation but nevertheless represents an advantage provided by evolution to enable a pathogen to adjust rapidly to the hostile environment normally presented by its natural host.

B. Genetic Exchange in Bacteria

The exchange of genetic material between bacterial cells is known to occur by transformation, conjugation, and transduction. Although bacteria of any given species do not exchange genetic information by all three mechanisms, cells of all species exchange genetic material by at least one of the three mechanisms. Studies of gene transfers between bacteria have made possible the mapping of some bacterial chromosomes.

1. Transformation

The exchange of genetic information by the transfer of naked DNA from one cell to another is called *transformation*. This phenomenon was first described in an *in vivo* experiment in mice, with pneumococci. Subsequently, the results of *in vitro* experiments established that bacteria of other genera can also exchange genetic information by this means. Short segments of donor DNA are taken into recipient cells and combined with the recipient chromosomes. Because the piece of DNA taken up by the recipient cell is small, only a few genes are transferred, a circumstance which has greatly aided in mapping the chromosomes of some bacteria.

Transformation provides a means for assaying the biological activity of DNA and consequently of relating the specific activity of a mutagen with alterations in DNA produced by the mutagen. In addition, it provides a useful tool for determining the effect of common chemicals on DNA function. Transformation is also a promising means for assessing the functional ability of DNA that has been synthesized *in vitro*.

2. Conjugation

Bacteria of some species exchange genetic information by a form of sexual recombination, in which "male" cells conjugate with "female" cells. During conjugation a part of, or sometimes even the entire, chromosome of the donor male bacterium is transferred to the female recipient. Subsequent genetic recombination of the DNA results in incorporation of the transferred genes.

Elucidation of the genetic elements that control bacterial conjugation has led to a better understanding of reactions between chromosomes and extrachromosomal elements. Obviously, bacterial conjugation is a useful tool with which to study genetics in general and bacterial genetics in particular. The direct transfer of hereditary characteristics from one bacterium to another is of great importance in medicine as well; e.g., the transfer of antibiotic resistance.

It is appropriate that a discussion of conjugation begin with the *E. coli* F factor (fertility or sex factor) since no other fertility factor model is so well understood. The F factor of *E. coli* is an episome consisting of a piece of DNA about the same size as bacteriophage λ (i.e., about 1% of the size of the bacterial chromosome). The term *episome* is used to designate a genetic element which can exist within a given population of bacteria either autonomously (i.e., apart from the bacterial chromosome) or as an integrated element physically inserted into the bacterial chromosome. Episomes are considered to be nonessential to cell survival under normal conditions. Thus, it should be readily apparent that the bacteriophage λ is an example of an episome (see Chapter 3).

Genetic elements which are known to exist only in the autonomous form and are not known to be capable of integrating with the chromosome are called *plasmids*. The distinction between episomes and plasmids is not always meaningful. For example, a single mutation involving the alteration of a single base pair can lead to a variant of phage λ which is not able to become a prophage; consequently this mutant of phage λ should be called a plasmid. According to these definitions, the F factor is an episome in *E. coli* but a plasmid in those *Salmonella* spp. into whose chromosome the factor cannot integrate.

a. Autonomous F Factor. In *E. coli* the autonomous form of the F factor evidently replicates in approximate synchrony with the bacterial

chromosome. Cells with an autonomous F factor are called F⁺ ("male")
and those without are termed F⁻ ("female").

The functions controlled by F factors are not well understood. In addition to controlling its own autonomous replication, an F gene directs the synthesis of a product called *F protein*, which is a constituent of *F pili*. Although a bacterium may have many pili of various kinds, a given F⁺ cell usually does not possess more than a few F pili and these are longer than hold-fast pili. Mating between F⁺ and F⁻ cells occurs by attachment of the pilus of the F⁺ cell to the F⁻ cell. Genetic exchange involves a one-way transfer of DNA from the F⁺ cell to F⁻ cell with the pilus serving as a conduit for the transfer.

The DNA component which is transferred most efficiently from F⁺ to F⁻ cells is the F factor itself. Upon acquiring the F factor the F⁻ cell becomes an F⁺ cell. It has been demonstrated that a brief exposure of an F⁻ population to a few F⁺ cells causes a rapid conversion of essentially the entire population to F⁺ cells. This is feasible because newly formed F⁺ cells can in turn transfer the F factor to F⁻ cells. It is believed that the F factor itself is replicated at the time of transfer and that possibly the energy associated with replication is the driving force for DNA transfer.

The weight of experimental evidence supports the concept that an autonomous F factor can also "mobilize" the transfer of other bacterial DNA from F⁺ to F⁻ cells. However, the transfer of other bacterial DNA through the mediation of an autonomous F factor is inefficient compared to the transfer of the F factor itself. The primary means by which bacterial DNA is transferred when male and female cells are mixed will be discussed below.

Autonomous F factors are easily deleted from F⁺ cells by a variety of agents such as UV irradiation and acridine dyes. A cell which loses its F factor is said to have been "cured," and such cells become typical F⁻ cells capable of acting as recipients during conjugation.

b. Integrated F Factor. In a population of F⁺ cells there are always a few cells in which the F factor has become integrated into the bacterial chromosome. Cells with integrated F factor are called *Hfr* (*high frequency of recombination*) *cells*. The integrated form of F is stable, and such cells can be obtained in pure culture. Like F⁺ cells, the Hfr cells produce F pili. However, in common with cells lysogenic for a bacteriophage, it is found that Hfr cells are immune to the autonomous form of homologous F factor. In other words, an autonomous F factor cannot be perpetuated in a cell which has an integrated F factor.

The most striking feature of F factor integration is that the transfer of chromosomal DNA from Hfr to F⁻ cells is much more efficient than the transfer from F⁺ to F⁻ cells. In fact, it is generally believed that most of the transfer of bacterial DNA which occurs when F⁺ and F⁻ cells are mixed is mediated by the few Hfr cells found in most F⁺ populations.

The way in which bacterial DNA is transferred from an Hfr to an F⁻

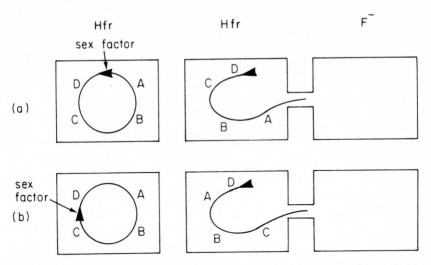

Figure 4-1. Conjugation between Hfr and F⁻ strains of *Escherichia coli*. The two parts of the figure demonstrate the effect of location of the integrated F factor on the origin and direction of transfer.

cell depends on where and how the sex factor is integrated into the bacterial chromosome. Unlike phage λ, which can integrate at only one site, the F factor can integrate at any one of a number of different locations. Furthermore, depending on the particular site at which the sex factor is integrated, F can be oriented in either direction. In Figure 4-1 the F factor is depicted as an arrow, which can be pointed (or oriented) in either a clockwise (Fig. 4-1b) or a counterclockwise (Fig. 4-1a) direction. This is important because it determines the direction in which the bacterial chromosome is transferred to recipient cells.

It is believed that during conjugation the chromosome breaks at the site (the origin) of integration of the F factor, and the gene originally next to it enters the recipient cell first. Replication of the bacterial chromosome begins at the origin and the DNA is transferred as a single, continuous strand. In Figure 4-1a the order of transfer of the genes would be A, B, C, D and in Figure 4-1b the order would be C, B, A, D. The probability that a recipient gene will acquire the leading gene may, under ideal conditions, be as high as 25%. The farther a gene is from the leading end of the chromosome (i.e., from the origin) the less its chances of transfer. The time required for transfer of an entire chromosome of *E. coli* is about 90 minutes under ideal conditions. Because the link between conjugating male and female bacteria is fragile and easily disrupted, transfer of the entire bacterial chromosome is uncommon. Therefore, the transfer of the integrated F factor at the very end rarely occurs, and most recipient cells remain F⁻.

c. Intermediate F Factor. On occasion, the integrated F factor leaves the bacterial chromosome and carries with it a piece of adjacent bacterial DNA. The bacterial DNA acquired by a departing F factor is usually adjacent to the head end of the episome (as depicted in Figure 4-1). There is some evidence to support the idea that when a departing episome acquires a piece of bacterial DNA it leaves behind some episomal DNA; hence the terms *intermediate* or *substituted* F factor. A cell with an intermediate F factor is called an F′ ("F prime") cell. The intermediate sex factor, including the bacterial genes it carries can be transferred to a female with an efficiency which resembles the transfer of an autonomous F episome. Except for the genes attached to the sex factor itself, F′ cells do not mediate the transfer of bacterial genes with a high efficiency.

The cell which acquires an intermediate F factor becomes diploid for the region of the chromosome carried by the intermediate F. The bacterial genes carried by the intermediate F, in rare instances, can undergo genetic recombination with the homologous genes in the bacterial chromosome but more often the cell survives as a partial diploid. The intermediate F is somewhat unstable and F′ cells are easily cured of their fertility factor. It is of singular importance that the F′ particle bears a close resemblance to certain episomes which mediate the rapid transfer of multiple drug resistance among enteric pathogens (Chapter 18).

3. Transduction

Certain bacteriophages are able to carry bacterial genes from one bacterium to another by a process known as *transduction*. There are two types of transduction: specialized and generalized.

Specialized transduction will be mentioned only briefly. Occasionally when phage DNA, such as that of phage λ, is excised from the bacterial chromosome an error is made. Excision of phage λ may result in a piece of bacterial DNA remaining attached to the excised λ DNA while a piece of λ DNA is left behind. These hybrid particles are defective and are called λ*dg*; they are defective because they lack the λ functions which are left behind. They also carry the adjacent bacterial genes which control the ability to ferment the sugar galactose. Phage λdg bears a certain resemblance to the intermediate sex factors just discussed. A number of other bacteriophages have also been found which are able to transduce only those genes which are located near the site of phage attachment.

Of broader interest is the observation that certain bacteriophages are able to transfer any gene from one host cell to another by a process known as *generalized transduction*. The simplest and most widely accepted explanation of the mechanism of generalized transduction is that during the assembly-line production of mature phage particles, a phage head can occasionally be filled with a piece of bacterial DNA rather than phage DNA. Thus, the production of generalized transducing particles is caused by a sort of "phenotypic mixing phenomenon" in which a piece of bacterial DNA has replaced phage DNA in an otherwise normal phage particle. The transducing particles have the same host range as the phage. The probability that a given gene will be accidentally incorporated in a phage head and eventually transferred to a recipient cell is approximately equal for most genes. However, some factors (mostly unknown) can lead to a greater probability of a particular gene being picked up and transferred.

Transduction is known to occur among bacteria of many genera and therefore may be the most important mechanism of genetic exchange among bacteria in nature. Transduction is known to be an important mechanism of transfer of drug resistance between certain types of pathogens.

C. Control of Genetic Expression

As previously mentioned, not all bacterial genes function simultaneously. Rather, it has been observed that genes which control the individual steps in a particular metabolic pathway are often transcribed or (alternatively repressed) *en bloc*. This form of gene regulation is quite important to the energy economy in a bacterium since, on the one hand, it enables the cell to "switch on" blocks of genes when they are needed, and, on the other hand, to "switch off" genes when they are not needed. Two metabolic pathways, whose control mechanisms have been well studied, should serve to explain some of the principles of gene regulation.

Wild-type *E. coli* can utilize the disaccharide lactose as a source of energy because it is able to manufacture two enzymes. One of these enzymes, called *β-galactosidase*, splits lactose into glucose and galactose, and the other, called *lactose permease*, promotes the entry of lactose into the cell. The regulatory mechanism whereby *E. coli* makes copious amounts of β-galactosidase and lactose permease in the presence of lactose and almost none in the absence of lactose depends on a regulation unit called the *operon*.

Figure 4-2a illustrates the genes in the lactose operon as well as the mechanism by which the operon is repressed in the absence of lactose. A regulator gene codes for a repressor which attaches to the operator gene, thereby preventing the initiation of transcription of the operon's genes by the cell's RNA polymerase.

Figure 4-2b illustrates what happens when lactose is present. Lactose attaches to and, as a consequence, inactivates the repressor. Therefore, transcription of the β-galactosidase and lactose permease genes is coordinately repressed in the absence of lactose and coordinately derepressed in the presence of lactose.

In the lactose system, lactose is referred to as an *inducer* since it induces the production of the enzymes required for the fermentation of lactose. The overall process of enzyme production by adding lactose is called *induction* or *induced enzyme formation*. Similar terminology has already

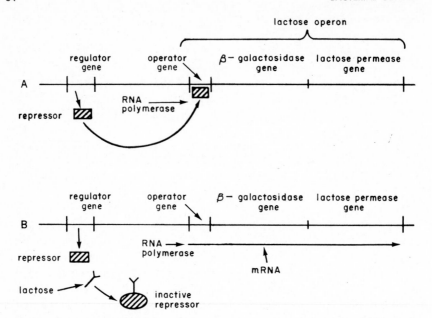

Figure 4-2. The lactose operon. (A) The repression of messenger RNA synthesis by repressor substances. (B) The induction (derepression) of the lactose operon caused by the inactivation of repressor by an inducing agent (lactose).

been introduced in Chapter 3 to describe the induction of a prophage (via its derepression) by an inducing agent.

The basic function of the operon is to coordinate repression or derepression of transcription of genes involved in a metabolic pathway. This principle is not only used by cells for degradative (catabolic) pathways but also for biosynthetic (anabolic) pathways.

When wild-type *E. coli* cells are supplied with a surplus of exogenous tryptophan the cells cease making tryptophan. Figure 4-3a illustrates the fact that a regulatory gene makes an inactive or *aporepressor*, which is unable to prevent the transcription of the genes in the tryptophan operon. Figure 4-3b illustrates that a surplus molecule of tryptophan which is either supplied exogenously or made endogenously can act as a *corepressor* (or *effector*). Acting together, the aporepressor and tryptophan form a full-fledged repressor capable of switching off the transcription of the genes in the tryptophan operon. This phenomenon is usually referred to as *repression* in contrast to the phenomenon of induction which has just been discussed in reference to lactose fermentation.

Finally, it has been found in tryptophan biosynthesis that the end product (i.e., tryptophan) can react with and inactivate the first enzyme in the biosynthetic pathway (enzyme E1 in Figure 4-3a). This phenomenon is called *end product* (or *feed back*) *inhibition.* Thus, *E. coli* has two

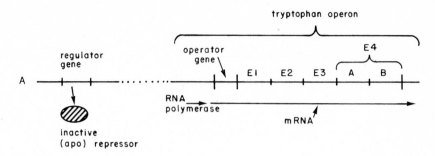

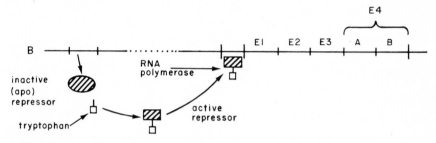

Figure 4-3. The tryptophan operon. (A) The inability of aporepressor to prevent messenger RNA synthesis. (B) The activation of aporepressor by tryptophan leading to the repression of the synthesis of messenger RNA.

mechanisms to prevent the production of tryptophan when tryptophan is present in excess: end product inhibition and repression.

There are many other examples of gene regulation. In most of the systems studied, the operon or some variation of the operon controls the system. The ability of a cell to control coordinately the transcription of the genes which direct the elements of a given metabolic pathway represents an important means by which the cells can rapidly adapt to a hostile environment. For example, certain cells carry the genetic potential to produce penicillinase, an enzyme which inactivates the antibiotic penicillin. The price the cells have to pay to possess the potential to produce penicillinase is merely the energy and raw materials needed to replicate the specific genes necessary for the enzyme's production. When placed in the presence of penicillin, the potentially resistant cells are able to reorder their energy priorities and produce penicillinase thus permitting survival of the cells.

D. Some Examples of the Application of Microbial Genetics to Problems in Medical Microbiology

Many aspects of microbial genetics are important to medical microbiology from both a practical and theoretical standpoint. Several interesting applications of microbial genetics to medicine are presented below:

1. Mutation

Mutations among microbes of medical importance can lead to confusion in diagnosis as well as problems with chemotherapy. A notable mutation among pathogens is from antibiotic sensitivity to resistance. Mutation to drug resistance is apparently a natural evolutionary event which will constantly complicate therapy and require a continuing search for new antimicrobial drugs. However, it is the responsibility of every physician to be fully aware that the overuse and misuse of antibiotics can increase the chances that drug-resistant strains will be selected.

Since mutations are relatively rare, the possibility that an organism will mutate simultaneously to resistance to more than one antibiotic is extremely rare. Hence within the limits set by drug antagonism, it is possible in special instances to avoid selection of drug-resistant mutants of bacteria by treating the patient simultaneously with more than one antibacterial agent (Chapter 6). Alternatively, since resistance to high levels of certain antibiotics is sometimes acquired in a step-wise fashion and furthermore, because of the phenomenon of phenotypic lag, it is often possible to avoid the selection of drug-resistant mutants by utilizing a high concentration of a given antibiotic from the first moment of treatment.

2. Genetic Exchange

A complete understanding of the attributes of microbes which convey pathogenicity must include knowledge of the genetic characteristics of the organism. Thus far only one species has been intensively studied, *E. coli*, and even in this instance only about 10% of the genes have been characterized and mapped! Extensive "genetic engineering" has been accomplished with *E. coli*. It is conceivable that the knowledge gained with this organism will make it possible to reduce the pathogenicity of various microbes. It may also be possible through the techniques of genetic engineering to "create" new and more effective vaccine strains which will lack pathogenicity but will induce maximal immunity.

References

Hayes, W.: *The Genetics of Bacteria and Their Viruses*. 2nd ed. New York: John Wiley and Sons, 1968.
Stent, G. S.: *Molecular Genetics*. San Francisco: W. H. Freeman and Company, 1971.
Watson, J. D.: *Molecular Biology of the Gene*. 2nd ed. New York: W. A. Benjamin, 1970.

Chapter 5

Sterilization and Disinfection

In view of the exceedingly large numbers of diverse microorganisms that populate our environment, the need for controlling them under many circumstances is obvious. Not only must disease-producing microbes be controlled but also those responsible for food spoilage and deterioration of various other materials. Common techniques that are employed for controlling microorganisms include sterilization of surgical instruments with heat (autoclaving), application of disinfectants on skin before surgery, canning techniques for preserving foods, use of fungicides to prevent material deterioration, and the use of chemotherapeutic agents to eradicate disease-producing microbes.

Sterilization procedures must destroy all forms of microbial life because the term *sterile* literally means the absence of all life. In this regard, microorganisms vary markedly in their resistance to various adverse environmental conditions. Bacterial spores are the most resistant forms of life, and techniques employed for sterilization must be designed to destroy this unique resting stage of microorganisms which characterizes the genera *Bacillus* and *Clostridium*. Spores will survive drying indefinitely, whereas some vegetative bacterial cells die quickly and others survive for varying, but limited, periods. Techniques used by the canning industry are specifically designed to kill spores with minimum alteration of the food products.

Most of our basic concepts concerning sterilization emerged from the innovative experiments of Pasteur which ultimately disproved the dogma of spontaneous generation in 1864. However, as late as 1876, Bastian published experimental results which opposed Pasteur's earlier claim that contaminated urine "sterilized" by boiling remained free of growth on subsequent incubation. Bastian declared that if the urine were made alkaline prior to boiling, growth often took place. Pasteur repeated the experiment and was forced to admit the truth of Bastian's claims. Two possible explanations could have accounted for the results: (1) *the urine was sufficiently acid so that it did not support the growth of the bacteria present,* or (2) *boiling was more effective in the acid than alkaline range of pH employed, particularly with respect to bacterial spores.*

As a consequence of this experience, Pasteur adopted the practice of heating fluids to 120°C by using steam under pressure and thus introduced the autoclave into the laboratory. In addition, he initiated the practice of sterilizing glassware by dry heat at 170° C. Tyndall, who observed that vegetative bacteria were easily destroyed by boiling, developed a sterilization procedure consisting of repeated heatings with appropriate incubation intervals between them. Such intervals allowed the heat-resistant spores to germinate into vegetative cells which were susceptible to killing at 100° C. This method, which was first described by Tyndall in a letter to Huxley in 1877, is still known as *tyndallization*. Present sterilization methods are based on the above observations together with a more exact knowledge of the heat resistance of bacterial spores. For example, it is well known that spores are more susceptible to heat in an acid medium than in a neutral or slightly alkaline medium.

Compared to moist heat (steam), hot air has low penetrability and heat transfer is relatively slow. In particular, dry heat is relatively ineffective if articles are wrapped with heat-insulating material.

In choosing a sterilization procedure, the type of item to be sterilized and convenience are considered as well as the cost and efficiency of the method.

A. Death Curve of Populations of Microorganisms

When populations of microorganisms are subjected to the common sterilization procedures, they are killed exponentially (Fig. 5-1). Accordingly, the number of bacterial cells dying in each time interval is a function of the number of survivors present. The exponential death process can be expressed by the following formula:

$$S = S_o e^{-kt}$$

S_o is the number of bacteria surviving at 0 time, and S represents the number of survivors at a later time t. The rate of exponential death is expressed by the term -k when ln (S/S_o) is plotted vs time.

It can be seen in Figure 5-1 that it took 30 minutes to reduce the population of bacteria from 10^3/ml to 10^0/ml. Therefore only one organism/ml was viable after 30 minutes of sterilization. Based on the exponential death rate function, there would be 10^{-1} organisms/ml at 40 minutes and 10^{-2} organisms/ml at 50 minutes of sterilization. This means that after 40 minutes one viable organism would be present in 10 ml and at 50 minutes only one organism would be viable in 100 ml. After 120 minutes of sterilization only one organism should be viable in 1000 liters. As a general rule a reduction of this magnitude can be considered a safe and practical sterilization procedure in most instances. It should be apparent that killing microorganisms is basically a problem of statistics and a sizable margin of safety must be built into any sterilization procedure.

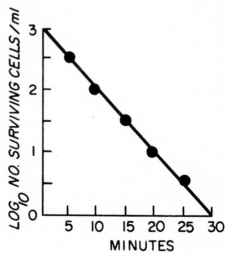

Figure 5-1. Exponential death curve of bacteria subjected to common sterilization procedures.

B. Sterilization by Heat

Heat may be employed in several ways for sterilizing objects. (1) *Incineration* can be used to sterilize transfer loops, coverslips, and so forth. (2) *Hot air*. Objects are usually heated at 160° to 170° C for 1 to 2 hours. This method is commonly used for glass Petri dishes, flasks, test tubes, pipets, and glass syringes. Obviously, most liquids cannot be sterilized by this method. (3) *Steam under pressure (autoclaving)* is the most effective practical method for heat sterilization. Exposure to steam in an autoclave at 15 pounds pressure (121° C) for 20 minutes will kill all forms of life. Steam under pressure has high penetrability and is particularly effective since it condenses on a cool object to release 596 cal per gram (heat of condensation). This condensation allows more steam to make contact with the objects being sterilized and as a result, the process of heat transfer continues until temperature equilibrium is reached. (4) *Flowing live steam* under ambient atmospheric pressure is highly effective against vegetative bacteria but is not a reliable method for killing bacterial spores unless the time-consuming tyndallization technique is used. At sea level, the boiling temperature attained approaches 100° C, but at high elevations the boiling point of water is so reduced that this technique is relatively ineffective. (5) *Boiling water* has been used to prepare objects, such as syringes and instruments, for minor surgery. As one would expect, this technique is not reliable for killing spores and should not be used when an autoclave is available. (6) *Pasteurization* is a process whereby a substance is heated to accomplish the killing of nonsporing pathogens or certain organisms that cause spoilage of milk or food products. In the case of milk, the holding process consists of heating at 62.5° C for 30 minutes and then cooling quickly. Milk may also be "flash pasteurized" by heating it in a thin layer for 3 to 5 seconds at 74° C. Pasteurization is useful for killing important pathogenic microorganisms that may be shed into milk by infected cows or may gain entrance into milk during its processing and distribution. However, pasteurized milk is *not sterile* since spores and certain nonsporing microbes such as *Streptococcus lactis* usually survive this treatment.

C. Sterilization by Filtration

There are many types of filters on the market which remove bacteria from liquids and accordingly are useful for "sterilizing" solutions containing heat-sensitive materials, such as serum proteins. Since viruses usually pass through such filters, the materials filtered are only "sterile" with respect to nonviral agents. The early filters were prepared from special purified clays. Subsequently, filters composed of asbestos pads were devised. Still later, fritted glass filters composed of masses of very finely porous Pyrex glass were developed. All of these filters have pore sizes which exceed the size of bacteria. Accordingly, the effectiveness of these filters does not result from sieve action but by adsorption of the bacteria due to differences between the respective electrical charges of the bacteria and filter material.

More recently, filters in the form of membranes composed of cellulose acetate or similar substances, each having a uniform porosity, have been made. These filters are available with porosities ranging from 0.005 to 1.0 μm and depend on sieve action almost exclusively for their effectiveness. A 0.22 μm filter removes bacteria, whereas the smallest pore size filters available retain the smaller viruses. The filter is mounted in a special apparatus and sterilized prior to use.

Membrane filters are especially useful for isolating and identifying organisms from water and air. The organisms retained by the filter are transferred with the filter to appropriate growth media.

D. Gas Sterilization

Under special circumstances, gases have been employed for sterilizing mattreses, bed clothing, heat-labile objects such as plastics, and even entire rooms or buildings.

1. Ethylene Oxide

Ethylene oxide (CH_2OCH_2) has a boiling point of about 11° C. It is usually mixed with 80 to 90% CO_2 to minimize its explosiveness, or it can be used as an 11% concentration in halogenated petroleum. The mixture is fed into an enclosed chamber resembling an autoclave in order to control humidity, temperature, and pressure. Ethylene oxide is a highly effective microbicidal agent and functions by alkylating protoplasmic nitrogenous components. However, it does not alter most organic materials that would be damaged by heat or moisture. It has good penetrability and dissipates readily from the sterilized material.

Ethylene oxide readily penetrates polyethylene wrapping material used for disposable items, but cellulose acetate, polyvinylidene chloride, and polyester wrapping materials are less permeable and should not be used.

2. Betapropiolactone

Betapropiolactone ($(CH_2)_2CO$) is a liquid at 20° C which may be stored at 4° C. It has been used to sterilize vaccines and tissue grafts. It must be used in a closed chamber where temperature and humidity can be controlled. Exposure for 2 to 3 hours at concentrations of 2 to 5 mg/L of air is a highly effective sterilizing procedure. Betapropiolactone is more active than ethylene oxide; it is noncorrosive and noninflammatory but has weak penetrability. It is generally recommended as a disinfectant for rooms.

3. Formaldehyde

Formaldehyde (CH_2O) has been used to a limited extent as a gaseous sterilant. Its sterilizing activity is due to its reactivity for amino groups in protein molecules. For example, in the disinfection of rooms, it has been recommended that 1 ml of formalin (37.5% formaldehyde) be vaporized for each cubic foot of space with an exposure time of 10 hours at 70° F and 50% relative humidity. A major limitation of the procedure is that the room must be aired for several days to remove the unpleasant odor.

Melamine formaldehyde can be used as a source of formaldehyde gas in special applications for sterilizing items after packaging. A strip of paper impregnated with melamine formaldehyde is incorporated during the packaging process of needles, blades, and plastic ware. The packages are heated to 50 to 60° C to release formaldehyde within the package from the melamine polymer. Effectiveness of this type of sterilization is monitored by exposing paper strips containing 10^5 to 10^6 bacterial spores to an identical packaging and heating process.

E. Disinfectants

In some textbooks the term *disinfection* is defined as "the destruction of potential pathogens on inanimate objects," whereas the term *antisepsis* is defined as "the destruction of such microbes in surface wounds or on body surfaces." In this chapter *disinfection* will be used in the general sense, namely to denote the destruction of any microorganism that is capable of producing an infection regardless of its location. If a disinfectant is lethal for bacteria or fungi, it is referred to as being *bactericidal* or *fungicidal*. If it prevents multiplication, it is commonly referred to as being *bacteriostatic* or *fungistatic*. The most useful disinfectants have broad-spectrum bactericidal or fungicidal activity.

There are two general groups of disinfectants. The toxicities of disinfectants of the first group are sufficiently low so that they can be used topically on skin and open wounds. In this application they are commonly referred to as *antiseptics*. However, topical disinfectants in this category are too toxic for systemic (parenteral) use and should not be confused with chemotherapeutic agents which can be administered systemically as well as topically. Disinfectants of the second group are generally too toxic for topical application on skin but are useful for disinfecting liquids and inanimate objects.

Standardization of disinfectants with respect to their effectiveness is a difficult problem. The use of the *phenol coefficient* for standardizing disinfectants represents an attempt to rate them by comparing their activities with those of phenol under standard conditions. For example if a disinfectant has a phenol coefficient of 3, it is 3 times as effective as phenol when compared in a standard bactericidal test. Unfortunately the activities of disinfectants vary greatly depending on a number of environmental conditions. Consequently, the phenol coefficient is only a rough estimate of the effectiveness of an agent; under field conditions the estimate may be completely erroneous. For example, the presence of excessive organic material can markedly alter the efficiency of many disinfectants and, as a consequence, the effectiveness of a disinfectant must be certified under actual field conditions.

1. Some Compounds That Are Used to Disinfect Skin and External Wounds

a. Iodine. A 2% tincture of iodine is useful for small cuts and abrasions as well as for reducing the number of bacteria on skin prior to venipuncture or surgery.

b. Betadine. The trade name of a commercially available iodophor, Betadine is gaining popularity as a preoperative antiseptic. It has the advantage of being highly bactericidal, nonirritating, and nonstaining.

c. Merthiolate. Merthiolate (a trade name) is an organic mercurial; it is fairly effective for skin wounds and normal skin. Its bacteriostatic properties reside in the ability of mercury to react with the thio groups of proteins, thus inactivating bacterial enzymes. Thio groups of the host can reverse its bacteriostatic activity.

d. Silver Nitrate. Silver nitrate is commonly used in a 1% aqueous solution for application to infant's eyes at birth to prevent infection and guard against blindness of the newborn due to *Neisseria gonorrhoeae* (Chapter 13). Silver ions have the property of combining with and inactivating enzymes.

e. Hexachlorophene. A chlorinated biphenol with surface-active properties which disrupt the cellular membrane, hexachlorophene has low toxicity and is bactericidal in low concentrations. This compound is commonly used in concentrations ranging from 1:1000 to 1:10,000 to irrigate surgical wounds and is usually incorporated into surgical soaps. The residual hexachlorophene helps suppress the growth of skin bacteria during and following surgery.

f. Detergents. There are cationic, anionic, or nonionic detergents. The cationic compounds (for example, Zephiran chloride) are the most effective disinfectants of this group; these are ammonium halides in which the hydrogen atoms have been replaced by organic radicals. The cleansing action of detergents and their ability to disrupt bacterial membranes contribute to their effectiveness as bactericidal agents. Their nontoxicity permits their use on food utensils and as a general preparatory agent for surgery.

g. Ethyl Alcohol and Isopropyl Alcohol. Both ethyl and isopropyl alcohols are commonly used in a 70% concentration; higher concentrations are less effective. Their bactericidal activity is inactivated by mucus or pus, and they are not effective against bacterial spores. However, these alcohols are moderately effective against vegetative bacteria on skin, especially in combination with green soap. The action of alcohols involves their capacity to precipitate cellular proteins.

2. Some Chemical Agents for Disinfecting Liquids and Inanimate Objects

Since toxicity is usually not a problem, many of the disinfectants commonly used to kill microorganisms on inanimate objects are either too toxic for human use or are used in concentrations exceeding those which can be safely used on skin or minor wounds. Many of the disinfectants listed above can also be used on inanimate objects.

a. Wescodyne.   Wescodyne (a trade name) is a commercially available iodophor which combines the cleansing action of a nonionic detergent with the bactericidal action of iodine. This compound is recommended over alcohol for sterilizing and storing thermometers.

b. Phenol.   Phenol (C_6H_5OH) in a 1% solution kills essentially all vegetative forms of bacteria in 20 minutes. A 5% solution, which is commonly used to disinfect surgical instruments and excreta, will kill bacterial spores in a few hours. Its effectiveness is altered only slightly by organic matter.

c. Cresols.   A mixture of cresols emulsified in green soap is sold under the trade name of Lysol. Lysol is about 4 times as effective as phenol. Ortho-, meta-, and paracresols are employed in a mixture known as tricresol, which is also more effective than phenol.

d. Mercuric Chloride.   When used under optimal conditions at a concentration of 1:1000, mercuric chloride is a powerful germicide. Mercuric ions form mercaptides with sulfhydryl groups which inactivate bacterial enzymes. However, the activity of mercuric chloride is markedly reduced by the presence of organic matter.

e. Chlorine.   Chlorine is commonly used to disinfect drinking water and water in swimming pools. It is important to monitor the free chlorine content and maintain effective concentrations. Chlorine gas added to water at a pH above 2.0 forms hypochlorous acid and hydrochloric acid. The hypochlorous acid (HOCl) is the bactericidal agent and acts through its oxidizing capacity. Another source of chlorine is NaOCl (sodium hypochlorite) which is available in grocery stores under the trade name of Clorox.

f. Cationic Detergents.   Highly effective as general disinfectants, cationic detergents are extensively employed to cleanse and disinfect food utensils. Concentrations as low as 1 ppm are effective and leave a residue which extends the reaction time.

g. Formalin.   Formalin (formaldehyde in solution) is a potent antimicrobial agent due to its high reactivity with proteins. It can block free amino groups at pH 9.5, reacts with the nitrogen of the imidazole ring of histidine at pH 6.0, and is fixed to amide and guanidyl groups at pH 5.0 or below.

F. Radiation

1. Ultraviolet Light

Ultraviolet light has moderate microbicidal activity when applied properly. Its effectiveness is limited by its extremely low penetrability. It can penetrate quartz but not glass. The wave length commonly used is about 2537 Å. Ultraviolet light is useful for *reducing* the population of airborne microorganisms in operating rooms, tissue culture rooms, and "sterile" rooms. It is also used widely in meat-packing houses and bakeries for controlling molds. The action of ultraviolet light is due directly to the formation of pyrimidine dimers from adjacent monomers on the same DNA strand and indirectly to the production of peroxides in the medium which act as oxidizing agents. The dimers may be mutagenic or lethal for bacteria. Resistance to pyrimidine dimers depends on the effectiveness of enzyme repair systems.

2. Gamma Radiation

Gamma radiation generated by cobalt 60 is effective for sterilizing packaged plastic wares such as plastic Petri dishes. It has been used for sterilizing dressings, catheters, and syringes and could find a special application in preserving foods except for the disagreeable flavors resulting from this procedure. About 2.0 to 2.5 $\times$ 10^6 rads are required to reduce microbial populations by a factor of 10^7.

3. High-energy Electrons

High-energy electrons have been used to sterilize plastic and rubber articles. Linear accelerations in the range of 1 to 5 MeV are used for this purpose.

G. General Considerations

Personal biases influence the selection of a general disinfectant for use on skin surfaces. Preparations containing hexachlorophene, organic iodine solutions, or cationic detergents are most often selected for preoperative skin preparation. On the other hand, minor skin abrasions are commonly cared for by cleansing thoroughly with soap and water and protecting the area from subsequent contamination.

Cationic detergents may be chosen to disinfect areas such as table tops because they do not have the unpleasant odor of phenol or cresol. Regardless of the agent used it is important to allow sufficient time for the agent to act in order to be effective. *Merely wiping a clinical thermometer with an iodophor like Wescodyne just prior to its use for each of a series of patients is not an acceptable practice.* Adequate exposure of an object to a disinfectant must always be allowed.

If the types of organisms contaminating an object or solution were known, it would be possible to select the least drastic of the sterilization methods that would be effective. In practice, however, one must assume that spores are present; accordingly the method chosen is not directed toward a particular organism but against all organisms or at least all pathogenic organisms that may be present on the item. In many instances, surgical instruments could be sterilized with either the autoclave, the hot air oven, the gas sterilizer, or by gamma radiation without harming the instruments. However, autoclaving is the most practical means for ensuring the sterility of such objects.

References

Lowbury, E. J. L., Lilly, H. A., and Bull, J. P.: Methods for disinfection of hands and operation sites. Brit. Med. J. 2:531, 1964.

Perkins, J. J.: *Principles and Methods of Sterilization in Health Sciences.* Springfield, Ill.: Charles C. Thomas, 2nd edition, 1969.

Tulis, J. J.: Formaldehyde gas as a sterilant. International Symposium on Industrial Sterilization, Amsterdam, September 26-27, 1972.

Chapter 6

Antimicrobial Chemotherapy

In the course of past centuries man accidentally discovered a few useful agents for preventing and treating the infectious diseases which afflicted him. One example is quinine, the antimalarial agent present in the bark of the cinchona tree. Also the early Chinese used moldy soybean curd to treat boils and wore sandals covered with mold to control foot infections.

Before the age of science, discovery of antimicrobial agents was purely accidental or the result of undirected trial and error. Apparently the first systematic search for an antimicrobial drug was made by Paul Erhlich at the beginning of this century. Using the knowledge that salts of heavy metals were useful for treating surface lesions of syphilis, he set as his goal the synthesis of a relatively nontoxic compound which would be highly lethal for *Treponema pallidum*. His discovery of salvarsan in 1910 was a crowning success and ushered in the chemotherapeutic era with the great hope that agents effective against essentially all pathogens would soon be discovered. However, in following years most of the drugs tried proved to be too toxic. Moreover, the belief of that time, which is no longer tenable, that the basic biochemical activities of microbes and mammalian cells are essentially identical, provided no rational basis for synthesizing compounds with selective toxicity for pathogens.

The first systematic search for natural antibiotics which was made by Gratia and Doth about 1924 resulted in the discovery of actinomycetin. Subsequently, Fleming observed marked inhibition of *Staphylococcus aureus* on a plate contaminated with a penicillium mold, which led to the discovery of the "miracle drug" penicillin—a discovery which reawakened interest in the potential of antimicrobial chemotherapy.

A. Concepts of Selective Toxicity

The term *antibiosis* was first defined by Vuillemin in 1889 as a condition "in which one creature destroys the life of another in order to sustain his own." Based on this principle, many useful antimicrobial agents have been isolated from culture filtrates of soil organisms such as members of the genera *Bacillus, Penicillium,* and *Streptomyces.* In addition, a few substances of biological origin have been modified chemically either to extend their spectrum of activity, to enhance activity by way of the oral route, or to improve stability.

In the selection of any antimicrobial drug for systemic use, the most important requirement is that it is more toxic for the microbe than for host cells (selective toxicity). Ideally, such a drug should have *no* toxicity for the host, but this has been rarely achieved. Since cell walls of bacteria are chemically unique, drugs which inhibit cell-wall synthesis have essentially no toxicity for mammalian cells. Accordingly, the penicillins fulfill this requirement better than most antibiotics available.

Many useful drugs have been synthesized based on exact knowledge of their potential for acting specifically against some vital biochemical step in the metabolism of the microbe. A search for new and more effective drugs is continuously under way because of the constant threat of emergence of drug-resistant strains (Chapter 4) and special problems of therapy associated with certain drug-resistant organisms, such as members of the genera *Proteus, Pseudomonas, Staphylococcus,* and *Klebsiella.*

The most effective antibacterial drugs are those that are *bactericidal,* because successful therapy may be achieved with these drugs even if host defense mechanisms are impaired. In the case of extracellular parasites, a *bacteriostatic* drug can only be highly effective when defense forces such as phagocytosis continue to function normally. Diseases caused by intracellular parasites (tuberculosis, brucellosis, typhoid fever, typhus, etc.) do not respond to chemotherapy as rapidly as diseases caused by extracellular parasites because most antimicrobial drugs do not readily penetrate host cell membranes. For example, streptomycin does not penetrate the phagosomes of macrophages infected with tubercle bacilli nearly as well as isoniazid. Consequently, isoniazid is a more efficient therapeutic agent for tuberculosis than streptomycin.

B. Mechanisms of Action of Antimicrobial Agents

There are 5 major mechanisms by which antimicrobial agents can inhibit or kill microorganisms. They may: (1) inhibit the assembly of a critical metabolite (sulfonamides); (2) inhibit cell-wall synthesis (penicillin); (3) irreversibly damage the cell membrane (polymyxin); (4) inhibit protein synthesis (tetracyclines, erythromycin, Rifampin); or (5) inhibit nucleic acid metabolism (griseofulvin).

C. The Common Antibacterial Drugs

1. The Sulfonamides

Prontosil, which was described by Domagk in 1935, marked the beginning of the era of widespread antibacterial chemotherapy. Prontosil *per se* was not active but released sulfanilamide *in vivo* which was the active moiety. Subsequently many sulfonamide compounds were synthesized in attempts to improve the antibacterial action of the basic molecule. These compounds rapidly penetrate the blood-brain barrier and have been used extensively in the treatment of meningococcal meningitis. They are also used for treating trachoma and are reasonably effective for preventing re-

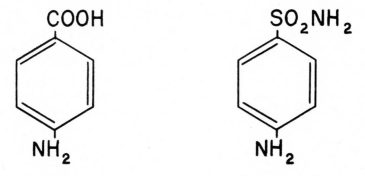

p-Aminobenzoic Acid   Sulfanilamide

Figure 6-1. The structural similarity of PABA and sulfanilamide explains the basis of competitive inhibition of folic acid synthesis.

curring β-hemolytic streptococcal infections in patients with rheumatic fever.

The sulfonamides act by competing (competitive inhibition) with para-aminobenzoic acid (PABA) (Fig. 6-1) thus aborting the biosynthesis of folic acid by the bacterial cell. Their selective action is based on the principle that they do not inhibit mammalian cells which utilize preformed folic acid but inhibit bacterial cells that depend on folic acid assembled intracellularly.

Disadvantages of the sulfonamide drugs include: (1) they are only bacteriostatic; (2) they have a limited antibacterial spectrum; (3) drug-resistant strains of bacteria develop readily; and (4) they may, on rare occasions, cause side effects such as aplastic anemia, thrombocytopenia, granulocytopenia, and periarteritis nodosa due, in part, to their tendency to sensitize the host (see *Fundamentals of Immunology*).

2. The Sulfones

Although diaminodiphenyl sulfone (DDS), a relative of the sulfonamide drugs, is currently the drug of choice for the treatment of leprosy, Rifampin shows great promise.

3. Para-aminosalicylic Acid (PAS)

This drug, in combination wtih isoniazid or streptomycin, is widely used in the treatment of tuberculosis. In common with the sulfonamides its mode of action is based on competition with PABA. Other drugs, such as ethambutal and Rifampin, are finding increased use as replacements for PAS.

4. Isoniazid (INH)

Isoniazid, a bactericidal drug, is used exclusively for the treatment of tuberculosis (Fig. 6-2). It may be given alone as a chemoprophylactic drug to individuals who are recent "tuberculin converters," or in combination with p-aminosalicylic acid or Rifampin to patients with clinical tuberculosis. Isoniazid penetrates macrophages and can be bactericidal to mycobacteria within phagosomes of macrophages providing the organisms are

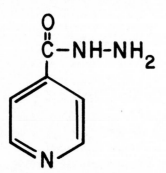

Figure 6-2. Structure of isoniazid.

actively metabolizing. Isoniazid is not effective against the atypical myco-bacteria (Chapter 29).

5. The Penicillins and Cephalosporins

The natural penicillins are highly effective against all gram-positive cocci except enterococci and penicillinase-producing staphylococci. In addition, they are active against gonococci, meningococci, and *Treponema pallidum* as well as some actinomycetes. All penicillins have a β-lactam-thiazolidine ring which is conjugated to different side chains (Fig. 6-3.) Two natural penicillins are depicted in Figure 6-4.

Several semisynthetic penicillins have been produced by controlling the synthesis of the nucleus, 6-aminopenicillanic acid without the customary

Penicillin

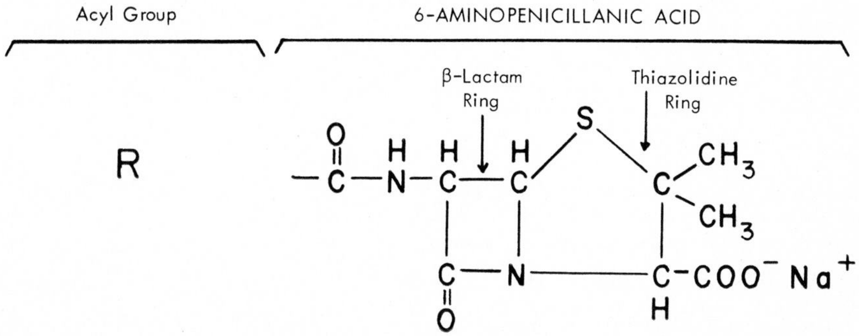

Figure 6-3. Basic structure of penicillin indicating the relationship of the acyl group to the 6-aminopenicillanic acid molecule. (Adapted from Adv. Intern. Med. *16*:373, 1970.)

Name	Characteristic	R Side Chain
Benzyl (G)	Susceptible to penicillinase. High activity against most gram-positive bacteria. Low activity against gram-negative bacteria; acid labile.	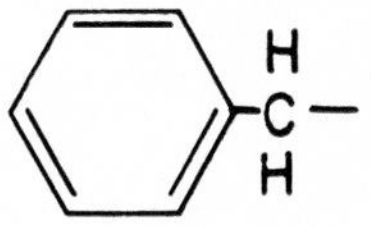
Phenoxymethyl (V)	Less susceptible to acid hydrolysis than G, susceptible to penicillinase.	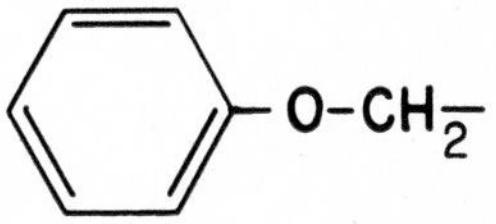

Figure 6-4. Characteristics and structure of the acyl groups of two natural penicillins. If corn steepliquor is supplied with β-phenylethylamine, penicillin G is produced, whereas, if phenoxyacetic acid is added, penicillin V is synthesized by *Penicillium chrysogenum*. Note site of attachment of acyl group to the 6-aminopenicillanic acid molecule in Figure 6-3. (Adapted from Adv. Intern. Med. *16*:373, 1970.)

Name	Characteristic	R Side Chain
Dimethoxyphenyl (Methicillin)	Penicillinase — resistant. Lower activity than Penicillin G. Acid-labile. Low protein binding.	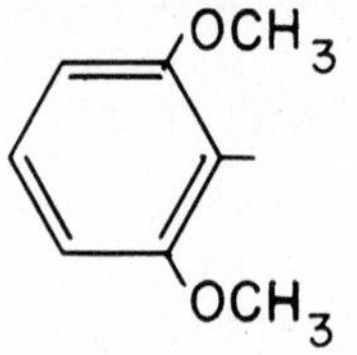
5 — methy — 3 phenyl — 4 isoxyzolyl (Oxacillin)	Penicillinase resistant. Acid-stable. High protein binding.	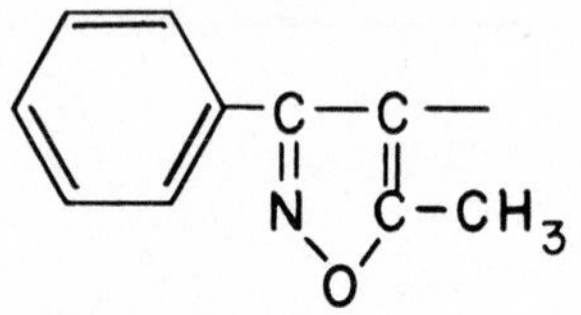
α Aminobenzyl (Ampicillin)	Penicillinase sensitive. Wider spectrum. Acid-stable.	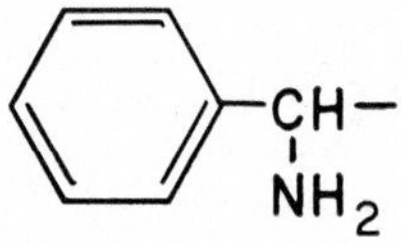
α Carboxybenzyl (Carbenicillin)	Wider spectrum — activity against Pseudomonas.	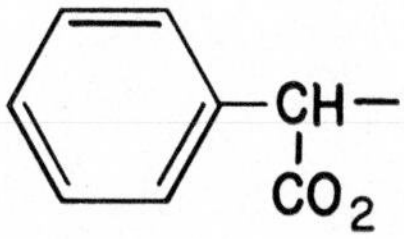

Figure 6-5. Characteristics and structure of the acyl groups of selected semisynthetic penicillins. Note site of attachment of acyl group to the 6-aminopenicillanic acid molecule in Figure 6-3. (Adapted from Adv. Intern. Med. *16*:373, 1970.)

side chains. The side chains are added by *in vitro* chemical techniques. One very important property of some of the semisynthetic penicillins is that they are resistant to penicillinase (methicillin, oxacillin). In the case of ampicillin and Carbenicillin, a broader antibacterial spectrum is expressed. Structural formulas of four semisynthetic penicillins are presented in Figure 6-5.

The basic mechanism of action of all penicillins is to block bacterial cell-wall synthesis. Accordingly, they are only bactericidal when the bacteria are actively growing and synthesizing new cell walls (Fig. 6-6).

The penicillins can be given either orally or intramuscularly. However, absorption through the gastrointestinal tract can vary, depending in part on their acid resistance. Careful consideration must be given to this point when oral penicillin is used for serious infections. Benzathine penicillin given by injection allows slow release of penicillin *in vivo* and is useful when levels must be maintained for extended periods as in prophylaxis for rheumatic fever. The major problem with penicillin is its tendency to induce hypersensitivity (see *Fundamentals of Immunology*).

The cephalosporins are similar to the penicillins except that they contain a nucleus which has a six-membered thiazolidine ring fused to a β-lactam ring; this makes them moderately resistant to penicillinase. Cephalo-

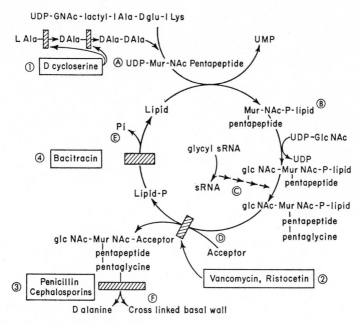

Figure 6-6. Schematic representation of the stages in the synthesis of bacterial cell wall to illustrate sites of action of some antimicrobial agents (follow from upper left, clockwise). (1) D-cycloserine inhibits alanine racemase and D-alanine-D-alanine synthetase. (2) Vancomycin and ristocetin inhibit transfer of disaccharide-peptide units from the lipid intermediate to the cell-wall acceptor. (3) Penicillin and cephalosporins irreversibly inhibit the transpeptidase and prevent the final cross-linking step. (4) Bacitracin inhibits dephosphorylation of the lipid pyrophosphate, which prevents regeneration of the phospholipid. (Reprinted with permission from Adv. Intern. Med. *16*:373, 1970.)

thin and cephaloridine, which are semisynthetic derivatives, have been found to be valuable clinically. Since these compounds are inactivated at pH of 4.5 or less they must be given by injection. Cephalexin and cephaloglycin are acid-resistant and readily absorbed in the gut so they may be given orally. These drugs are bactericidal and active against most of the common gram-positive organisms (Fig. 6-6). However, they are also effective in treating urinary tract infections because the levels reached in urine (300 to 500 μg/ml) are inhibitory for most gram-negative organisms.

6. The Aminoglycosides: Streptomycin, Kanamycin, and Neomycin

Streptomycin has been used primarily for treating tuberculosis, *Klebsiella* pneumonia, *Haemophilus influenzae* meningitis, tularemia, *Shigella* dysentery, and the common gram-negative urinary tract and systemic infections (Fig. 6-7). Streptomycin is moderately toxic and can cause damage to the 8th cranial nerve following prolonged therapy. Another disadvantage is that it cannot be given orally. When given with penicillin, a synergistic

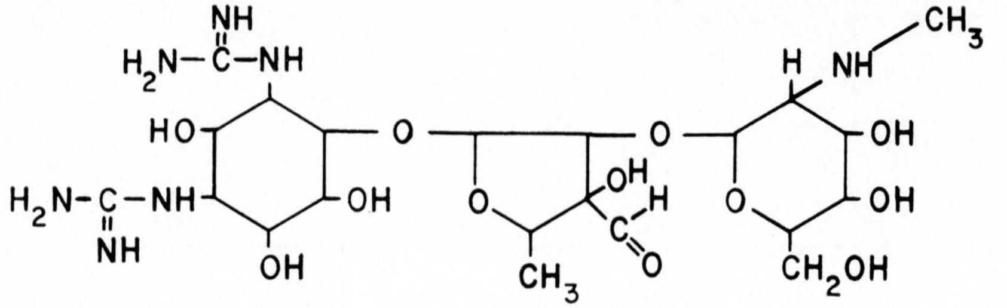

Figure 6-7. Structure of streptomycin.

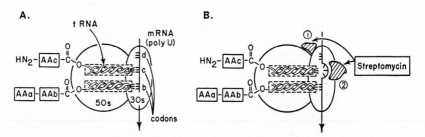

Figure 6-8. Schematic representation of the normal relationship of tRNA to the mRNA template and site(s) of action of streptomycin. (A) Normal relationship of the tRNA to the mRNA template. (B) The primary effect of streptomycin is on protein synthesis; this effect may be due to modification of the association of the 30S and 50S subunits, which results in the production of aberrant initiation complexes (1) or to distortion of the mRNA, with misreading of the genetic code (2). (Reprinted with permission from Adv. Intern. Med. *16*:373, 1970.)

action resulting from this combination provides a useful regimen for treating subacute bacterial endocarditis caused by enterococci. The primary effect of streptomycin is on protein synthesis (Fig. 6-8).

Kanamycin is more toxic than streptomycin; it is used primarily for short-term therapy of acute urinary tract infections.

Neomycin is poorly absorbed and is too toxic for routine systemic administration. However, it is effective for achieving gastrointestinal antisepsis prior to surgery.

7. The Tetracyclines

Chlortetracycline, oxytetracycline, and tetracycline are the generic names of three antibiotics having similar properties (Fig. 6-9). The tetracyclines are effective against most gram-negative organisms, and as a consequence they have replaced streptomycin and the sulfonamides for this application. They are also effective against mycoplasma, chlamydia, and rickettsia. Tetracyclines are generally ineffective against infections caused by members of the genera *Proteus, Pseudomonas* and *Salmonella*. They are readily

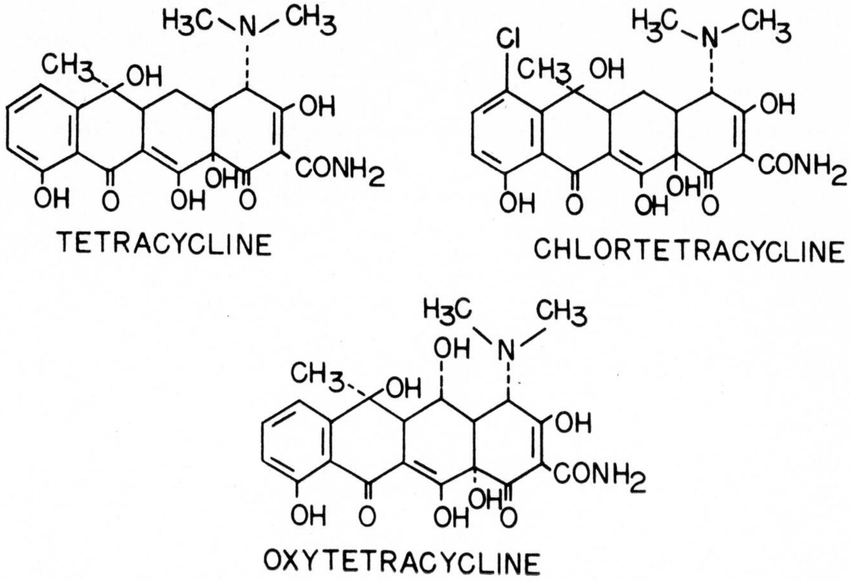

Figure 6-9. Structure of chlortetracycline, oxytetracycline, and tetracycline.

absorbed from the gastrointestinal tract but can alter the normal flora and give rise to intestinal disturbances and superinfection by opportunistic pathogens, especially if treatment is prolonged. The tetracyclines inhibit the binding of the aminoacyl-tRNA to the 30S subunit of the ribosome (Fig. 6-10).

8. Chloramphenicol

Chloramphenicol, a bacteriostatic compound, has the same antimicrobial spectrum as the tetracyclines (Fig. 6-11). However, in some patients it is toxic for bone marrow and can produce aplastic anemia. It is particularly effective for treating typhoid fever, *Haemophilus influenzae* meningitis, and rickettsial infections. Chloramphenicol must be administered in reduced dosages to infants because their detoxification system (glucuronide conjugation in the liver) is not fully developed. The drug is now prepared by chemical synthesis. Chloramphenicol inhibits the formation of peptide bonds (Fig. 6-10).

9. The Macrolides: Erythromycin and Oleandomycin

The macrolides have been effectively used to treat infections caused by penicillinase-producing staphylococci. However the penicillinase-resistant penicillins will probably soon replace these drugs for this application. In addition to erythromycin and oleandomycin, other antibiotics in this group include carbomycin and spiramycin. Erythromycin inhibits the translocation of the peptidyl-tRNA from acceptor to donor site (Figs. 6-10 and 6-12).

10. Lincomycin and 7-chloro Lincomycin

Lincomycin and 7-chloro lincomycin are bacteriostatic drugs which inhibit the formation of peptide bonds (Figs. 6-10 and 6-13). Their antibacterial spectrum is similar to that of erythromycin. They are effective against pneumococci, streptococci, staphylococci, and *C. diphtheriae*.

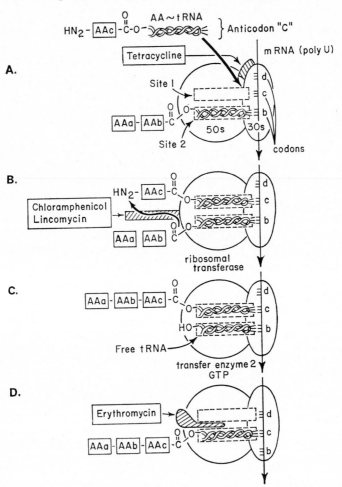

Figure 6-10. Schematic representation of the steps in the synthesis of the polypeptide chain to illustrate sites of action of some antibiotic agents. (A) Tetracycline inhibits the binding of the aminoacyl-tRNA to the 30S subunit of the ribosome. (B) Chloramphenicol and lincomycin inhibit formation of the peptide bond. (D) Erythromycin inhibits the translocation of the peptidyl-tRNA from acceptor to donor site. Erythromycin also competitively inhibits the binding of chloramphenicol to the 50S subunit and can displace bound lincomycin but not chloramphenicol. (Reprinted with permission from Adv. Intern. Med. *16*:373, 1970.)

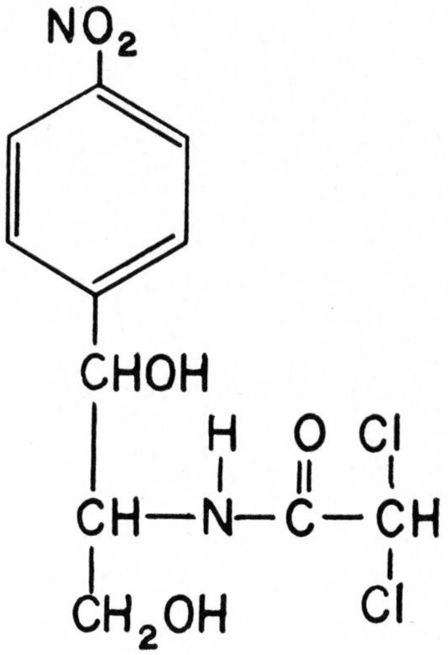

Figure 6-11. Structure of chloramphenicol.

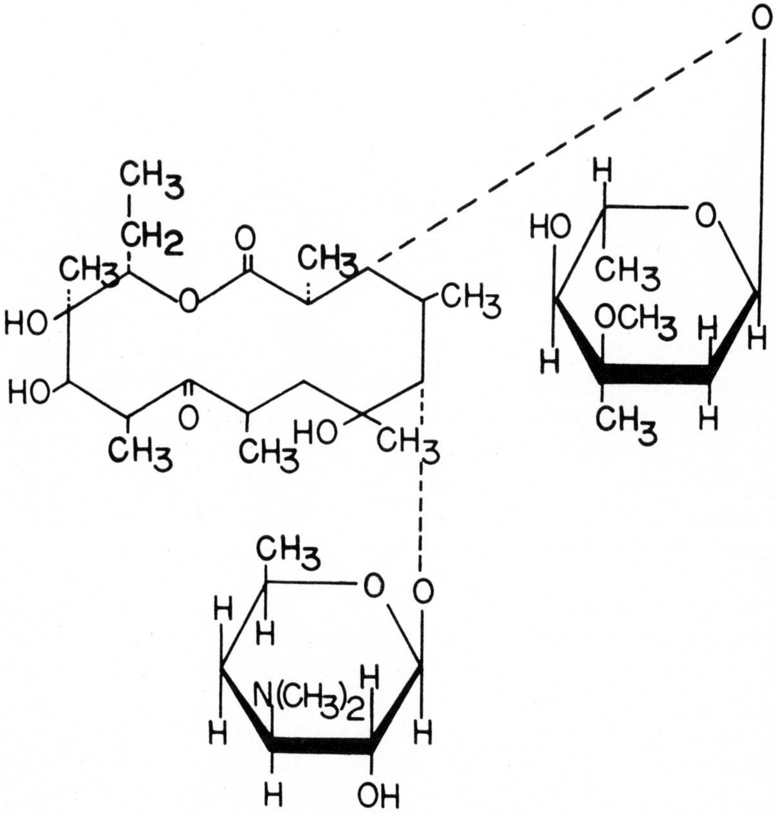

Figure 6-12. Structure of erythromycin.

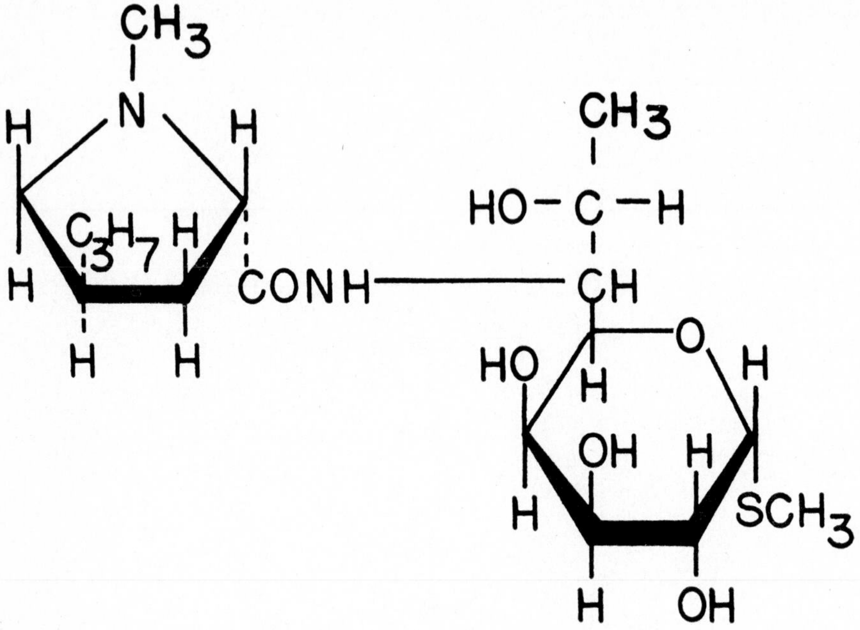

Figure 6-13. Structure of lincomycin.

11. Rifamycins

The rifamycin antibiotics are fermentation products of *Streptomyces mediterranei sp. n.* The rifamycins are ansa compounds consisting of a chromophoric naphthoquinone or naphthohydroquinone ring which is spanned by a long aliphatic bridge. Rifampin, an orally active semisynthetic derivative which has been used very extensively, is a 3-(4-methyl-piperazinyl)-iminomethyl derivative of rifamycin SV (Fig. 6-14). Clinically, rifampin has a wide spectrum of activity and is highly active against mycobacteria and gram-positive organisms as well as *Neisseria* and *Haemophilus.* These antibiotics specifically inhibit DNA-dependent RNA polymerase by blocking the RNA chain initiation steps. Cross-resistance with other antibiotics has not been detected.

12. Polymyxins: Polymyxin B and Polymyxin E

The polymyxins are basic polypeptides that irreversibly injure bacterial cell membranes. As one would expect, stationary phase cells are as susceptible as log-phase cells.

These drugs are relatively neurotoxic and nephrotoxic and are usually employed systemically only as a last-ditch stand against infections that are resistant to all other antibiotics. In some instances polymyxin B is the only effective agent for treating serious infections caused by *Pseudomonas ae-*

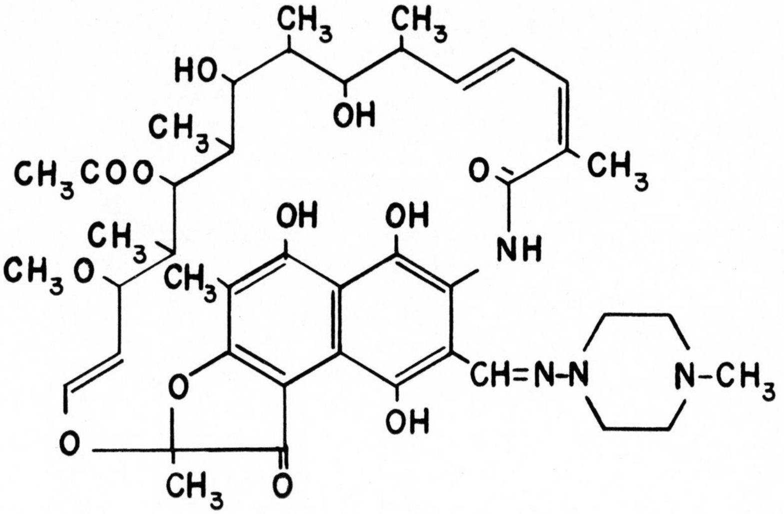

Figure 6-14. Structure of Rifampin.

ruginosa. It is also used for gastrointestinal antisepsis and for special topical applications. Polymyxin E (colistin) is dispensed as a methane-sulfonate complex for use against urinary tract infections.

D. The Common Antifungal Drugs

1. Amphotericin B

Amphotericin B is a complex polyene antibiotic produced by a species of *Streptomyces*. In spite of its relatively high toxicity, it is the most effective agent available for the treatment of disseminated coccidioidomycosis, blastomycosis, histoplasmosis, cryptococcosis, and candidiasis. Its mode of action involves membrane damage to the fungal cells.

2. Griseofulvin

This antibiotic is derived from certain species of the genus *Penicillium* (Fig. 6-15). It is active against dermatophytes (*Microsporum* and *Trichophyton*) but is inactive against bacteria and the fungi which produce systemic mycoses. The drug accumulates in the keratin layer which explains its selective action against dermatophytes. Its action depends on inhibition of nucleic acid synthesis of the dermatophytes.

E. Sensitivity Tests

The sensitivity of a microbial isolate (obtained from a patient) to chemotherapeutic agents under consideration can be determined in the laboratory by either the paper-disc method or by the more accurate tube-dilution tech-

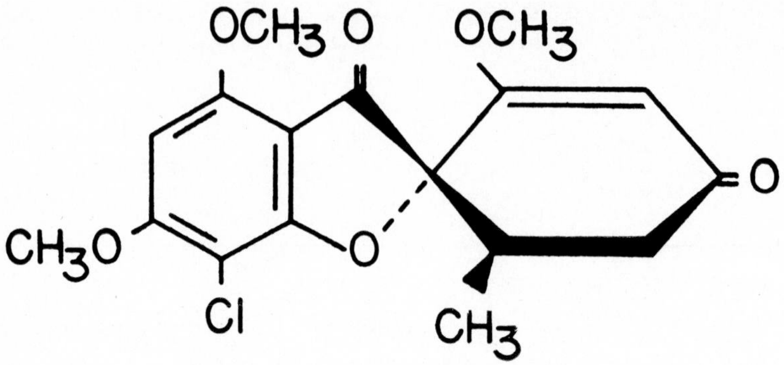

Figure 6-15. Structure of griseofulvin.

nique. The paper-disc method is the most commonly used method because of its relative simplicity. Standardized commercial discs containing known amounts of the respective antimicrobial agents are placed on agar plates seeded with the test organism. Upon incubation a clear zone surrounds the disc if the test organism is sensitive to the antimicrobial agent which diffused from the disc into the agar. The size of the zone of inhibition usually correlates with the degree of sensitivity of the microorganism. Verification of microbial sensitivities and drug potencies requires standard control curves plotting the size of inhibition zones vs drug concentration.

The tube-dilution technique can detect the smallest amount of antimicrobial agent that will inhibit the growth of a standardized inoculum of the test organism. This amount is referred to as the *MIC* (*minimal inhibitory concentration*) of the drug against the test organism. It is also possible to subculture the respective tubes from the test and determine the minimum concentration of antimicrobial agent which will kill (subcultures will have no growth) the test organism *in vitro*. This endpoint is referred to as the *MBC* (*minimal bactericidal concentration*) of the drug.

On certain occasions it is necessary to quantitate the level of a chemotherapeutic drug achieved *in vivo* in serum or plasma of the patient. This can be done by using a tube-dilution technique with a standard test organism.

F.   Considerations that Relate to Success or Failure in Chemotherapy

As a general rule, *successful antimicrobial chemotherapy depends on host defense mechanisms acting in concert with the antibacterial action of the drug.* For example, if abscesses are present, even bactericidal drugs are relatively ineffective; this is probably due largely to lack of multiplication of microorganisms within abscesses and/or to the presence of dead leucocytes which form a barrier to the penetration of the drug. However, if such abscesses are drained, chemotherapy usually becomes highly effective.

Chemotherapy is relatively ineffective when foreign bodies (bone spicules, sutures, splinters of wood, etc.) *are present in a lesion.* Somehow, foreign bodies protect bacteria from phagocytosis causing the persistence of multiple foci of infection.

Obstruction of any organ drainage system impairs the cellular defenses and complicates chemotherapy. Accordingly, bacterial infections associated with obstruction of urinary or respiratory tracts tend to persist in the face of intensive chemotherapy. Usually a cure is effected only when the foreign body is removed or the obstruction is relieved.

In general, *any disease which impairs the immune mechanisms of the host will impair the effectiveness of chemotherapy.* For example, disease states such as agranulocytosis, leukemia, uremia, and diabetes mellitus which depress host resistance compromise the success of chemotherapy.

G. The Problem of Superinfections

Most antimicrobial drugs alter the delicate balance of the normal flora which in turn disturbs the equilibrium of microbial antagonism between indigenous organisms. This can lead to the emergence and dominance of certain indigenous organisms which can act as opportunistic pathogens (*Pseudomonas aeruginosa, Candida albicans, Proteus* sp. and some strains of *Staphylococcus aureus*). If these organisms are drug-resistant they can markedly complicate therapy. Broad-spectrum antibiotics are most likely to create such problems, especially when therapy is prolonged.

H. The Problem of Drug Resistance

The emergence of drug-resistant strains is an ever-present problem. In this regard, it should be emphasized that antibacterial drugs do not cause mutations but instead select resistant mutants that develop spontaneously. This is most likely to occur with opportunistic pathogens and organisms which are the most prevalent in the environment. It is of interest that some microorganisms such as *Diplococcus pneumoniae* and *Streptococcus pyogenes* (group A) have not developed appreciable resistance in spite of having been exposed to many years of chemotherapy. This suggests that, in the case of some species, loss of virulence goes hand in hand with mutation to drug resistance. In addition to the emergence of mutants that are resistant to antibiotics, resistance can be acquired as a consequence of episomal transfer (Chapter 4) which can result in the simultaneous acquisition of resistance to more than one drug.

I. General Axioms Pertinent to Chemotherapy

1. Actively multiplying organisms are more susceptible to bactericidal drugs than nonmultiplying organisms.

2. When a bacteriostatic drug is used, duration of therapy must be sufficient to allow cellular and humoral defense mechanisms to "eradicate" causative organisms.

3. If possible, bactericidal drugs should be used to treat infections of the endocardium or the meninges. The host defenses are relatively ineffective in these sites, and the dangers imposed by such diseases require prompt eradication of the organisms.

4. Chemotherapy is relatively ineffective against organisms present in abscesses, lesions with foreign bodies, cavitary lesions, and organ systems in which obstruction of duct systems exists.

5. Chronic bacterial diseases caused by intracellular parasites require prolonged therapy to allow cellular immune mechanisms to assist in the eradication of the infecting organisms.

6. Combined therapy is used in special cases (1) to prevent emergence of resistant strains (INH plus PAS in tuberculosis), (2) to take advantage of bactericidal synergism (penicillin plus streptomycin to treat bacterial endocarditis), and (3) to treat rare emergency cases during the period when an etiological diagnosis is still in progress.

7. Bacteriostatic drugs such as sulfonamides or the broad-spectrum antibiotics may interfere with the bactericidal action of penicillin; accordingly, this combination of drugs should be avoided in treating pneumococcal meningitis or bacterial endocarditis, where the bactericidal action of penicillin is necessary.

8. Without adequate laboratory diagnostic evidence, "upper respiratory infections" should not be treated on a routine basis with antibacterial drugs because 95% of these infections are caused by viral agents.

References

Bauer, A. W., Kirby, W. M. M., Sherris, J. C., and Turck, M.: Antibiotic susceptibility testing by a standardized single disk method. Amer. J. Clin. Path. *45*:493, 1966.

Ericsson, H. M., and Sherris, J. C.: Antibiotic sensitivity testing. Acta Path. Microbiol. Scand. Suppl. 217 (Section B), 1971.

Franklin, T. J., and Snow, G. A.: *Biochemistry of Antimicrobial Action.* New York: Academic Press, 1971.

Garrod, L. P., and O'Grady, F.: *Antibiotics and Chemotherapy.* 3rd ed. Baltimore: The Williams & Wilkins Co., 1971.

Kagan, B. M.: *Antimicrobial Therapy.* Philadelphia: W. B. Saunders Company, 1970.

Martin, E. W.: *Hazards of Medication: A Manual on Drug Interactions, Incompatibilities, Contraindications and Adverse Effects.* Philadelphia: J. B. Lippincott Company, 1971.

Pestka, S.: Inhibitors of ribosome function. Ann. Rev. Microbiol. *25*:487, 1971.

Strominger, J. L., and Tipper, D. J.: Bacterial cell wall synthesis and structure in relation to the mechanism of action of penicillins and other antibacterial agents. Amer. J. Med. *39*:708, 1965.

Swenson, R. M., and Sanford, J. P.: Clinical implications of the mechanism of antimicrobial agents. Adv. Intern. Med. *16*:373, 1970.

Wehrli, W., and Staehelin, M.: Actions of the rifamycins. Bacteriol. Rev. *35*:290, 1971.

Weinstein, L.: Chemotherapy of microbial disease. In *The Pharmacological Basis of Therapeutics*. L. S. Goodman and A. Gilman, eds. New York: The Macmillan Company, 1965.

Weiser, R. S., Myrvik, Q. N., and Pearsall, N. N.: *Fundamentals of Immunology*. Philadelphia: Lea & Febiger, 1969.

Chapter 7

Principles of Host-Parasite Interactions

A. Interactions between Nonpathogenic Parasites and their Hosts, 85
B. Selective Attachment of Bacteria to Mammalian Cells, 85
C. Interactions between Pathogenic Parasites and their Hosts, 86
D. Evolutionary Development of Pathogenic Microorganisms, 87

The fetus is anatomically well protected from invasion by parasites normally encountered or carried by the mother during pregnancy and, in the large majority of instances, the fetal compartment remains sterile throughout pregnancy. There are only a few parasites that readily invade the fetus to cause congenital infections, such as the rubella virus and *Treponema pallidum*.

Accordingly, parasitism of the human host normally begins when the neonate acquires the normal microbial flora. After birth the gastrointestinal tract of the newborn rapidly becomes colonized with *Escherichia coli*, enteric streptococci, *Bacteroides* sp., and lactobacilli. The mucous membranes of the mouth and nasopharynx soon become colonized with staphylococci, lactobacilli, neisseriae, and α-hemolytic streptococci and the skin with staphylococci and corynebacteria.

During fetal development, the mother transfers her representative spectrum of IgG Abs to the fetus which provide the neonate with an important form of passive immunity until active acquired immunity is established. In general, this form of passive immunity is remarkably effective and plays a highly important role in preventing some of the normal flora organisms from invading the neonatal host and causing disease.

The neonate is capable of producing IgM immediately after birth, whereas competence to synthesize IgA develops at about 2 to 3 weeks after birth. In the case of IgG, synthesis begins when the neonate is 4 to 6 weeks old. Cell-mediated immunity can also be induced shortly after birth. It should be emphasized that immune responses are comparatively weak during the first year of life and moreover that passively transferred maternal IgG Abs can specifically dampen the immune response of the neonate. As soon as passively acquired maternal IgG declines to a low level (at 6 to 12 months) due to normal catabolism, the infant reaches an "immunological null period" which is gradually overcome as microbial Ags are encountered. Accordingly, the early years of life are normally plagued with numerous infections until the antigenic spectrum of the common infectious agents has been experienced. With increasing age, the immune response becomes stronger and more effective. This is largely due to accumulative and reinforcing experiences with an increasing number of immunogens of the parasites that are encountered. As a consequence, the incidence of various infections drops markedly when the human host reaches adulthood. During this period, the normal flora maintains a state of constant parasitism with only minor variations.

Evidently microbes of the normal flora exist in equilibrium and regulate each other's growth; if this equilibrium is upset as a consequence of chemotherapy, one species of the normal flora often gains ascendency and causes disease. The normal flora can interfere with colonization and/or invasion by some pathogenic microorganisms and, under some circumstances, can probably induce partial immunity against pathogens as a result of cross-reacting immunogens.

A.   Interactions between Nonpathogenic Parasites and their Hosts

The most common form of parasitism involves members of the normal flora which are classed as *nonpathogens* with respect to a normal healthy host. Man naturally encounters many other nonpathogenic parasites from external sources which colonize his body only temporarily and seldom, if ever, cause infectious disease. It is probable that when such microbes penetrate integuments, the resulting infection is usually inapparent because immunity is soon acquired and the microorganisms are eradicated. Certain soil mycobacteria (scotochromogens) are examples of organisms having such a relationship with a human host.

It should be emphasized that the apparent stability of host-parasite interactions involving nonpathogenic parasites depends on normally functioning immune mechanisms, both innate and acquired. However, if an individual is immunologically deficient, the so-called nonpathogenic parasites can assume the role of "opportunistic" pathogens. For example, iatrogenic manipulation of the host response with immunosuppressive drugs often results in infection by organisms of the normal flora. Also, congenital or acquired obstruction of a tubular structure such as a ureter or a bronchus can interfere with normal defense mechanisms of the structure; this interference in turn predisposes to local infection with microorganisms of the normal flora or other microorganisms of low virulence.

B.   Selective Attachment of Bacteria to Mammalian Cells

The normal flora organisms appear to attach selectively to certain epithelia in the human host. For example, *Strep. salivarius* and *Strep. sanguis* adhere readily to the epithelial cells of the tongue and cheek but do not adhere well to teeth. In contrast, *Strep. mutans* adheres poorly to the epithelia on the cheek and tongue but has high avidity for teeth. Certain microorganisms also selectively colonize the mucosal epithelia. It appears that surface properties of bacterial cells mediate the attachment to specific types of cells. Whereas pili appear to play an important role in attachment of some virulent organisms, other factors must be responsible for attachment of nonpiliated indigenous microbes. It has been proposed that mucopolysaccharides on the surface of normal flora organisms may have specificity for attaching to superficial epithelium in the stomach and intestine. Environmental compatibility together with some type of specialized attachment mechanism probably accounts for the specific distribution pattern of indigenous organisms.

C. Interactions between Pathogenic Parasites and their Hosts

By definition, a *pathogen* is "a parasite which is capable of producing apparent illness in a significant number of healthy individuals who have not encountered the parasite previously or who have no significant acquired immunity to the parasite."

The primary requirement for perpetual propagation of a pathogen is that it has a susceptible host that permits the parasite to multiply, escape, and infect new hosts. Since essentially none of the highly pathogenic microorganisms for which man is the natural host is a member of the normal flora, they are forced to rely principally on carrier states in order to persist in nature. With the exception of a few saprophytic organisms that can act as facultative parasites to cause disease (such as certain soil fungi), the vast majority of pathogenic microorganisms perpetuate themselves by serial passage in natural hosts, the reservoirs being either patients with actual infection or carriers. For the perpetuation of the parasite, it is noteworthy that a host-parasite equilibrium must exist which allows the parasite to propagate in individual hosts without destroying all or nearly all of the host population. In this regard, long-established host-parasite relations tend to evolve toward a state of "perfect" parasitism such that the host provides a perpetual subsistence for the parasite in the face of a decreasing level of pathogenesis. The relationship between the host and his normal microflora exemplifies a type of perfect parasitism.

In some instances, *unnatural* hosts may be fortuitous victims of a parasite and, accordingly, are termed *accidental hosts* or *incidental hosts*. Since in most instances accidental hosts fail to transmit the parasite to other hosts, they are referred to as *terminal hosts*. Since unnatural hosts do not exert selective pressure on the evolution of the parasite, such host-parasite relations, by chance, may be devastating for the host. In fact, the majority of highly fatal human infectious diseases involve man as an unnatural host, e.g., rabies, plague, tularemia.

Host-parasite interactions may also involve vectors such as arthropods. For example, *Rickettsia rickettsii,* the agent of Rocky Mountain spotted fever, is transmitted by ticks within a population of natural wild animal hosts. In addition, the tick can function as a vector to transmit the disease to unnatural hosts (such as man infected by the bite of a tick). Since the rickettsiae multiply in the tick and can be transmitted transovarially, the combination of the infected animal and infected tick serves as a dual linked reservoir system in nature.

There are a number of important variables that determine the outcome of infection. Some of these are: (1) age of the host, (2) physiologic state of the host, (3) immunocompetence of the host, either genetic or acquired, (4) previous antigenic experience of the host, (5) anatomic defects of the host, (6) physical injury or trauma to the host, (7) portal of entry of parasite, (8) size of the infecting dose of organisms, (9) physiologic state of the parasite, and (10) virulence of the parasite.

D. Evolutionary Development of Pathogenic Microorganisms

It would be expected that the least pathogenic microorganisms might be highly susceptible to the innate nonspecific humoral systems of defense such as lysozyme and the serum beta-lysin system (see *Fundamentals of Immunology*). *Sarcina lutea* (sensitive to lysozyme) and *Bacillus subtilis* (sensitive to β-lysin) are examples of organisms which would fit this category. The next hierarchy of pathogenic microorganisms to evolve would be expected to be resistant to the extracellular system of defense (both nonspecific and specific) and, in addition, resistant to phagocytosis in the absence of specific opsonizing Ab. *Diplococcus pneumoniae* is an example of this type of host-parasite relationship. It is noteworthy that *D. pneumoniae,* an extracellular parasite, is fully susceptible to the normal intracellular bactericidal mechanisms once the organisms have been ingested by phagocytes.

In the course of evolution, a few bacterial parasites have emerged that produce disease solely because of the synthesis of potent exotoxins. However, it is of singular interest that bacteria in this category of extracellular parasites, as a rule, do not invade deeply into healthy tissues. For example, *Corynebacterium diphtheriae* causes only a superficial localized infection in the pharynx but synthesizes a potent toxin that can exert serious systemic effects. In this case, immunity is effected simply by specific Abs (antitoxin) that neutralize the toxin. It should be emphasized that the local secretion of toxin in the pharynx probably interferes with local antibacterial defense mechanisms thus allowing the local infection to flourish. However, antibacterial defenses prevent *C. diphtheriae* from invading and extending the infection to the blood stream or the lower respiratory tract.

The ultimate evolutionary step reached by microorganisms has involved not only resistance to the humoral systems of defense, but also resistance to the normal baseline phagocytic systems of defense. *Mycobacterium tuberculosis,* which can be referred to as a *facultative intracellular parasite,* is a classic example of an organism reaching this stage of parasitism. Characteristically, the chronic granulomatous diseases (tuberculosis, brucellosis, histoplasmosis, etc.) are chronic and granulomatous because of a persisting intracellular infection of mononuclear phagocytes. The lesion in these host-parasite interactions is composed primarily of macrophages, epithelioid cells, giant cells, and lymphoid cells.

Mononuclear phagocytes in a normal animal are essentially incapable of resisting the intracellular growth of virulent tubercle bacilli. Furthermore, the polymorphonuclear phagocytes probably fail because their life span is too short to allow them to injure or destroy an organism with such challenging substrates and biochemical armor as those possessed by virulent tubercle bacilli. Accordingly, among the bacteria and fungi the ultimate in parasite evolution has resulted in microorganisms with complex cell walls and surface macromolecules that make them refractory to the normal bactericidal and/or digestive processes of the phagocytic cell systems, as well as to humoral elements. It is also probable that some pathogenic intracellular parasites possess toxic moieties which disrupt the chain of events leading to the development of an effective phagolysosome or block the differentiation and maturation of macrophages.

Evidently a successful host response to pathogenic intracellular parasites commonly depends on a lymphocyte-mediated mobilization and activation of the macrophage system. Current concepts suggest that the thymus-dependent immune lymphocytes (T lymphocytes) that mediate delayed sensitivity undergo blast transformation in the presence of Ag and, as a consequence, secrete mediators which mobilize macrophages and accelerate their maturation, thus leading to an accumulation of "super" macrophages. It has been suggested that once macrophages are activated, their total effector response is nonspecific. Whereas, this idea is tenable in the experiment in which BCG-activated macrophages are challenged with *Listeria monocytogenes,* it does not hold in the experimental situation in which BCG-activated macrophages are challenged with *Francisella tularensis.* In this latter case, there must be a component of specific immunity which interplays with the basic lymphocyte-macrophage system of cellular immunity. It is likely that in the specifically immunized host, the macrophages are somehow immunologically protected from the toxicity of this highly pathogenic microorganism. It is also likely that Abs passively associated with the macrophage mediate the protective component of immunity in this case.

There is a final category of parasites which evidently grow extracellularly but appear to be controlled by the environment generated by cellular immune mechanisms. In this group, *Actinomyces israelii* multiplies extracellularly, yet immunity appears to be of a cellular nature. This naturally raises the question as to whether a local cellular immune reaction can create a hostile microenvironment for an extracellular parasite. This principle could apply in the immune response against many types of parasites including certain fungi that grow extracellularly.

The host's adaptation to the evolutionary changes in microorganisms has evidently taken place largely through the development of the specific immune response. Whereas microorganisms have probably acquired increased virulence by selection and mutation or genetic transfer via episomes or transduction, the mammalian host has responded by evolving a highly effective immune system that can: (1) neutralize toxins, (2) neutralize viral infectivity, (3) kill some bacteria extracellularly involving nonspecific and/or specific humoral components, (4) enhance phagocytosis (opsonins), (5) enhance the mobilization of phagocytes, and (6) enhance the capacity of mononuclear cells to kill microorganisms (lymphocyte-macrophage cellular immune system).

The total immune response represents an interplay of special combinations of immune mechanisms which involve both baseline constitutive and acquired systems. For example, opsonic action can combine with cell-mediated immunity, and antitoxic immunity can interplay with opsonic action and phagocytic destruction of the offending parasite. It is possible that the forces of cell-mediated immunity can exert an important adjunct action on humoral immunity even against the so-called extracellular parasites.

In summary, in normal hosts, most infections are inapparent. A few parasites are capable of producing self-limiting disease with recovery mediated by the immune response (e.g., salmonella gastroenteritis). Only a small minority of parasites can produce serious progressive disease leading to irreversible damage or even death of the host. In this latter category, physicians are obliged to intercede by vaccinating susceptible individuals and by providing passive immunity and/or chemotherapy.

References

Allansmith, M., McClellan, B. H., Butterworth, M., and Maloney, J. R.: The development of immunoglobulin levels in man. J. Pediat. *72*:276, 1968.

Claflin, J. L., and Larson, C. L.: Infection-immunity in tularemia: Specificity of cellular immunity. Infect. Immun. *5*:311, 1972.

Craddock, C. G., Longmire, R., and McMillan, R.: Lymphocytes and the immune response. New Eng. J. Med. *285*:324, 1971.

Douglas, S. D., and Fudenberg, H. H.: Genetically determined defects in host resistance to infection: cellular immunologic aspects. Med. Clin. N. Amer. *53*:903, 1969.

Hirsch, J. G.: Antimicrobial factors in tissues and phagocytic cells. Bacteriol. Rev. *24*:133, 1960.

Mackaness, G. B.: Resistance to intracellular infection. J. Infect. Dis. *123*:439, 1971.

Miller, J. F. A. P.: Immunity in the foetus and the newborn. Brit. Med. Bull. *22*:21, 1966.

Pearsall, N. N., and Weiser, R. S.: *The Macrophage.* Philadelphia: Lea & Febiger, 1970.

Rowley, D.: Phagocytosis and immunity: the carrier state and cellular immunity. Experientia *22*:9, 1966.

Smith, H., and Pearce, J. H., eds.: *Microbial Pathogenicity in Man and Animals.* Cambridge: Cambridge University Press, 1972.

Sterzl, J., and Silverstein, A. M.: Developmental aspects of immunity. Advances Immunol. *6*:337, 1967.

Suter, E., and Ramseier, H.: Cellular reactions in infection. Advances Immunol. *4*:117, 1964.

Chapter 8

The Normal Microbial Flora

One of the most remarkable aspects of host-parasite relationships involves the wide array of microbes that colonize normal human beings from the moment of birth. In the course of evolution these microorganisms, which are termed the *normal microbial flora*, have adapted specifically to various parts of the body and represent persistent parasites of essentially every normal human being. It is of singular ecological interest that each animal species has its own characteristic natural microbial flora which is remarkably constant among individuals and that such flora become rapidly established in the newborn by contact with adults of the species. It is highly important that students of medicine understand the relationship between man and the microbes that normally inhabit the body because this relationship is an integral part of man's total ecology including the agents of infectious diseases. The following facts attest to the vital role that the normal microflora play in body economy. Members of the normal microflora (1) *can assume the role of pathogens if the host's defenses are defective*, (2) *can interfere with colonization and/or invasion by true pathogens*, (3) *can immunize the host against pathogens when related or cross-reacting Ags are shared, and* (4) *can be confused with the true etiologic agent of a disease because of their ubiquity on body surfaces and mucous membranes and the fact that many of them closely resemble pathogens.*

The normal microflora is comprised of those organisms which *universally* colonize various regions of the body and in a sense represent "standard equipment" of the normal healthy host; e.g., *Staphylococcus epidermidis* on skin or *Escherichia coli* in the intestinal tract. They are distinct from the so-called "transient flora" consisting of organisms that colonize only temporarily or on an intermittent basis. Members of the transient flora may include facultative parasites which normally exist as saprophytes, opportunistic pathogens, and true pathogens. A pathogen may establish a short-term or long-term carrier state in its host. The long-term carrier state of pathogens obtains because of acquired immunity of the host together with special anatomical or microenvironmental conditions which permit limited propagation of a pathogenic microorganism in a host for extended periods without any apparent harm; e.g., carriers of *Salmonella typhi* or coagulase-positive *Staphylococcus aureus*. The carrier state is the major means whereby pathogenic microorganisms persist in their natural hosts, the carrier functioning automatically as the reservoir of the infectious agent.

A. Distribution Patterns of the Normal Microbial Flora

The various microorganisms that consistently inhabit the skin, nose, pharynx, mouth, conjunctivae, lower intestine, external genitalia, and vagina are listed in Table 8-1. The flora of *skin* varies depending on the anatomical site. As a rule *Staph. epidermidis* and *Corynebacterium acnes* are the most abundant inhabitants of skin. The latter organism is normally found in sebaceous glands and hair follicles. *Mycobacterium smegmatis* is normally present on the external genitalia and adjacent skin.

TABLE 8-1

Microorganisms Found Consistently[1] on Various Integuments of the Human Body

---

SKIN:

Staphylococcus epidermidis	*Pityrosporum ovale* (scalp and
Corynebacterium acnes	other skin areas)

CONJUNCTIVA:

Corynebacterium species[2]	*Haemophilus* species

NOSE:

Staphylococcus epidermidis	*Streptococcus mitis*
Corynebacterium species	*Streptococcus salivarius*
Haemophilus species	*Moraxella lacunata*

MOUTH:

Staphylococcus epidermidis	Anaerobic micrococci
Streptococcus salivarius	*Streptococcus mitis*
Lactobacillus acidophilus	Anaerobic streptococci
Corynebacterium species	*Neisseria* species
Actinomyces bifidus	*Bacteroides* species
Leptotrichia buccalis	*Actinomyces israelii*
Treponema dentium	*Fusobacterium fusiforme*
Mycoplasma species	*Candida albicans*
Spirillum sputigenum	

TABLE 8-1 *(Continued)*
Microorganisms Found Consistently[1] on Various Integuments of the Human Body

PHARYNX:

Streptococcus salivarius	*Streptococcus mitis*
Neisseria species	Anaerobic streptococci
Corynebacterium species	*Veillonella alcalescens*
Fusobacterium fusiforme	*Bacteroides* species
Treponema dentium	*Vibrio sputorum*
Klebsiella aerogenes	*Actinomyces israelii*
Proteus species	*Haemophilus* species

LOWER INTESTINE:

Streptococcus mitis	Anaerobic micrococci
Streptococcus faecalis	*Streptococcus salivarius*
Lactobacillus species	Anaerobic streptococci
Escherichia coli	*Clostridium* species
Pseudomonas aeruginosa	*Alcaligenes faecalis*
Bacteroides species	*Klebsiella aerogenes*
Mycoplasma species	*Fusobacterium fusiforme*
Candida albicans	

EXTERNAL GENITALIA:

Staphylococcus epidermidis	*Streptococcus* species
Streptococcus faecalis	Anaerobic streptococci
Escherichia coli	*Spirillum sputigenum*
Bacteroides species	*Treponema dentium*
Mycobacterium smegmatis	*Candida albicans*
Fusobacterium fusiforme	*Mycoplasma* species

VAGINA:

Anaerobic micrococci	*Mima vaginicola*
Neisseria species	*Escherichia coli*
Mima polymorpha	*Treponema dentium*
Haemophilus vaginalis	*Mycoplasma* species
Streptococcus faecalis	

[1]This list is not intended to contain all of the organisms of the normal microbial flora.
[2]More than one species.

Within 12 hours after birth α-hemolytic streptococci are found in the upper respiratory tract and become the dominant organism of the oropharynx. Other nonpathogenic organisms that become permanent residents in the mouth and throat include coagulase-negative staphylococci, neisseriae, lactobacilli, *Bacteroides,* corynebacteria, and spirochetes. In addition, species of *Haemophilus, Actinomyces,* and *Mycoplasma* are usually present in a large majority of healthy individuals. As a rule α-hemolytic streptococci predominate in the pharynx and coagulase-negative staphylococci predominate in the nose. It is of interest that the normal lower respiratory tract is bacteriologically sterile even though the trachea may contain numerous bacteria. This exemplifies the remarkable defense system presented by the lung involving alveolar macrophages and mucociliary clearance.

The surface of the esophageal wall usually contains only the bacteria swallowed with saliva and food. Because of low pH the stomach is virtually sterile except during the early intervals after eating. In patients with carcinoma of the stomach or achlorhydria due to pernicious anemia, the stomach literally becomes a fermentation vat attesting to the role of HC1 in maintaining a low population of organisms in the normal stomach.

The number of bacteria increases progressively from a point below the duodenum to the colon, being comparatively low in the small intestine. The maximum number of bacteria exists in the contents of the colon and can approach 10^{10}/gm of feces. In breast-fed infants lactobacilli predominate in the feces, evidently as the result of environmental conditions created by ingested human milk rich in lactose. As the consequence of a more diverse diet, a relative increase in numbers of *E. coli, Bacteroides* sp, clostridia, and enterococci occurs. Members of the genus *Bacteroides* represent the most numerous organisms in the adult colon.

The vagina becomes colonized with lactobacilli immediately after birth followed by staphylococci, enterococci, and diphtheroids. With the onset of puberty and the child-bearing years, lactobacilli predominate in the vagina, allegedly because of the high glycogen content of the epithelial cells. Lactobacilli are probably responsible for the acidity of vaginal secretions during the child-bearing age. The onset of the postmenopausal period is attended by a drop in the numbers of lactobacilli and the return of the prepubertal flora.

The normal urethra is usually sterile above the urethrovesicular junction. A few bacteria from the external mucous membranes of the genitalia may contaminate the lower segment of the urethra.

Small numbers of organisms such as diphtheroids, *Haemophilus* sp, neisseriae, non-hemolytic streptococci, and coagulase-negative staphylococci can be isolated from the conjunctivae.

A discussion of the principle of selective attachment of bacteria to mammalian cells is presented in Chapter 7. Whereas the mechanisms operative in attachment are not known with certainty, it is likely that components on the bacterial surface are, in part, responsible for the special distribution pattern of indigenous microbes. In this regard, it must be emphasized that the microorganisms must also find the habitat of their choice compatible with their survival.

B. Possible Benefits of the Normal Microbial Flora

Microorganisms of the normal flora appear to exert mutual control on each other through some type of microbial antagonism. Bacterial antagonism presented by the normal flora also appears to play a role in controlling implantation and colonization of pathogenic microorganisms. It is well recognized that if the gastrointestinal flora is reduced by treatment with streptomycin, experimental animals will exhibit a marked increase in their susceptibility to *Salmonella enteritidis* introduced by the oral route.

In addition, the normal microflora can provide an important stimulus to the development and maturation of the organ systems responsible for acquired immunity. In particular, endotoxin may influence the immunologic response of the host and enhance the activity of some of the immunologic systems.

The normal microflora of the intestinal tract can contribute vitamin K and several B vitamins which could be beneficial under some circumstances.

C. Potential Liabilities of the Normal Microbial Flora

Normal flora microorganisms can assume the role of serious opportunistic pathogens when host defense factors are depressed or the equilibrium of the flora is altered by prolonged antibiotic therapy. It has been suggested that endotoxins produced by the normal flora of the intestinal tract effect chronic low-grade toxicity. This is based on the observation that animals raised on diets that suppress endotoxin-producing organisms grow faster than animals on standard diets.

It has also been observed that when penicillinase-producing staphylococci are associated with chronic gonococcal urethritis, they may interfere with the capacity of penicillin to eradicate the gonococci.

There is an accumulating body of evidence which suggests that certain streptococci can induce the formation of plaque, a deposit of microbial dextrans and organisms on teeth. It has been proposed that anaerobic streptococci convert sucrose to dextrans which in turn are fermented by the cariogenic streptococci and possibly lactobacilli present in the plaque with resulting acid demineralization of the enamel. In addition, proteolytic organisms, including actinomycetes and bacilli, apparently produce damage to the dentin. Undoubtedly, genetic, hormonal, and nutritional factors are important in this disease.

D. Shifts in the Normal Microbial Flora as a Consequence of Changes in the Environment

Special manipulations that select for particular organisms can have a marked influence on the so-called normal flora. For example, penicillinase-producing *Staph. aureus* is not a member of the normal flora and commonly colonizes fewer than 20% of the members of a healthy population. However, in some hospital populations (employees and patients) colonization with *Staph. aureus* may range from 50 to 100%. This increased colonization rate is due to the high prevalence of the organism in the hospital environment which in turn results from the high incidence of staphylococcal infections and carriers. These hospital strains of *Staph. aureus* are capable of colonizing a large percentage of individuals in the hospital environment so long as they are abundant in the environment, but are not capable of maintaining this state when staphylococcus-infected patients are moved out of the hospital. In other words, these strains of staphylococci have not evolved to the point where they are as well equipped for permanent colonization of normal individuals as *Staph. epidermidis*. This principle applies to other microorganisms and has led to much confusion as to what organisms should be classified as normal flora. A similar principle obtains when army recruits experience increased colonization rates of *Neisseria meningitidis* and *Streptococcus pyogenes* group A as the result of barracks life coupled with sporadic infections by the above organisms. Changes in diet also can cause temporary alterations in the flora of the gut.

References

Miller, C. P., and Bohnhoff, M.: Changes in the mouse's enteric microflora associated with enhanced susceptibility to salmonella infection following streptomycin treatment. J. Infec. Dis. *113*:59, 1963.

Morris, A. L., and Greulich, R.: Dental research: the past two decades. Science *160*: 108, 1968.

Rosebury, T.: *Microorganisms Indigenous to Man*. New York: McGraw-Hill Book Company, 1962.

Chapter 9 | Principles of Pathogenesis and Modes of Transmission of Infectious Diseases

Pathogenesis literally means "the genesis of disease." Hence, *pathogenicity* refers to the capacity of an agent to produce disease, and *the term* pathogen *is used to designate a parasite which commonly produces disease.* Except for a few potential pathogens that normally propagate in soil or organic material (facultative parasites), the majority of pathogens depend on at least one natural host for their propagation. By definition, a pathogen must be able to produce disease in a significant number of individuals who have not encountered the parasite before or who have inadequate acquired immunity to the parasite; for continued perpetuation a pathogen must have a portal of exit from the infected natural host and must be able to reach and infect new natural hosts (communicability or transmissibility).

Nonpathogens are organisms which seldom or never produce disease under normal conditions. Whether an organism produces disease depends on the host as well as on the organism; for example, pathogens usually fail to produce disease in immune individuals, whereas nonpathogens produce disease only in immunologically compromised or deficient individuals. Microbes which are not natural pathogens for a given host species, because they lack a system to transmit the parasite from one individual to another, may be highly pathogenic if administered artificially; e.g., experimental tuberculosis in the guinea pig.

Virulence is a term having two alternate usages, one as a synonym for *pathogenicity* and the other to designate degrees of pathogenicity possessed by different strains of a given species of microbe. It has been suggested that the term *pathogenicity* be used to designate the degree of disease produced by different species of microbes and that the term *virulence* be used to designate degrees of pathogenicity of different strains of a given species of microbe. However, in accordance with the dictates of common usage, the terms *virulence* and *pathogenicity* will be used synonymously in this text.

A. Infection vs. Colonization

Many microbes can propagate on the surface of external integuments for long or short periods without producing clinical evidence of injury. This host-parasite relation is referred to as *colonization*. The normal flora organisms of the healthy host are examples of permanent colonization; they do not usually penetrate the external integuments and seldom reach subepithelial tissues or the blood stream unless local defenses are depressed or a mechanical break of the external integuments occurs. Whenever a microbe, including a normal flora organism, gains entrance to subepithelial tissues and grows, the condition is referred to as *infection*. Providing that body defenses do not arrest the growth of the organism, the initial state before evidence of injury occurs, called *silent* or *inapparent infection,* can progress to *clinical* or *apparent infection.*

B. Attributes of Parasites Which Contribute to Pathogenicity

1. Invasiveness

With few exceptions, microbial parasites must penetrate external integuments and multiply within tissues in order to produce disease. In the case of actual wounds and abrasions, the mode of entry is obvious; however, most infections occur without readily discernible breaks in integuments. In this regard, microscopic breaks in certain integuments are probably frequent, such as in the mucosae of the alimentary tract, which are constantly subjected to the abrasive action of foods. In addition, it appears that some bacteria may be carried through certain mucosae by phagocytes, whereas others pass directly through epithelial cells. Apparently, penetration of integuments by some microbes requires considerable time; hence, the capacity to penetrate integuments often demands that the organisms tolerate local conditions and colonize.

A remarkable observation, the importance of which has been recognized only recently, is that many, if not most, of the normal microbial flora of the mucosal epithelia and the pathogens that attack such epithelia have adsorption affinities for particular epithelia which enable them to attach specifically; e.g., *Bordetella pertussis* to respiratory epithelium and *Shigella dysenteriae* to the epithelium of the colon. Such attachment permits the organisms to colonize and, in the case of pathogens, to produce disease either with or without subsequent invasion into subepithelial tissues. Without attachment, colonization and disease production by some microbes might not occur. One way by which the normal flora may oppose colonization by pathogens is that of preempting receptor sites on epithelia; another is by antibiosis.

Certain pathogens, such as *Bord. pertussis,* attach to but do not invade the epithelium; others attach to and invade only cells of the epithelial layer (*Sh. dysenteriae*); and still others breach the epithelium and reach subepithelial tissues (*Salmonella typhi*).

Although the surface properties of bacteria and epithelia that cause specific adsorption are not known, it is probable that host cells have receptors and that the envelopes, capsules, or pili of bacteria contribute to attachment. For example, attachment of *Vibrio cholerae* to gut epithelium is mediated by pili. In the case of *Sh. dysenteriae,* which selectively attaches to and invades colonic epithelium, it is probable that the organism in some unique fashion excites its own engulfment by colonic epithelial cells. In this regard, it is of interest that avirulent strains of *Sh. dysenteriae* lack the capacity to penetrate colonic epithelium.

In some circumstances organisms colonize in large numbers on integuments and, evidently as a result, produce sufficient injury to the epithelium to incite inflammation and produce "breaks" through which they pass. Once they penetrate an external integument, organisms tend either to remain localized or to be swept passively with the lymph flow to the lymph nodes; some species of microbes have a marked tendency to enter lymphatic channels and pass rapidly to the draining *lymph nodes* and beyond. For example, *Treponema pallidum* spreads from the point of entrance with extreme rapidity via *lymphatics* and lymph nodes to reach blood and distant organs in a matter of minutes to hours.

A few species of pathogens which localize on but do not penetrate surface integuments or penetrate superficially may nevertheless be highly fatal because of locally produced toxins; e.g., *V. cholerae* and *Corynebacterium diphtheriae*. Still other organisms grow within the integument and do not produce systemic injury; e.g., *Epidermophyton floccosum*.

2. Multiplication and Spread

Multiplication of organisms within tissues depends on their abilities to satisfy their biophysical and biochemical needs in host microenvironments and at the same time to evade, resist, or suppress host defenses, both natural and acquired. Most microbes do not grow *in vivo* at maximum rates attainable *in vitro* either because of host defenses or because of unfavorable changes they induce in the microenvironments they inhabit. Host environments include not only extracellular and intracellular environments in healthy tissue but also environments within lesions including abscesses and areas of necrosis, such as may occur in the center of a tubercle. Since host microenvironments and defenses vary markedly among animal species and among individuals of a species, it is evident why patterns of disease vary widely.

a. Adequacy of Nutritional Factors Supplied by the Host. Most pathogens can evidently meet their nutritional needs within the extracellular environment of the host; however, in a few instances, specific nutritional needs are not adequately met. For example, it has been found that the placentae of ungulates, which are susceptible to abortion by *Brucella abortus,* contain erythritol, an important growth factor for the organism, whereas the placentae of resistant species of animals lack erythritol. Iron shortage *in vitro* is known to enhance the formation of several bacterial toxins; e.g., toxins of *C. diphtheriae, Clostridium tetani, Clostridium perfringens,* and the *Staphylococcus aureus* enterotoxin. However, iron influences host-parasite relations in various ways, and the role of free iron in infectious diseases is not fully understood. The oxygen tension in tissues is also an important environmental variable for some pathogens. Growth requirements of a pathogen are not necessarily limited to basic nutritional needs but may include special precursors or cofactors needed for synthesizing virulence factors such as capsules or toxins.

The ability of intracellular parasites to satisfy growth needs within intracellular environments is crucial to their persistence. Although it is difficult to envision what the nutritional conditions within the intracellular microenvironments of various cells might be, they are presumably austere within the intact phagosome of "professional phagocytes," at least for most organisms.

b. Antimicrobial Factors in the Extracellular Environment. Specific humoral defenses such as the antibody-complement system or nonspecific humoral factors such as lysozyme or beta-lysin can be markedly antibacterial for some microorganisms. Tissue breakdown products resulting from cell death or excesses of cell metabolites which may accumulate at sites of inflammation or ischemia can also exert marked antibacterial activity.

c. Antimicrobial Factors in Intracellular Environments. Bacteria seldom gain entrance into cells other than professional phagocytes, presumably because they lack means for active penetration or the capacity to excite phagocytosis by the host cell. Environments within normal phagocytes are hostile to most pathogenic bacteria and only a few species, the so-called intracellular parasites, can survive in these environments for periods sufficient to produce disease.

Polymorphonuclear and mononuclear phagocytes differ markedly with respect to the microbes they can engulf and inhibit or destroy. Certain organisms can actually be protected as a result of being phagocytized by macrophages because they escape phagocytosis by neutrophils which would otherwise destroy them; e.g., *Yersinia pestis.* Other organisms, such as *Mycobacterium tuberculosis,* are more resistant to destruction by neutrophils than macrophages. However, since neutrophils are short-lived cells, the protection they afford tubercle bacilli is likewise short-lived; consequently, at any given time after infection, the majority of ingested tubercle bacilli seen in tissues are usually within macrophages. It is probable that engulfed tubercle bacilli resist the neutrophil because of some property of their lipid-rich cell wall, which resists degradation by enzymes within the phagolysosome.

The antimicrobial activities of phagocytes are presumed to result largely from lysosomal components discharged into the phagosome, which probably often act in concert rather than singly. It is also possible that metabolic products of the phagocyte enter the phagosome and act in combination with lysosomal constituents to bring about the demise of the parasite. For example, certain oxidases acting in the presence of H_2O_2 can kill bacteria *in vitro*. It has been postulated that metabolic activation of phagocytes results in the generation of H_2O_2 which presumably would be available for this bactericidal system.

3. Factors Responsible for Evasion or Depression of Host Defenses

Substances responsible for evasion or depression of host defense activities have been called *aggressins* or *virulence factors*. Undoubtedly, virulence factors that permit the early lesion to flourish often differ from factors that cause death of the host. Little is known about the nature of virulence factors directed at nonspecific humoral agents of defense, such as beta-lysin and lysozyme. However, products of virulent strains of certain organisms have been noted to protect avirulent strains against destruction by antimicrobial serum components. More is known about virulence factors which protect organisms against engulfment by phagocytes. Their action is one either of repelling or injuring the phagocyte or of shielding the organism against intracellular killing. For example, the organism may produce a substance which blocks chemotaxis or opposes engulfment, as in the case of the capsule of *Diplococcus pneumoniae;* the organism may produce a substance which kills or injures phagocytes by acting extracellularly (streptolysin O) or intracellularly (streptococcal NADase) or the organism may alter the cell in some manner which prevents fusion of lysosomes with the phagosome. The properties of capsular materials which account for resistance to engulfment have not been defined; they could be physical, such as surface tension effects. Whereas nonpathogenic bacteria tend to be engulfed, killed, and destroyed by phagocytes, most pathogenic bacteria either resist phagocytosis or resist destruction by phagocytes after engulfment.

Depression of host defenses as the result of microbial aggressive activity can be either local or systemic. Examples of substances that produce local aggressive effects are numerous and will not be considered in detail here; they include antiphagocytic surface components and leukocidins, etc. For example, *Staph. aureus* produces both leukocidin, which destroys phagocytes, and another substance, "protein A," which combines with the Fc portion of immunoglobulin thus interfering with its opsonic activities. Most organisms produce more than one substance that could oppose local host defenses and since these substances often act in concert, it has been exceedingly difficult to delineate their possible roles in depressing local defense; to wit, hyaluronidase, coagulase, staphylokinase, staphylococcal leukocidins, streptokinase, streptolysins and M proteins of streptococci, and the proteolytic enzymes of the clostridia.

Systemic depression of host defense as the result of microbial aggressive activity may be specific and/or nonspecific and may occur during infection. Fortunately, marked nonspecific systemic immunodepression seldom occurs as the result of infection; an individual suffering from one infectious disease is commonly able to mount a near normal immune response to another. An exception is the increased susceptibility of patients with viral influenza to staphylococcal pneumonia. Another example is lepromatous leprosy which apparently imposes a measurable nonspecific depression of delayed sensitivity and cell-mediated immunity, as indicated by milder tuberculin reactions, failure to develop full contact hypersensitivity to chemical sensitizers, and lowered capacity to reject skin allografts, etc. However, the change is not so profound that it significantly reduces the immunity of such patients to other diseases, such as tuberculosis.

Absence or marked suppression of specific immune responses, especially of cellular immune responses, to Ag(s) of the infecting agent is well documented. The reasons for these defects are obscure but could result from genetic incompetence, antigen mimicry, immunologic tolerance, immune deviation, or competition of Ags.

4. Patterns of Spread of Organisms From Sites of Infection

Dissemination of organisms from a focus of infection is opposed by various mechanisms of defense including inflammation, arrest in lymph nodes, and blood clearance involving circulating phagocytes and fixed phagocytes of the reticuloendothelial system (RES) (*Fundamentals of Immunology*). Although most bacteria gain entrance into the circulation via the lymphatic system, *they may sometimes enter the blood directly* as, for example, when a lesion, such as a caseating tubercle, ruptures into a vein. Spread within cavities and organs can likewise occur by rupture of a lesion into a duct, a tube, or a cavity. Spread from an infected cavity to the blood stream often is more rapid than via lymphatic routes.

The *lymphatic system* exerts a powerful localizing influence on the spread of microbes and only a few organisms such as *T. pallidum* can readily pass through the lymphatic system to the blood.

The *blood circulatory system* likewise has great powers for localizing bacteria, and it is only when highly virulent organisms are able to colonize and grow at foci in the circulatory system that a secondary progressive bacteremia occurs.

The *central nervous system* is not readily invaded by most bacteria because of a certain degree of gross and histologic isolation (the so-called "blood-brain barrier") which even restrains macromolecules, including Abs. The *placenta* also offers marked resistance to transgression by most bacteria.

Bacterial products, including enzymes and toxins, may promote spread of infecting agents. Although much has been written about such substances, including hyaluronidases, fibrinolysins, and collagenases, there is little certainty that they play important roles in spread of infection. Instead the tendency to spread may be strongest among organisms which produce the least tissue injury early in infection and thus escape the localizing effects of inflammation; e.g., *T. pallidum.*

The *forces of acquired immunity* that obviously play an important role in restricting the spread of infection include hypersensitivity reactions, opsonins, antitoxins, and bacteriolysins.

Selective localization of pathogens may occur at various loci on integuments or, following blood-borne spread, at various sites in tissues and organs. Different organisms show uniquely different patterns of localization; for example, *Mycobacterium leprae* tends to invade nerves and *M. tuberculosis* rarely localizes in thyroid, pancreas, or heart. The reasons for selective localization within tissues and even within cells are largely obscure but probably relate either to the ability of the organism to tolerate, suppress, or escape defense forces at such sites and/or because local environments best provide the biophysical or biochemical needs of the organism. For example, *Mycobacterium balnei* cannot grow above 34° C and hence only grows and produces lesions in "cool areas" of the body. Another example of the effect of the physical environment on localization is *Cl. tetani,* which will only grow in anaerobic areas; e.g., wounds where the blood supply is deficient. An additional example of selective localization is offered by the strains of *Escherichia coli* that possess the K antigen, and as a result are able to invade the kidney, presumably due to their high resistance to phagocytosis and C lysis.

5. Microbial Factors Responsible for Injury

When infection has progressed to the point at which clinical disease is evident, it is obvious that the host has sustained appreciable injury. However, the events leading to such injury are often exceedingly complex and usually involve both primary effects of microbial activities or products and secondary effects involving the liberation of harmful host mediators or tissue components. *From a theoretical standpoint, there are several major ways, both direct and indirect, by which a parasite might injure its host.* It could produce a toxin which could cause local injury or diffuse to cause systemic injury; it could compete with host cells for some vital nutrient; it could produce injurious metabolic products; it could block vessels or injure cells by physical effects; it could release inflammatory substances which by producing clots, swelling, and scarring may block channels (vessels, ducts, airways, gut, etc.) or produce pressure damage to vital organs; it could cause excessive accumulation or proliferation of host cells to the point where pressure and crowding-out effects cause injury; finally, by synthesizing Ags, it could so stimulate the immune response that harm would result from hypersensitivity reactions, especially those involving delayed hypersensitivity, Ag-Ab complexes, and possible autoimmune phenomena.

Since *host responses alone could totally account for the injury produced in infection,* the virulence of an organism could be independent of any toxins it might produce and result solely from its ability to evade host defenses and multiply to achieve a certain numerical threshold.

Whereas, in subsequent chapters, clear examples of harm resulting from each of the ways cited above will emerge, it is noteworthy that there is no single infectious disease in which all of the precise mechanisms responsible for injury are known; this is especially true at the cellular and biochemical levels.

The extent to which organisms grow in the body does not correlate with the extent of injury or disease produced. Organisms which can produce potent toxins or incite exaggerated allergic responses can cause injury all out of proportion to the extent of their growth.

Bacterial toxins are divided into two categories: the protein *exotoxins* which are, with certain exceptions, the extracellular products of gram-positive bacteria, and *endotoxins,* which are complex lipopolysaccharide constituents of the cell walls of gram-negative bacteria. In general, exotoxins, which are usually secretion products of viable bacteria, are strongly antigenic, highly toxic, easily converted to toxoids, readily neutralized by antibodies, relatively heat-labile, and highly selective with respect to the tissues and cells they affect. In contrast, endotoxins, although antigenic, are relatively heat-stable, relatively less toxic, not convertible to toxoids, poorly neutralized by Abs and, irrespective of their source, have similar toxicities for various tissues and cells.

Most bacterial exotoxins are enzymes. Certain of them are the most potent lethal poisons known; for example, type D botulinum toxin is 3 million times more toxic than strychnine. Tetanus toxin is so potent that the amount that can kill a patient is far short of the amount necessary to immunize. Several of the bacterial exotoxins such as *Cl. perfringens* toxin are secreted as inactive "protoxins" and are rendered toxic by proteolytic enzymes which split off small fragments of the protoxin. A number of exotoxins, such as staphylococcal leukocidin, are composed of two or more molecular components which act synergistically.

An interesting development in recent years has been the discovery of *an increasing number of instances in which the synthesis of bacterial exotoxins depends on lysogeny.* For example, certain toxins of *Staph. aureus, Streptococcus pyogenes,* and the toxins of *C. diphtheriae* and *Cl. botulinum* types C and D, are produced only by lysogenic strains of organisms. However, not all lysogenic strains are toxinogenic and not all strains artificially lysogenized by toxinogenic phages become toxinogenic. Thus the production of some bacterial exotoxins is a fortuitous result of parasitism by phage. Consequently it is reasonable to expect that the panel of toxins produced by strains of organisms of a species could change with the evolution of phage-host relationships and in some instances could account for changes in bacterial pathogenicity and disease patterns; indeed this may have occurred in the case of scarlet fever which appears to be less common and less severe than in past decades.

The profound selective toxicity of bacterial exotoxins is another of their remarkable properties. Some are effective against one animal species and not another; one may attack epithelium, whereas another may attack only nerves. As an extreme example of selectivity, the alpha toxin of *Staph. aureus* attacks rabbit neutrophils but not human neutrophils! The mode of action of exotoxins is largely obscure, even in the case of the much-studied neurotoxins. For example, the fixation of tetanus toxin to ganglioside has given no clue to its mode of action at the molecular level.

Endotoxins are constituents of the cell walls of both pathogenic and nonpathogenic gram-negative bacteria. They are complexes containing polysaccharide, protein and lipids; at least two lipids, referred to as *A* and

B, are present. The toxic moiety appears to be associated with lipid A which is complexed to both the protein and the polysaccharide (Chapter 2). Endotoxins stimulate the RES and various hormone and enzyme systems, including the enzymes responsible for fibrinolysis. Depending on dosage and timing they can produce leukocytosis or leukopenia, fever, stimulation or breakdown of defense systems, hemorrhage, and severe injury of cells of various organs, as well as shock. Although complexing of endotoxin with Abs appears to speed its clearance from blood by the RES, it is uncertain whether frank neutralization of toxicity occurs. There is recent evidence that an Ab directed against the lipid structure can be produced which may have antitoxic activity. *The contribution of endotoxins to the pathogenesis of infectious diseases remains controversial.* However, it seems probable that endotoxins are liberated from infecting gram-negative organisms and that they contribute substantially to pathogenesis.

The role of toxins in the pathogenesis of bacterial diseases has been clearly established in only a few instances (e.g., diphtheria and tetanus); however, toxins of various types probably play an important role in the pathogenesis of most infectious diseases. The importance of establishing the precise roles of bacterial components, including toxins, in pathogenesis and of elucidating their mechanisms of action cannot be overemphasized, for if such goals could be accomplished, rational and new approaches to the control of bacterial diseases would be at hand.

It is commonly very difficult to establish the role of a toxin, or indeed any factor, in the pathogenesis of an infectious disease, let alone elucidate its mode of action. The marked capacity of bacteria to undergo phenotypic shift with changes in environment means that *in vitro* behavior is not a dependable criterion of *in vivo* behavior. Hence, failure to demonstrate a toxin by *in vitro* culture does not prove that a toxin is not produced *in vivo;* the truth of this statement has been well demonstrated in the case of anthrax. Also a lack of correlation between toxin production and virulence does not prove that the toxin does not contribute importantly to pathogenesis since some other factor, such as capsule production, may be the dominant factor in virulence. Likewise, failure of a toxin to produce symptoms and lesions characteristic of the disease does not prove that it is unimportant in pathogenesis since toxins can contribute to pathogenesis by acting in concert with other microbial products. Although neutralization of toxin and prevention of disease by antitoxin support the role of toxin in tissue injury, it is always possible that the toxin behaves solely as an aggressin to enable the organisms to invade and makes no major contribution to injury, particularly at the systemic level; such may be the case in gas gangrene in which antitoxin may prevent infection but is of little or no therapeutic value in the face of an established clinical infection.

Other pathophysiologic effects are evident in infectious diseases, but little is known about the mechanisms involved. For example, if pneumococcal septicemia progresses too far, the disease is fatal even if the bacteria are killed with massive doses of penicillin. *In effect the patient may die "bacteriologically cured."* Apparently, pneumococci can cause some type of irreversible physiologic derangement.

It is also well recognized that *many intracellular parasites such as Francisella tularensis, Rickettsia prowazekii* and *Rickettsia rickettsii express marked toxicity for normal macrophages.* For example, it has recently been observed that *R. prowazekii* disrupts the phagosome of the macrophage and prevents an effective phagolysosome from forming. Apparently injury is due to a toxin associated with the living rickettsiae since macrophage death from engulfed organisms can be prevented by pretreating the rickettsiae with specific antiserum. In addition, this type of membrane damage does not occur in immune hosts. Such observations suggest that there are probably many microbial components, still to be identified, that can exert deleterious effects on the host.

6. Relation of Virulence Factors to Immunogens

It is probable that virulence is seldom if ever limited to a single unique microbial attribute even though the lack of but one such attribute may render the organism incapable of producing disease, as in the case of the avirulent pneumococcus which lacks a capsule. Obviously the pneumococcus must possess other "virulence" attributes which enable it to injure its host. It is only by a comparative study of the capacity of virulent and avirulent organisms and their products to cause injury or alter the course of infection that any of the various factors of virulence can be identified.

Virulence factors are not always immunogenic; for example, the hyaluronic acid of the capsule of *Strep. pyogenes* is antiphagocytic and represents a virulence factor, second only to M protein, but is chemically identical with animal hyaluronic acid and does not stimulate Abs or immunity. Many lipids, because of their chemical nature, are nonantigenic, and still other substances may resemble host Ags so closely that they fail to stimulate an immune response or do so but weakly (antigen mimicry). Consequently, in the search for virulence factors and immunogens, it should be kept in mind that any given organism may possess one or more virulence factors and that a virulence factor is not necessarily an immunogen in the sense that it will stimulate specific immunity.

C. Host Factors Which Contribute to Pathogenesis

For the most part Ab-mediated hypersensitivity reactions with attending inflammation are probably beneficial to the host; an exception may be the lesions produced by soluble Ag-Ab complexes, although even in this instance it is difficult to rule out potential beneficial effects, such as limitation of spread of infection resulting from thrombosis of vessels, etc.

1. The Acute Abscess

The acute abscess is a striking example of a lesion representing in large part a host contribution to pathogenesis. An acute abscess resulting from infection represents the outcome of the local accumulation of large numbers of closely packed neutrophils attracted to the site of infection by chemotactic products of bacteria and injured tissue as well as by the split products of C resulting from Ag-Ab reactions. Although neutrophils are short-lived cells, their death tends to be hastened in the abscess by overcrowding and in many instances by bacterial toxins. The release of large amounts of lysosomal enzymes (hydrolases) from dying neutrophils, together with bacterial toxins and lack of adequate blood supply and nutrition, leads to local destruction of tissue. *Pus,* which represents the partially liquified remains of dead leukocytes and necrotic tissue, is the hallmark of the acute abscess.

In terms of host protection, the attraction of neutrophils to the site of infection to form the abscess is usually beneficial because of its value in localizing the infection. Although the pus formed may not provide a particularly good environment for the growth of most microbes, it is at the same time not a menstruum into which living leukocytes can migrate readily and carry on further phagocytosis. Hence, organisms often persist and even grow within pus, remote from host defense forces; it is only when a progressing abscess ruptures spontaneously or is surgically drained that rapid healing can occur. Abscesses in certain sites may favor spread rather than localization of infection (e.g., the palm of the hand) because pressure forces the pus along fascial planes and tendons with extension of the infection. The abscess also presents problems with respect to chemotherapy since it may not be readily penetrated by drugs and, in addition, the nonmultiplying organisms contained are not susceptible to those antibiotics that demand bacterial cell wall synthesis for their activity (Chapter 6).

In the case of a foreign body, such as a contaminated splinter, pus formation aids in its elimination by local sacrifice of tissue and discharge through the skin. *Thus the abscess can be an asset or a liability depending on the size and location of the lesion.*

2. Delayed Sensitivity and the Allergic Granuloma

Delayed hypersensitivity contributes importantly to the lesions of chronic infectious diseases and to immunity. For example, the very composition of the tubercle, an "immune structure," is undoubtedly in large measure determined by delayed hypersensitivity. On the other hand, delayed hypersensitivity reactions can cause severe local injury to endothelium and destruction of many tissues, especially in chronic granulomatous diseases such as tuberculosis. With respect to the overall welfare of the host, the inflammation and local destruction of tissue involved in delayed hypersensitivity reactions are usually beneficial.

The allergic granuloma, which is characteristically produced by intracellular parasites, is a highly effective anatomic structure of immunologic defense. Lymphokines generated by lymphocytes in the granuloma undoubtedly exert a marked regulatory influence on cellular events within the granuloma, an influence which continues so long as Ag persists locally to sensitize and activate lymphocytes. Lymphokine production is presumed to stem from the triggering of sensitive lymphocytes of the granuloma by Ag diffusing from the infecting organisms. It can be envisioned that lymphokines attract lymphocytes and macrophages to the lesion by chemotaxis and that arriving macrophages, under their influence, tend to become immobilized, activated, and fused to form giant cells. Cytophilic Abs are probably produced locally by stimulated lymphocytes and may contribute to the antimicrobial activities of macrophages. It is also possible that macrophages may be transformed into epithelioid cells under the influence of lymphokines. Epithelioid cells, by their strong tendency to adhere to one another, and the fusion of macrophages around organisms to form giant cells exert a strong localizing influence on the infecting agent. Moreover, even when necrosis of epithelioid cells occurs, growth of organisms is restricted in the resulting caseous material because of its inherent properties, including low oxygen tension. It is only when restraining forces fail and the granuloma enlarges and ruptures that serious harm to the host results due to pressure effects, loss of vital tissue, hemorrhage, and spread of infection. *Thus delayed hypersensitivity reactions associated with granulomata may be beneficial or harmful depending on the magnitude and location of the lesions.*

Amyloid disease sometimes follows chronic infections, such as tuberculosis, leprosy, and staphylococcal osteomyelitis. Although the mechanisms concerned in its genesis are obscure, it is possible that in chronic infections it results from some accompanying derangement in the immune response.

3. Immune Complex Disease

Immune complex lesions can occur in man as the result of either acute or chronic infections. Ideal conditions for the development of systemic immune complex disease should be those favoring the development of harmful soluble Ag-Ab complexes in the blood; namely, conditions in which the complexes are formed in the region of Ag excess. Theoretically, these conditions should occur in situations in which Ab production is weak, and the supply of Ag is abundant and continuous. However, the pathogenesis of immune complex disease is more complicated than is generally believed and may vary with the nature of Ag and the nature and avidity of Ab. It is not unexpected that immune complex disease occurs as a complication of infectious diseases; the surprise is that it is not manifested or recognized more often.

Soluble immune complexes tend to be deposited along basement membranes in blood vessels, including those of the glomerulus where they accumulate as "lumpy deposits" on the epithelial aspect of the basement membrane.

Acute post-streptococcal glomerulonephritis in man, a sequela of acute streptococcosis, is one model purported by some investigators to be the result of circulating complexes of streptococcal Ag and specific Ab. Although the lesions conform morphologically to immune complex disease in the experimental animal model using pure foreign protein as Ag, there is still doubt that post-streptococcal glomerulonephritis in man is a simple Ag-Ab complex disease, and the nature of the Ag(s) in the complexes remains a matter of dispute (Chapter 11). There is recent evidence that immune complex glomerulonephritis occurs in a number of infectious diseases, including bacterial endocarditis, malaria and possibly secondary syphilis.

Vasculitis, including polyarteritis nodosa, which sometimes occurs as the result of diseases such as streptococcosis and tuberculosis, probably represents an immune complex disease (*Fundamentals of Immunology*). The frequent occurrence of polyarteritis nodosa in patients with circulating complexes of Australia Ag and Ab lends additional support to the pathogenetic role of immune complexes in infectious diseases. In any event, the high concentration of microbial Ags at the sites of local lesions, together with microbial toxins that increase vascular permeability and thus promote penetration of vessel walls by immune complexes, should provide ideal circumstances for the development of immune complex vasculitis.

Rheumatic fever, a sequela of streptococcal pharyngitis, probably represents still another model of immunologic injury and is thought by some investigators to result from antistreptococcal Abs which cross-react with related Ags of heart muscle (Chapter 11). One alternative theory is that the lesions of rheumatic fever result from the local deposition and prolonged persistence of highly toxic and allergenic components of streptococcal cell walls.

Another possible mechanism of injury is that bacterial Ags may adsorb to cells and thus render them susceptible to cytotoxic damage by Ab and C.

4. Immediate Hypersensitivity Reactions

Immediate hypersensitivity reactions due to IgE antibodies are not known to contribute importantly to pathogenesis, although this is a possibility. By increasing vascular permeability, they could promote penetration of immune complexes into vessel walls and contribute to immune complex disease.

5. Fever

The term *fever* is used to designate high body temperature resulting from a disturbance in the thermoregulatory center in the brain. Such disturbances are due to direct injury of the brain or to blood-borne *endogenous pyrogens*. Although many, if not all, cells contain endogenous pyrogens, they are most abundant in neutrophils and macrophages. Fever commonly accompanies any bacterial infection of substantial nature, and the course of the fever is often characteristic of the particular infection. Apparently in fevers of infection, the humoral agents, which act on the thermoregulatory center in the brain, are exclusively the endogenous pyrogens liberated from stimulated or damaged cells, particularly leukocytes. Microbes bring about the release of endogenous pyrogens in various ways including direct stimulation and injury to cells and tissues by "toxins," commonly referred to as "bacterial pyrogens," as well as by hypersensitivity reactions.

The most-studied bacterial pyrogens, the endotoxins of gram-negative bacteria, act principally on neutrophils and macrophages to cause them to release endogenous pyrogens.

Fever is accompanied by numerous other symptoms and alterations, including changes in circulation and respiration. Fevers of infection seldom exceed 104 to 105°F for any extended time. In pneumococcal pneumonia temperatures of about 104°F are common and persist for several days. Temperatures of 105°F and above, due to any cause, are dangerous if they persist for any extended time and may lead to death or permanent brain damage. At 106°F and above, the thermoregulatory center probably soon breaks down and delirium, coma and death often occur; this is encountered especially in heat stroke. Brain damage due to hyperthermia probably results from unbalanced metabolism induced by the elevated temperature.

*Although it is tempting to speculate that fever should represent a general defense mechanism, no sound support for this hypothesis has been advanced.** Whereas its harmful effects are evident, fever is not known to bolster host defenses and its possible beneficial effects on the course of infection have not been documented. In the few diseases caused by temperature-sensitive organisms, such as syphilis and gonorrhea, temperatures high enough to arrest the organism do not develop and the only known beneficial effects of temperature in these two diseases have resulted from high temperatures induced by artificial means, a former therapeutic practice.

6. Septic Shock

The term septic shock *is used to designate a clinical state associated with infection;* it is characterized by circulatory collapse with hypotension, respiratory distress, and mental abnormalities. It usually develops rapidly,

---

* Fever is reported to be beneficial in certain virus infections.

is commonly attended by bacteremia, and is often fatal. The condition is usually caused by gram-negative bacteria and in these instances is generally thought to result principally from the effects of endotoxin. However, this is uncertain and at present the term *septic shock* is used loosely to designate a condition which will probably prove to be the end result of many and different chains of pathogenetic events.

D. Transmission of Infectious Agents

1. Modes and Routes of Transmission

In order to persist in nature a parasite must have some means whereby it can leave one host and infect a new host. This requires a suitable portal of exit from the donor host, who may be either a carrier or an individual with clinical diseases, and a portal of entry into the new host. *Reservoirs* (sources) of infecting agents range from patients and carriers to biological vectors, such as insects, in which the agent can multiply, and to soil in the case of certain facultative pathogenic parasites.

Portals of entry and exit include the (1) respiratory tract, (2) alimentary tract, (3) genitourinary tract, (4) skin, and (5) conjunctivae. Infectious agents may be transmitted by (1) aerosols, (2) contact, (3) fomites (inanimate objects), (4) ingestion, (5) mechanical vectors, (6) biological vectors, and (7) placental passage.

It is readily apparent that the host-parasite cycle must be highly specialized in order to accommodate the exacting combinations of circumstances necessary for transmission of an infectious agent, including the ability of the agent to survive the various rigors of the external environment. For example, most agents that cause respiratory infections are transmitted almost exclusively by fresh *aerosols* (droplet nuclei) passing from a donor to a susceptible individual within the aerosol trajectory range generated by coughing, sneezing, and talking. This includes the organisms responsible for streptococcal sore throat, tuberculosis, mycoplasma pneumonia, and pertussis. It is only in a few instances that infection is frequently the result of inhalation of microbes carried in airborne dust particles, such as the etiologic agents of psittacosis and smallpox. Such organisms must obviously withstand drying under atmospheric conditions.

Examples of microbes commonly transmitted by *contact* include *Fr. tularensis* (handling infected rabbits) and *Neisseria gonorrhoeae* (usually sexual contact). *Fomites* can be involved if an appropriate object becomes contaminated, and contact is made by the new host within a suitable period of time; e.g., smallpox and anthrax.

Ingestion of food or drink is a common means of transmission of the organisms responsible for a number of diseases, including typhoid fever, bovine tuberculosis, and cholera.

Vectors, such as certain arthropods, may transmit infectious agents solely by mechanical means (mechanical vectors) or in addition serve as reservoirs in which the organism multiplies (*biological vectors*). Flies are important as mechanical vectors in the transmission of *Sh. dysenteriae* from contaminated feces to food. In many diseases biological vectors serve as an integral part of the host-parasite cycle because the vector provides an important site for propagation of the parasite. An example of a disease in which a biological vector is important in disease transmission is Rocky Mountain spotted fever, which is transmitted to man by the bite of ticks infected with *R. rickettsii.*

In a few instances infection is passed from the mother to offspring *in utero;* e.g., congenital syphilis and granulomatosis infantiseptica due to *Listeria monocytogenes.*

2. The Role of the Carrier in Transmission

The majority of pathogenic bacteria that have man as their natural host can establish the chronic carrier state in man. *Indeed most of such pathogens would fail to persist in nature if they lacked the ability to establish the chronic carrier state, inapparent infection which can activate to clinical disease or chronic disease.* In other words, it is probable that pathogenic bacteria that have man as their sole natural host seldom if ever persist in nature solely by passage from one acutely infected person to another. Consequently, knowledge of the factors which determine inapparent infections and the carrier state is important for understanding herd immunity and designing measures for controlling transmission of infectious agents. *Many bacteria that are carried tend to induce specific immunity,* which may ultimately eliminate carriage of the organism in question; e.g., *D. pneumoniae* types. In other instances *the carried organisms tend to become less virulent* due to immune elimination of highly virulent over less virulent mutants; e.g., *Strep. pyogenes.*

Carrier studies of *C. diphtheriae* have been particularly enlightening. Since immunity to the toxin discourages carriage of the organism as well as clinical disease, long-continued mass immunization of a population with toxoid reduces the carrier rate and the incidence of disease to extremely low levels and finally to extinction. Extinction of the organisms occurs because in a highly immune population the number of individuals who will assume carriage of the organism is so few that the chain of passage of the organism among such individuals is broken. The same breaking of the chain of passage can take place in other diseases in which carriers and active disease are rare but in which inapparent infections that occasionally activate occur; e.g., tuberculosis in developed countries. *Public health measures to increase herd immunity and prevent infection can effectively accomplish virtual extinction of many infectious diseases within a population.*

The carriage of certain bacteria occurs even if the carrier has significant immunity to the microbe. Organisms in certain anatomic sites (*Sal. typhi* in the gall bladder) are apparently protected from immune mechanisms. Special genetic abnormalities of anatomic structures may also favor the persistence of microorganisms and account for the long-term carrier state in certain individuals. The importance of the carrier state in the perpetuation of a human pathogen becomes obvious in those instances where man is the only natural host.

E. Criteria for Establishing the Etiologic Agent of an Infectious Disease

Although Henle (1840), Koch's teacher, was the first to propose criteria for establishing etiologic agents of infectious disease, their validity awaited the proof provided by Koch (1884) and thereafter were called "Koch's Postulates." In substance they were stated essentially as follows:

(1) The particular infecting microbe must be found in all cases of the disease, preferably in locations and numbers which would explain the lesions and symptoms of the disease.

(2) The organism must be grown in pure culture in order to prove that it is an independent, animate particle.

(3) Inoculation of the pure culture into a healthy host must reproduce the disease, including the presence of the same organism in the lesions.

Koch's postulates have proved to be highly useful for establishing the causative agents of many diseases. Even though it is not possible to satisfy all of Koch's postulates in every instance, the etiologic agent can often be established with reasonable certainty; e.g., leprosy. Although the causative organism of leprosy has never been cultured, it appears to be one of the mycobacteria as judged by all other criteria. It is the only agent that is constantly present in abundance in the lesions of the disease and causes a disease in animals resembling, in certain measure, human leprosy; there is little doubt that it is the cause of leprosy.

References

Bloom, B. R.: In vitro approaches to the mechanism of cell-mediated immune reactions. Advances Immunol. *13*:102, 1971.

Florey, H. W.: *General Pathology.* 4th ed. Philadelphia: W. B. Saunders Co., 1970.

Germuth, F. G., Jr., Senterfit, L. B., and Dressman, G. R.: Immune complex disease. V. The nature of circulating complexes associated with glomerular alterations in the chronic BSA-rabbit system. Johns Hopkins Med. J. *130*:344, 1972.

Gocke, D. J., Hsu, K., Morgan, C., Bombardieri, S., Lockshin, M., and Christian, C. L.: Vasculitis in association with Australia antigen. J. Exp. Med. *134*:330s, 1971.

Gutman, R. A., Striker, G. E., Gilliland, B. C., and Cutler, R. E.: The immune complex glomerulonephritis of bacterial endocarditis. Medicine *51*:1, 1972.

Smith, H.: Microbial pathogenicity in man and animals. 22nd symposium of the Society of General Microbiology. England: Cambridge Univ. Press, 1972.

Weiser, R. S., Myrvik, Q. N., and Pearsall, N. N.: *Fundamentals of Immunology.* Philadelphia: Lea & Febiger, 1969.

Zabriskie, J. B.: The role of streptococci in human glomerulonephritis. J. Exp. Med. *134*:180s, 1971.

Chapter 10

Diplococcus

The genus *Diplococcus,* a member of the family *Lactobacillaceae,* contains but a single species of significant medical importance to man, *Diplococcus pneumoniae,* the most common cause of lobar pneumonia. It is also known by the name *Streptococcus pneumoniae* because of its close taxonomic relation to the streptococci. Five other species, all anaerobes of little or no medical importance, are normal inhabitants of the mouth and intestinal tract.

Diplococcus pneumoniae is a pyogenic extracellular pathogen and is frequently carried in the upper respiratory tract (URT) of man, its principal natural host. Pneumococci have been isolated irregularly from horses, cattle, dogs, monkeys, guinea pigs, and rabbits. Although epizootics of pneumococcal disease occasionally occur in laboratory animals such as rats, guinea pigs, and monkeys, it is notable that such outbreaks tend to be narrowly limited to certain serologic types (type 19 for the guinea pig and type 2 for the rat). No animal is known to be an important reservoir of infection for man.

Diplococcus pneumoniae was discovered independently by Pasteur and Sternberg in 1881. It is classified on the basis of serologic types originally designated by Roman numerals.

A. Medical Perspectives

Prior to the development of therapy with specific antiserum in the early 1930s and later with drugs, the pneumococcus was a major cause of death. The organism produces infections in various organs and tissues, the most common and serious being bronchopneumonia and lobar pneumonia. Whereas pneumococcal bronchopneumonia is largely confined to the very young, the aged, and the debilitated, epidemic lobar pneumonia occurs most frequently in healthy young adults, especially males. In decades past it took a terrible toll of lives in this group; for those in the prime of life Osler called it "Captain of the Men of Death." The case fatality rate ranged from 20 to 40% or more and exceeded 50% in the case of infection due to organisms of type 3. Current therapeutic practices have reduced the case-fatality rate to about 5%; and except for type 3 infections, uncomplicated cases, if treated early, can usually be saved. However, because diagnosis is frequently delayed and because complicating disease is often present, pneumococcal infections remain a major cause of serious illness and death; deaths from pneumonia alone in the USA are estimated to be about 25,000 annually.

It is of singular importance that although treatment of patients with pneumococcal meningitis or bacteremic pneumonia may be "bacteriologically successful," i.e., most or all of the organisms are killed within a matter of hours, such patients often die later, apparently of delayed toxemia. Consequently future possibilities for lowering mortality rates must hinge not only on earlier diagnosis and treatment, vaccines and chemoprophylaxis, but on devising therapeutic means for counteracting the toxemia involved.

One of the most remarkable team achievements in medical history was the elucidation of the major virulence mechanism involved in pneumococcal infection. This was accomplished by a succession of investigators during the 1920s and 1930s at the Rockefeller Institute for Medical Research, including Dochez, Avery, Heidelberger, Goebel, MacLeod, and McCarty. They made major contributions toward establishing that the antiphagocytic capsule of the pneumococcus is the major determinant of virulence and that acquired immunity results from opsonizing Ab directed at the particular polysaccharide making up the capsule of the infecting organism. *Thus the type-specific capsular polysaccharide was found to be both the principal virulence factor and immunogen.* In addition, their studies on the phenomenon of Griffith's transformation of serologic types of pneumococci led to the discovery that DNA can serve as a transforming agent and opened the field of molecular genetics. The findings of this group of investigators provided the basis for specific serum treatment of lobar pneumonia instituted in the 1930s. Ironically, this long-awaited advance in therapy was quickly supplanted by sulfonamide treatment and later by treatment with penicillin and other antibiotics.

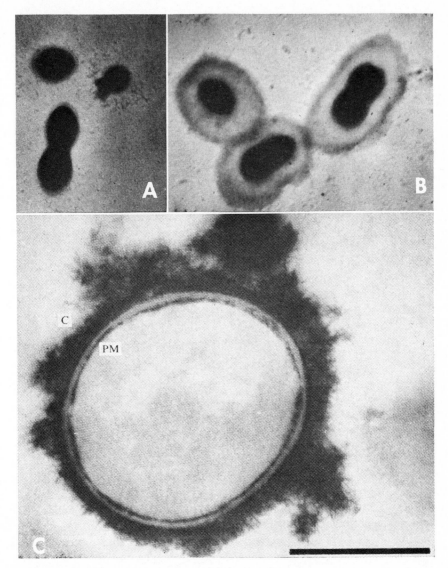

Figure 10-1. Demonstration of capsules on *Diplococcus pneumoniae* and capsule swelling in the presence of specific anticapsular antibody. *A, D. pneumoniae* Type 1 (note normal capsule) × 10,500; *B, D. pneumoniae* Type 1 incubated 3 minutes with specific anti-Type 1 capsular antibody (note swelling of capsule) × 10,500. (Mudd, S., Heinmets, F., and Anderson, T. F.: J. Exp. Med. *78:*327, 1943.) *C, D. pneumoniae* stained with ruthenium red depicting the capsule (C) and plasma membrane (PM). Marker represents 0.5 μm. (Springer, E. L., and Roth, I. L.: J. Gen. Microb. *74:*21, 1973.)

B. Physical and Chemical Structure

Diplococcus pneumoniae is typically an encapsulated, gram-positive, lance-shaped coccus usually positioned in pairs with tips pointing outward. *In vivo* the organism may occur singly and in chains, as well as in pairs. In common with other pathogenic cocci it is nonsporing and nonmotile.

Aside from the unexplained toxicity it exerts during infection, the most notable attribute of the pneumococcus is its enormous capsule which swells upon the addition of specific antiserum (Fig. 10-1). Based on antigenic differences in their capsular polysaccharides some 85 distinct serologic types of pneumococci have been described. The capsular material is soluble in water and hence is sometimes referred to as "soluble specific substance" (SSS). Capsule size is directly related to the rate of polysaccharide synthesis because capsular material passes into solution in the surrounding menstruum; hence capsules shrink as cultures age and synthesis slows. There is limited antigenic relatedness between the capsular polysaccharides of some of the different types and between pneumococcal polysaccharides and polysaccharides from other sources. For example, type 14 polysaccharide cross-reacts with Abs specific for the blood group A substance.

The cell wall of *D. pneumoniae* contains a Forssman-like carbohydrate substance (C-substance) which is species specific, and M proteins which are analogous to the M proteins of *Strep. pyogenes*. Since neither C nor M antigens of the pneumococcus exert appreciable antiphagocytic activity, anti-M antibodies and anti-C antibodies play no significant role in immunity.

An abnormal beta-globulin called "C-reactive protein" is present in the serum of a variety of patients with acute inflammatory diseases, which reacts with pneumococcal "C substance" to form a precipitate. The possible significance of the occurrence of this protein in disease is not known.

C. Genetics

One type of genetic variation among pneumococci is concerned with the amount of capsular polysaccharide produced, a property which generally correlates directly with virulence. Most encapsulated strains tend to produce colonies with smooth surfaces and outlines (S colonies), whereas strains lacking capsules tend to produce rough colonies (R colonies). A special form of extreme roughness occasionally occurs due to extensive chaining of organisms and may sometimes be seen among encapsulated as well as nonencapsulated strains. Mutation from S to R and from R to S occurs and can be readily demonstrated. Since one or a few S organisms will infect and kill a mouse, mutation from R to S is easily demonstrated by injecting a large dose of R organisms into the animal's peritoneum. Whereas the R organisms are rapidly phagocytized and killed, the few S mutants present soon grow and can be recovered in pure culture.

A culture of pneumococci liberates DNA which can penetrate other pneumococci, including those of a different strain, and impose constitutional genetic change in the recipient. The first DNA-induced change studied was concerned with the transformation of a rough nonencapsulated strain of the pneumococcus to a smooth encapsulated strain. For example, when DNA extracted from an encapsulated type 3 organism was added to a nonencapsulated strain previously derived from a type 2 strain, the nonencapsulated strain was transformed to an encapsulated type 3 strain. Strains possessing more than one polysaccharide type in their capsules occur naturally on rare occasions, presumably as the result of transformation. Transformation has since been shown to involve many other genetic traits, including the quantity of capsular substance produced, resistance to therapeutic drugs, and so forth. Transformation has been demonstrated experimentally in the mouse and presumably occurs naturally in human beings.

D. Extracellular Products

Growing pneumococci liberate an *oxygen-sensitive hemolysin* pneumolysin, which causes alpha hemolysis on blood agar, as well as capsular polysaccharide and the enzyme, neuraminidase.

The capsular polysaccharide is produced in great abundance and, being soluble, reaches the blood in such large amounts that it can often be detected in the serum and urine of patients with lobar pneumonia. However, it is not toxic for animals, even when given in large doses.

Autolysis of organisms releases a "purpura-producing factor" which causes local hemorrhage when injected into the skin of rabbits. It has also been observed that high concentrations of pneumolysin are dermotoxic and lethal. Some strains are reported to produce a leukocidin in small amounts. Neuraminidase is induced *in vitro* by glycoproteins, glycolipids, and other sialic acid containing compounds; it is lethal for weanling mice and at present is the only strong candidate for explaining the irreversible toxicity and death sometimes resulting from human pneumococcal infections. It is antigenic and induces the production of neutralizing Abs.

E. Culture

The pneumococcus requires relatively complex media for growth. It is a facultative anaerobe lacking catalase and peroxidase; consequently it is commonly grown on media containing red blood cells, a rich source of catalase, in order to prevent the accumulation of toxic levels of the metabolite, hydrogen peroxide. The organism also stores best in media rich in blood and can be maintained at 4°C in such media for months. Its growth range is 25° to 42°C.

Being a member of the Family *Lactobacillaceae,* the pneumococcus is characterized by the production of large amounts of lactic acid which is growth inhibitory unless highly buffered media are employed. The organism is notorious for the readiness with which it undergoes spontaneous lysis due to activation of autolytic enzymes; when the phase of exponential growth is passed, the organism rapidly becomes gram-negative and lyses. This results in loss of turbidity in liquid cultures and shrinking of the central portions of old colonies on solid media which lends to them a "checker-like" appearance. Although the mechanisms which promote autolysis are not known, surface-active agents, such as bile salts, trigger lysis and are the basis of the so-called "bile solubility tests" used in laboratory diagnosis to aid in differentiating pneumococci from alpha-hemolytic streptococci. Any suspected organism which is "bile-insoluble" is usually not a pneumococcus. The media commonly employed for growing pneumococci include blood agar and beef infusion broth containing 10% serum or blood and a reducing agent such as thioglycollate. When grown aerobically on the surface of blood agar, virulent encapsulated strains produce medium-sized (0.5 to 3 mm) round, glistening colonies which are initially dome shaped and become surrounded by a greenish-brown zone of partial hemolysis containing red cell ghosts (alpha hemolysis). Small amounts of CO_2 stimulate growth, and some strains have been reported to require 20% CO_2 for primary isolation. Organisms which produce unusually thick capsules, particularly those of type 3, form relatively large mucoid colonies.

F.   Resistance to Physical and Chemical Agents

Pneumococci are "less than average" with respect to resistance to most physical and chemical agents. They are especially susceptible to soaps. Although they are susceptible to a number of antibiotics including tetracyclines, erythromycin, lincomycin, and particularly penicillin, it is notable that mutants tend to develop resistance to most antibiotics except penicillin. It is only recently that strains have been described which have increased resistance to penicillin. The pneumococcus is highly susceptible to ethylhydrocupreine hydrochloride, whereas the alpha-hemolytic streptococci are not. This is the basis of the "optochin test" for differentiating between the two organisms.

G.   Experimental Models

Injected organisms are pathogenic for mice, rats, rabbits, dogs, and subhuman primates, the mouse and rabbit being the most susceptible. The mouse is commonly used for virulence tests; one to 5 organisms given intraperitoneally usually cause death within 16 to 48 hr. Organisms of a few types, including encapsulated type 14, have limited virulence for the mouse which serves to illustrate that, with certain types at least, important virulence factors other than capsular polysaccharide exist and that virulence factors vary with the host species.

Disease closely simulating lobar pneumonia in man has been produced in dogs and subhuman primates. Birds, such as pigeons, are highly resistant because they possess natural opsonins, presumably acquired by natural exposure to cross-reacting Ags.

H. Infections in Man

Currently 80% of all bacterial pneumonias are caused by the pneumococcus and 75% of cases of pneumococcal pneumonia in adults are due to 10 types; namely, types 1, 2, 3, 4, 5, 7, 8, 12, 14 and 19 (50% are due to types 1 and 2 alone); in children the most common types are 1, 6, 14, 19 (also 5 and 7 in earlier reports). The prevalence of types causing disease varies with time and geographical area. The high-numbered types are, in general, less virulent, and bacteremia seldom occurs in infections caused by types above type 33. *In type 3 pulmonary infections with bacteremia the mortality exceeds 50% even with treatment!* In a small percentage of cases mixed infections with more than one type of pneumococcus or with the pneumococcus and *Klebsiella pneumoniae* occur. Such cases obviously present problems in both diagnosis and management.

Most pneumococcal infections result from organisms carried by the individual in his respiratory tract. The lung is the most common site of infection; predisposing causes include measles, respiratory virus infection, asthma with excessive mucus, alcoholism, malnutrition, fatigue, dusty atmosphere, toxic gases, congestive heart disease, or other pulmonary disease. Lung infection in the form of either lobar pneumonia or bronchopneumonia often leads to serious complicating infections at other sites, either by direct extension (empyema, pericarditis) or via the blood stream, with resulting endocarditis, meningitis, or arthritis. Endocarditis and meningitis are almost always fatal unless treated. Meningitis can sometimes result from direct extension of infection from the mastoid or from organisms invading through anatomic defects, such as those caused by basal skull fractures experienced even years earlier. Primary otitis media, an unusually common infection in young children, and mastoiditis are often due to *D. pneumoniae*. Another type of infection, peritonitis in female children, evidently occurs as the result of direct invasion of the organisms from the vagina, where they are sometimes carried.

Lobar pneumonia is the only pneumococcal infection that will be discussed in detail. Over 95% of cases of lobar pneumonia are of pneumococcal causation and presumably result most frequently from highly virulent indigenous or carried organisms to which the individual lacks adequate specific acquired immunity.* Most cases of pneumococcal pneumonia arise in the wake of viral influenza or the common cold, the majority being among otherwise healthy adults, particularly young men. Since late therapy often fails, early diagnosis and treatment are of the utmost importance. The disease is sudden in onset and is commonly heralded by chills, leukocytosis, plateau fever, prostration, cough, tenacious rust-colored sputum (often streaked with blood), and frequently, stabbing unilateral pleural pain. Excessively sticky sputum is usually due to infection with type 3 *D. pneumoniae* or *K. pneumoniae*. Early bacteremia occurs in about 25% of cases and is a serious prognostic sign. Hypoxia from impaired respiratory exchange is often so extreme as to require oxygen; congestive heart failure is a common complication. Icterus due to the combined effects of excessive red cell destruction and depressed liver function from anoxia sometimes occurs and is a grave prognostic sign. In untreated patients who survive, a sudden improvement of symptoms may occur (recovery by "crisis"), usually about the 7th or 8th day of illness (range 5 to 10 days), or the disease may gradually subside (recovery by "lysis"). Chemotherapy can, of course, produce artificial crisis (Section M).

The organisms which initiate infection are thought to invade directly through the bronchial tree. At onset the alveoli become filled with fluid rich in rapidly dividing pneumococci but largely lacking in host cells. Although the cause of sudden excessive edema is not known, the suggestion has been made that it may be an allergic response to proteins of the pneumococcus. The organisms spread by way of intercommunicating bronchioles and from alveolus to alveolus through communicating channels in alveolar walls (pores of Cohn) opened by the stretching effects of excessive fluid in the alveoli. The stage of edema is quickly followed by fibrin accumulation and infiltration of blood cells, especially red cells, lending the appearance and texture of liver (*stage of red hepatization*). During these early stages the organisms multiply to reach enormous numbers. Subsequently neutrophils infiltrate in large numbers, red cells lyse, and many pneumococci are phagocytized (*stage of gray hepatization*). In patients who recover promptly the organisms are largely eliminated by phagocytosis before the next stage (*stage of resolution*) occurs, during which fibrin is digested and neutrophils are replaced by a heavy influx of infiltrating macrophages. The latter help phagocytize the remaining pneumococci, red cells, dying neutrophils, and debris. Fluid is absorbed, and the lung returns to normal.

The rapidity and completeness of restoration of normal histology and function of the lung without scarring have long been a source of wonderment and probably rest on (1) lack of serious injury of alveolar walls by

---

* Lobar pneumonia is defined as "an inflammation of the lung in which the distribution of lesions involves one or more lobes or large portions of lobes, but not others."

the organism,* (2) rapid lysis of fibrin by enzymes liberated by dying neutrophils, thus thwarting the ingrowth of fibroblasts, and (3) good blood supply and lymphatic drainage, which maintain adequate nutrition. In some instances resolution does not occur, and the persisting fibrin is replaced by scar tissue which converts the affected lung into a dense semielastic tissue, a process termed "cornification." Chemotherapy tends to favor fibrosis, possibly by killing organisms, and thus minimizes the infiltration of neutrophils which contribute the enzymes responsible for fibrin digestion. In some cases of lobar pneumonia, especially involving children, alveolar walls may be ruptured by the extensive exudate with resulting emphysema. It is of singular interest that resolution of pneumococcal infection at other sites is less effective than in the lung and such lesions often require surgical drainage. Penicillin treatment of abscesses often fails, because in this lesion many of the organisms are not growing and phagocytosis is minimal, most of the leukocytes being dead. Shock in pneumococcal pneumonia is extremely difficult to manage and if present for any extended time is usually fatal. Early shock with its fall in temperature (pseudocrisis) may be mistaken for crisis. Although the death rate in pneumococcal pneumonia is highest when bacteremia occurs (about 18% even in treated cases), there is also, in general, a direct correlation between mortality and the mass of lung involved. The death rate in penicillin-treated patients with bacteremia rises from 7% in the 12 to 49 year age group to 28% in patients over 50 years of age!

I. Mechanisms of Pathogenicity

Pneumococcal pneumonia, indeed pneumonia due to many infectious agents, commonly results from a breakdown of one or more of the defense barriers of the lower respiratory tract, including the cough and epiglottal reflexes, the mucociliary escalator, the lymphatic drainage of the bronchi and bronchioles, and the macrophage defense of the alveoli. Lobar pneumonia evidently results from the aspiration of heavily contaminated secretions from the URT into the alveoli rather than from inhalation of contaminated sputum droplets or dust particles. During viral respiratory disease the URT secretions are usually excessive and are heavily contaminated with carried organisms. Since the secretions are thin in consistency, aspiration and drainage are apt to carry them to the terminal bronchioles and alveoli, especially if defenses are compromised in any way. In this regard it is of singular interest that the initial infection commonly begins in the lower lobes where aspirated fluids tend to settle. Prior inflammation accompanied by accumulation of edema fluid in alveoli is particularly predisposing to infection, presumably because the fluid serves as a good medium

---

* An exception to lack of injury sometimes occurs in type 3 infections in which there may be necrosis of alveolar walls.

for bacterial growth and hampers the phagocytic activities of resident alveolar macrophages. Experimental evidence supports this concept; normal lungs of animals are more resistant to intratracheal challenge than edematous lungs. It has been suggested that atelectasis may predispose to infection in both animals and man. Once infection begins, the influx of edema fluid into the alveoli is intense and carries the organisms centrifugally into adjacent alveoli through the opened channels between alveoli and communicating terminal bronchioles. As the result of bronchial spread, large areas of complete consolidation involving whole lobes or portions of lobes develop, which is in contrast to the patchy distribution of lesions seen in bronchopneumonia. Resident macrophages are apparently unable to arrest the unopsonized organisms by phagocytosis, and growth of pneumococci may not be contained by neutrophils until sufficient specific Ab accumulates to neutralize the large amounts of free solubilized capsular Ag present and accomplish specific opsonization. Agglutination of the organisms by Ab may help prevent their spread, but is a weak restraining force at best. Maturation of the lesion through its various stages occurs earlier at the initial site of infection than in peripheral areas of spread characterized by edema; consequently all stages of lesion development may be seen in the same lung until after final arrest takes place. Small numbers of organisms probably reach the blood in all cases of the disease, evidently by way of lymphatics draining the alveoli, but are only detected by blood culture when appreciable numbers are shed into the circulation. Persisting bacteremia indicates that organisms have not only reached the circulation but are growing in intravascular foci and have overwhelmed the forces which normally clear the blood of particulates. Early pleural involvement is common, probably as the result of lymphatic spread. Infections of the adjacent pleural and pericardial cavities may occur and represent serious complications. Empyema occurs in about 5% of cases.

Despite the fact that patients with pneumonia show evidence of marked "toxemia," no causative toxin has been implicated with certainty. Pneumococcal neuraminidase is toxic for experimental animals, and the possibility that it might be the important agent responsible for toxemia in human infections has not been ruled out.

Occasionally degeneration of renal tubules occurs, but the reason for this is not known. It is of interest that immune complex disease involving renal glomeruli does not occur despite the fact that enormous amounts of soluble Ag-Ab complexes are probably formed. This raises questions as to the localization pattern of these complexes and their capacity to fix C.

J. Mechanisms of Immunity

Since immunity is specific and long lasting, second attacks with organisms of the same type are rare. Both macrophages and neutrophils readily kill ingested pneumococci. Hence, the critical immune forces operating in the alveolus against invading pneumococci involve primarily opsonin-dependent phagocytosis. Whereas small amounts of natural complement-dependent polyspecific opsonins for pneumococci occur in most normal individuals, neither they nor the forces of surface phagocytosis serve to meet any substantial challenge on the part of invading organisms.

Healthy individuals lacking detectable specific anticapsular Ab can carry highly virulent organisms without developing lung infection. Since a few of the carried pneumococci must occasionally reach alveoli, macrophages, which are essentially the only phagocytes in normal alveoli, must effect the destruction of such organisms largely by surface phagocytosis and thus represent the effector cells of nonspecific antipneumococcal defense of the alveolus of the normal lung. In contrast, under the abnormal conditions existing at the time of infection, resident alveolar macrophages, unless assisted by substantial amounts of specific Ab, are evidently incapable of coping with large numbers of pneumococci present at the initiation of a progressive infection.

Once infection is established, macrophages evidently contribute less to total phagocytic defense than neutrophils, which mobilize, ingest, and kill pneumococci with remarkable facility in the presence of specific opsonins. Whereas surface phagocytosis is operative earlier in infection than specific opsonin-dependent phagocytosis, it is evidently insufficient to cope with an established infection. Consequently *the availability of adequate amounts of specific Ab is usually the critical factor determining the outcome of infection.* Enormous amounts of Ab are probably required to combine with available free Ag to the point where opsonization can occur. *Thus death or recovery may be likened to a race between the ability of the host to produce specific Ab and the organisms to produce capsular polysaccharide.* This is attested by the observations that free opsonins usually appear in the blood at or near the time of crisis, that the formerly used treatment with specific antiserum was effective, and that individuals lacking in the capacity to form Ab, such as patients with agammaglobulinemia, are highly susceptible to pneumococcal infection. The fate of Ag, the classes of Abs formed, their functions, and the dynamics of Ag-Ab interactions in lobar pneumonia have not been fully elucidated. With respect to the Abs produced and their functions, it has been claimed that in the mouse protection test IgM Ab is 100,000 times more effective than IgG Ab. Although this could explain why precipitin and agglutinin titers do not correlate well with mouse protection tests, there is no assurance that Abs of different immunoglobulin classes behave similarly with respect to pneumococcal immunity in mouse and man. The alleged role of IgA Abs in pneumococcal immunity in the mouse needs further investigation. It is conceivable that high avidity IgA Abs could assist by neutralizing circulating capsular polysaccharide thus leaving IgG or IgM Abs available for opsonization. It appears that IgA is not capable of functioning as an opsonin.

Pneumococcal polysaccharide is not readily destroyed by tissue enzymes and remains in the body for long periods. It readily produces immunologic tolerance, at least in the mouse. The possible implications of these properties of the polysaccharide with respect to human infections are not known. Tolerance obviously does not occur in patients who pass crisis and live or perhaps even in patients who die.

The basis of the Francis reaction is of theoretical interest. This is an immediate type of skin reaction induced by the intradermal injection of purified pneumococcal polysaccharide. It depends on the presence of free antipneumococcal Ab in serum and becomes positive about the time of crisis in patients who recover, but is seldom positive in those who die. The test is positive in convalescent patients and in some normal individuals. For some unknown reason it may be negative in some patients who develop serum Ab but who die later without undergoing crisis.

K. Laboratory Diagnosis

Although most cases of pneumococcal lobar pneumonia can be diagnosed easily by clinical findings and simple laboratory tests, others are difficult to diagnose, the most notorious being patients with infected pulmonary infarcts. Pneumonias due to staphylococci, Group A streptococci, and *Klebsiella pneumoniae* must always be considered. It is especially important to differentiate between pneumonia caused by *D. pneumoniae* and *K. pneumoniae* since the causative organisms differ markedly in their susceptibility to antibiotics. Differential diagnosis should include consideration of coexisting infectious disease and noninfectious conditions, such as congestive heart failure, pulmonary infarction, and atelectasis.

Whenever lobar pneumonia is suspected, sputum specimens should be stained and cultured, and blood should be inoculated into thioglycollate medium and plated on blood agar. Usually a Gram stain will permit a tentative diagnosis so that chemotherapy can be instituted; however, it is impossible to distinguish between *D. pneumoniae* and certain strains of alpha-hemolytic streptococci by the Gram stain alone. If antisera are available, the capsular swelling test on sputum is the most rapid and reliable test for early diagnosis.*

The sputum should come *from deep in the respiratory tract* and should be collected in a sterile jar at the bedside by the physician. Throat swabs, transtracheal aspiration, or lung puncture may be necessary in children. Swabs should be transported to the laboratory in a sterile medium to prevent drying, and cultures should be incubated in a CO_2 incubator, since 10% of newly isolated strains will not grow without added CO_2.

---

* Polyvalent antisera reactive against 82 types are now available in many institutions for diagnostic capsular swelling tests.

Blood agar is commonly used for streak plating. Colonies are small and should be observed with a dissecting microscope. Bile solubility tests and the optochin test are useful for identifying the pneumococcus.

The presence of pneumococci in blood or deep lung secretions secured by transtracheal or lung puncture is strong evidence that the pulmonary infection is of pneumococcal causation. Their presence in blood in appreciable numbers carries an unfavorable prognostic sign. Because of the high frequency of pneumococcal carriers, the presence of pneumococci in sputum is only of significance when the organisms are in great abundance and are accompanied by large numbers of neutrophils.

In difficult cases repeated examinations of sputum should be made using Gram, acid-fast, and negative stains. In some instances the mouse virulence test may be useful as a check on pathogenicity and to provide organisms for typing. The mouse inhibits the growth of most bacteria in sputum except the pneumococcus, which can usually be isolated in pure culture from the peritoneum or heart blood of the injected animals. Illness may become apparent as early as 5 to 8 hr. A few strains of pneumococci have limited virulence for mice and produce a more protracted infection.

L. *Therapy*

Although specific antisera and sulfa drugs were formerly used to treat pneumococcal pneumonia, penicillin has become the therapeutic agent of choice, and strains resistant to penicillin occur rarely, if ever. Other chemotherapeutic agents are less useful because resistant mutants commonly emerge.

Most cases of pneumococcal pneumonia respond dramatically to penicillin treatment, often with cessation of bacteremia within a few hours and passing crisis within 24 hours. Penicillin has reduced the overall mortality from about 30 to 5%. If fever persists in the face of penicillin treatment, it is probably "drug fever" due to hypersensitivity to penicillin rather than to the pneumonia itself. Despite successful antipneumococcal treatment, a few patients develop severe and often fatal secondary infections with organisms such as the staphylococcus.

Early treatment is of the utmost importance in order to stop the spread and growth of the organisms short of the point where toxemia is irreversible. Late treatment, especially of patients with bacteremia or meningitis, often fails despite rapid killing of the organisms, and it has been postulated that some unknown lethal substance or effect is produced by growing organisms which causes irreversible lethal injury. Obviously there is urgent need for better understanding of the cause of toxemia, for without such information there is no rational basis for improving therapy and little hope that the death rate can be reduced much below the present level of 5%.

M. Reservoirs of Infection

The principal, if not the sole, natural reservoir of human infections is man.

N. Control of Disease Transmission

The possession of type-specific Ab unquestionably conveys strong protection against infection and lessens the chance that the specific organism can establish the carrier state; individuals known to be immune to given types seldom become carriers of those types. Moreover, most carriers eventually become immune to the type(s) they carry and tend to free themselves of the carried organisms. Most normal individuals have low levels of specific Abs to a number of types, presumably as a result of carrier experience. The types of carried organisms change constantly, carried types being lost and new types acquired by chance through droplet transmission from other carriers. Convalescent patients seldom carry the causative type more than 2 to 3 weeks.

Acquisition of the carrier state by a nonimmune individual is apparently largely a matter of chance and commonly results from droplet transmission from other carriers rather than from patients. It is estimated that 40 to 70% of individuals are carriers at some time during each year and that during the peak period in late winter and early spring carrier rates often exceed 40%. Except for type 3, the carrier rate of highly virulent types is normally low. When the carrier rate in a population increases and when the carried organisms are highly virulent, the risk of an epidemic of lobar pneumonia is great, especially if an epidemic of a predisposing respiratory infection, such as viral influenza, occurs at the same time. *Whether or not an individual develops lobar pneumonia hinges on whether he is carrying a virulent strain of organism to which he is not immune at a time when his resistance becomes depressed.*

Since infection is commonly endogenous, effective control of pneumococcal pneumonia cannot be achieved by measures designed to prevent transmission of the disease from patients to healthy individuals, and stringent isolation of patients is only warranted when highly susceptible contacts are at risk, such as individuals with congestive heart failure, other pulmonary disease, debilitating illnesses, or immunosuppressed states. Potential methods for control of pneumococcal pneumonia are (1) prevention of predisposing illnesses, such as by vaccination against viral influenza, (2) active immunization with polyvalent pneumococcal vaccine containing specific polysaccharides representing the types commonly responsible for the disease in the geographic area, and (3) chemoprophylaxis with penicillin.

Both influenza vaccines and polyvalent pneumococcal vaccines are attractive measures for protecting highly susceptible individuals, such as patients with congestive heart failure, and for preventing or halting epidemics of lobar pneumonia. In view of the early proof that durable *immunity can be produced with polyvalent polysaccharide vaccines,* it is surprising and unfortunate that little effort has been made to introduce the practice of protective vaccination, and that commercial pneumococcal vaccines are not available.

References

Austrian, R., and Gold, J.: Pneumococcal bacteremia with especial reference to bacteremic pneumococcal pneumonia. Ann. Intern. Med. *60*:759, 1964.

Finland, M.: Recent advances in the epidemiology of pneumococcal infections. Medicine *21*:307, 1942.

Finland, M., and Sutliff, W. D.: Specific antibody response of human subjects to intracutaneous injection of pneumococcus products. J. Exp. Med. *55*:853, 1932.

Heffron, R.: *Pneumonia with Special Reference to Pneumococcus Lobar Pneumonia.* New York: The Commonwealth Fund, 1939.

Kearney, R., and Halliday, W. J.: Immunity and paralysis in mice: serological and biological properties of two distinct antibodies to Type III pneumococcal polysaccharide. Immunology *19*:551, 1970.

Kelly, R., and Greiff, D.: Toxicity of pneumococcal neuraminidase. Infect. Immun. *2*:115, 1970.

MacLeod, C. M.: Prevention of pneumococcal pneumonia by immunization with specific capsular polysaccharides. In *Infectious Agents and Host Reactions.* ed. by Mudd, S. Philadelphia: W. B. Saunders Co., 1970.

MacLeod, C. M., Hodges, R. G., Heidelberger, M., and Bernhard, W. G.: Prevention of pneumococcal pneumonia by immunization with specific capsular polysaccharides. J. Exp. Med. *82*:445, 1945.

White, B.: *The Biology of Pneumococcus: The Bacteriological, Biochemical and Immunological Characters and Activities of Diplococcus pneumoniae.* New York: The Commonwealth Fund, 1938.

Wood, W. B., Jr.: Cecil-Loeb *Textbook of Medicine.* 13th ed. ed. by Beeson and McDermott. Philadelphia: W. B. Saunders Co., 1971.

Chapter 11

Streptococcus

Streptococcus pyogenes, 131

Streptococci of Other Species, 151

The genus *Streptococcus,* of the family *Lactobacillaceae,* is comprised of a large number of species of saprophytes and of pathogenic and nonpathogenic parasites several of which are among the normal flora of the mouth and intestine of man. Streptococci are widespread in nature; some species are important in lactic acid fermentations, whereas others selectively parasitize and infect different animal hosts. Their taxonomy has been difficult and a complete and practical scheme of classification has not been devised. On a broad basis some authorities have divided all streptococci into those which are *alpha-hemolytic,* those which are *beta-hemolytic,* and those which are strict anaerobes.* *Gamma hemolysis,* an inappropriate term, is sometimes used to designate lack of hemolysis. The term *non-hemolytic* is also often used ambiguously to designate organisms which do not cause beta hemolysis, and thus includes the alpha-hemolytic streptococci! Division on the basis of hemolytic activities is unfortunate because the criterion of hemolysis varies widely among strains within a species and shows little correlation with other properties.

Current classification of streptococci, excluding those of the *viridans* and *anaerobic* groups, was established by Lancefield; it is based on distinctive group and type Ags. Serologic groups, which are designated by capital letters (A through O), are distinguished on the basis of antigenic differences in cell wall carbohydrate. Types within group A, which number about 55, are separated on the basis of antigenic differences of a protein in the cell wall designated "M protein" (see Section B).

Streptococcus pyogenes, often spoken of as "the group A streptococcus," is the most important species pathogenic for man; it causes over 95% of all streptococcal infections. Organisms of other species of streptococci particularly of groups C, D, G and O sometimes cause infection in man (Table 11-1). Of the various pathogenic streptococci only *Strep. pyogenes* will be discussed in detail.

Streptococcus pyogenes

A. Medical Perspectives

Streptococcus pyogenes has always been a constant cause of serious disease in man. Few organisms produce a wider variety of toxins or elicit a broader spectrum of lesions and sequelae. Clear descriptions of the distinct clinical entities caused by streptococci, *scarlet fever* and *erysipelas,* appeared in medical literature centuries before Billroth (1874) described "chains of globular microorganisms" in the lesions of erysipelas and Fehleisen (1882) reproduced erysipelas in volunteers with pure cultures of

* Streptococci which produce alpha hemolysis are sometimes grouped under the heading "viridans streptococci" because of a greenish color which develops in the zone of partial hemolysis. The term "beta hemolysis" is used to designate the clear zone type of hemolysis which results from the complete lysis of red blood cells.

TABLE 11-1
Lancefield Group Classification of Some Streptococci of Medical Importance

Group	Species	Habitat(s)
A	S. pyogenes	man
B	S. agalactiae	mastitis in cows, man
C	S. equisimilis	man and animals
	S. dysagalactiae	man and animals
D	S. faecalis	milk, man and animals
	S. durans	milk, man and animals
	S. zymogenes	man
	S. liquefaciens	man and animals
E		milk and swine
F	4 types	man
G	S. anginosus	man and dog
H	S. sanguis	man
K		man
L		man, dog, and pig
M		dog and man
N	S. lactis	milk
O		man

streptococci. *Rheumatic fever* (RF) and *glomerulonephritis,* serious sequelae of streptococcal infection, and the once deadly *puerperal fever* (commonly caused by *Strep. pyogenes*) were also recognized as clinical entities more than a century ago. The fascinating essays of Oliver Wendell Holmes and Semmelweis on the infectious nature of puerperal fever stand as classics in medical literature and are well worth the attention of any student of medicine.

Streptococcus pyogenes is no longer the dreaded pathogen it was as late as the early decades of this century, largely because of the advent of effective antibiotics. It is especially notable that in developed countries today streptococcal infections and their sequelae are not only less common but are less severe than during the last century. The precise reasons for these changes, which began before the advent of chemotherapy, are not known but probably include evolutionary changes in host and parasite as well as better nutrition and living conditions. *The most serious sequela of streptococcal infection is heart disease resulting from RF,* which has an incidence between 6 to 9 per 1000 among 18-year-olds in the USA. New cases are estimated to range from 50,000 to 100,000 annually. However, prior to the introduction of effective chemotherapy, streptococcal disease with its sequelae stood with tuberculosis and syphilis as the 3 most serious and important infectious diseases in the USA.

Although the future importance of infectious diseases cannot be predicted with any degree of certainty, there is no reason to believe that streptococcal diseases will return to their former high incidence or severity or become unmanageable, particularly so long as antibacterial drugs remain effective as prophylactic and therapeutic agents. Moreover, *there is the prospect that effective "vaccines" of M protein may soon be developed.*

Good examples of the effectiveness of penicillin against streptococci are the marked reduction in the incidence of repeated attacks of RF afforded by long-term penicillin prophylaxis and the marked lowering of the fatality rate in cases of streptococcal meningitis treated with the drug.

B. Physical and Chemical Structure

Streptococcus pyogenes is a gram-positive, nonmotile, nonsporing, commonly encapsulated, spherical to oval organism about 1 μm in diameter arranged in chains of varying length. The cells elongate in the axis of the chain prior to division. Since the cells usually fail to separate after division the chain grows in length with persisting cell wall material linking the cells together. Adherence is strongest immediately after division which leads to what appear to be chains of "diplococci." Since post-fission separation of cells results from enzymatic cleavage of cell wall materials, Abs against the surface M protein of the cell, which serve to mask the cell-wall substrates responsible for chaining, can prevent cleavage. This provides the basis for the "long-chain" serologic test used for detecting specific serum Abs against M proteins (anti-M Abs).

A schematized diagram of the surface structures of a streptococcal cell is presented in Figure 11-1. It should be noted that the outermost layer is

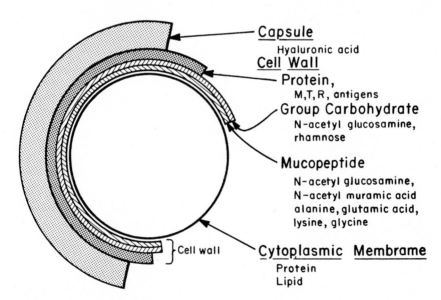

Figure 11-1. Composition of the cell wall of *Streptococcus pyogenes*. (Adapted from R. M. Krause, Bact. Rev. 27:369, 1963)

a capsule composed of hyaluronic acid, a nonantigenic substance which is antiphagocytic. In cultures the capsule can only be demonstrated in organisms a few hours old, in part because it is highly soluble in growth media, but principally because hyaluronidase, which hydrolyzes the hyaluronic acid capsule, is secreted by the organisms soon after the initiation of growth. Apparently capsules are better maintained *in vivo* than *in vitro*. Strains which produce little hyaluronidase and possess large capsules form relatively large *"mucoid"* colonies on blood agar which, as they age and dry, transform to flat wrinkled colonies (*matt colonies*). In contrast, strains which produce large amounts of hyaluronidase and accumulate little or no capsular material form small *glossy colonies*.

The second outermost surface layer of the cell is comprised of M, T and R proteins which extend through the capsule to the cell surface.* Apparently they are not structural components of the cell wall but following synthesis at the plasma membrane diffuse outward. They can be detected on the bacterial surface by agglutination tests with appropriate antisera, and when extracted in the soluble form can be identified by precipitin tests. Since the T and R Ags occur independently of M Ag and have not been shown to be medically important, they will not be discussed. Some of the M protein combines with cell wall components by primary chemical bonding.

The M protein (mol wt 40,000), which is highly resistant to acid and heat, is of paramount importance because it is the *sole "protective immunogen" and is the major determinant of virulence. Its antiphagocytic property is even stronger than that of hyaluronic acid;* moreover it precipitates fibrinogen and is toxic for platelets and secondarily for neutrophils which aggregate with the injured platelets. The M protein on the cell surface is readily accessible for linking with *specific Ab which tends to cancel out any protection against phagocytosis afforded by M protein* and possibly by the hyaluronic acid of the capsule as well. Moreover, most human sera contain an unidentified relatively heat-stable factor which counteracts the antiphagocytic activity of the hyaluronic acid capsule. Destruction of M protein by trypsin treatment which does not kill the organism greatly reduces its resistance to phagocytosis. Stripping the cell of both hyaluronic acid and M protein abolishes all resistance to phagocytosis. Whereas most strains of *Strep. pyogenes* produce but traces of proteinase during the late stages of growth, some strains produce such large amounts of this extracellular enzyme that they destroy their own M protein and certain other proteins as well. Since the proteinase is highly active at 37°C but not at 22°C, the capacity of strong proteinase-producers to synthesize M protein can be tested by incubating the cultures at 22°C to allow accumulation of the protein to detectable levels. *The M protein also endows the organism with the capacity to adhere to and colonize the mucosal epithelium of the upper*

* Another protein, M-associated protein (MAP) has been reported recently.

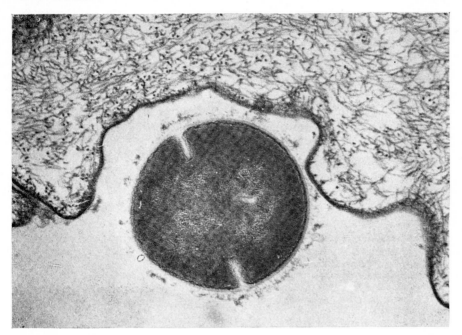

Figure 11-2. *Streptococcus pyogenes* strain ST A628 attached to the surface of a tongue epithelial cell of a germfree rat. The organism is surrounded by the M protein-containing surface fuzz, which appears to mediate its attachment to the epithelial cell membrane ($\times$ 80,000). (Ellen, R. P., and Gibbons, R. J.: M protein-associated adherence of *Streptococcus pyogenes* to epithelial surfaces: Prerequisite for Virulence. Infect. Immun. 5:828, 1972.)

respiratory tract (URT) (Figure 11-2). Thus adherence may be another attribute of M protein contributing to invasiveness and virulence. Since anti-M Abs of the class, secretory IgA, can block the adherence of streptococci to the mucosa of the URT, they may play an important role in immunity and resistance to carriage and infection by opposing colonization and invasion of tissues. *The M proteins of the different types of streptococci are antigenically distinct and immunity is type specific.*

The middle layer of the cell wall contains the "group specific" polysaccharide ("C-carbohydrate" Ag) which because of its cross reactivity with heart valve glycoproteins could play a part in the pathogenesis of RF. It is tightly bound to the underlying mucopeptide layer of the inner cell wall lying adjacent to the cytoplasmic membrane and protects it against lysozyme action. The cell wall mucopeptide Ag shows *in vitro* toxicity for neutrophils and cultured kidney cells and produces dermonecrosis. Recent animal work has shown that cell wall fragments of *Strep. pyogenes* containing the *C-carbohydrate-mucopeptide complex are singularly resistant to digestion by phagocytes and can persist* in tissues to produce chronic rheumatic fever-like lesions (Section H-8).

The cytoplasmic membrane contains Ags which cross-react with heart muscle and glomerular basement membrane, and transplantation-like Ags which speed allograft rejection in guinea pigs (Section H). A certain cytoplasmic component is reported to exert selective immunosuppression of B lymphocytes.

Highly pleomorphic forms of streptococci appear in ageing cultures and wall-less organisms (protoplasts) develop and grow in hypertonic media containing penicillin and lysozyme. Although such protoplasts multiply *in vitro* and have been observed in tissues of patients their possible role in disease production is unknown.

C. Genetics

Genetic variation is common among group A streptococci and involves many traits including the synthesis of extracellular products, the capsule, and cell-wall components, and colonial morphology and drug resistance. Variations in the production of hyaluronic acid capsules and M protein appear to be independent genetic traits. However, since both hyaluronic acid capsules and M protein are antiphagocytic and account for virulence, differences in virulence involve variations in one or both of these substances. For example, those organisms which possess an abundance of both substances are highly virulent, those deficient in one or the other substance are of intermediate virulence, and those deficient in both substances are of lowest virulence. As in the case of the pneumococcus, repeated culture *in vitro* favors overgrowth by nonencapsulated variants and contrariwise, low virulence organisms which lack hyaluronic acid capsules can be selectively suppressed by mouse passage to obtain more virulent encapsulated mutants. In like manner, low virulence strains lacking M protein can be converted to M protein-containing strains of higher virulence. *The natural selective pressure of immune forces is evident in man; for example in the face of developing immunity, carried organisms tend to lose their M protein and virulence, whereas epidemic strains which pass rapidly from one susceptible person to another are rich in M protein and are of high virulence.* Whether the loss of M protein during carriage may result from high proteinase-producing mutants appears not to have been thoroughly investigated.

Whereas resistance to certain chemotherapeutic agents, such as the sulfa drugs, develops readily, *strains resistant to penicillin do not emerge as the result of therapy, evidently because penicillin-resistant mutants are of low virulence.*

The production of the erythrogenic toxins responsible for scarlet fever is the outcome of lysogenization of streptococci by temperate bacteriophages, as in the case of *Corynebacterium diphtheriae*. However, unlike *C. diphtheriae,* which produces but a single toxin, 3 antigenically distinct erythrogenic toxins called A, B, and C are produced, presumably under the influence of different phages. Some strains produce both A and B toxins simultaneously. The quantity of erythrogenic toxin(s) produced by different strains of streptococci varies greatly but whether variations in toxic strength occur is not known. Lysogeny is common among group A streptococci, and it is probable that future studies will reveal that additional attributes of pathogenicity and virulence are controlled by phage.

D. Extracellular Products

Group A streptococci produce at least 20 antigenic extracellular substances, including many enzymes, a number of which have not been identified. Only those which show evidence of being medically important will be considered.

1. Erythrogenic Toxins

The erythrogenic toxins of group A streptococci mentioned above are low molecular weight proteins. Some groups C and G strains may produce toxins similar to if not identical with group A erythrogenic toxins. Erythrogenic toxins are destroyed by boiling and when injected into the skin of the "nonimmune" subject cause a delayed local erythema, which peaks at 24 hours (positive Dick test).* A scarletinal rash is produced when a large dose of toxin is administered systemically to a nonimmune subject. The toxins produce no reaction in an immune subject who possesses neutralizing antitoxin (negative Dick test). Although these toxins have many biological activities, their only known contribution to the pathogenesis of streptococcal disease is the production of a scarletinal rash. Whereas man is exquisitely sensitive to the toxin, most animals are highly resistant.

2. Streptolysin S and Streptolysin O

Two beta-hemolytic products, streptolysin S, a peptide, and streptolysin O, a protein, have been identified; the first is produced by essentially all strains and the second by the large majority of strains of *Strep. pyogenes.* Streptolysin O is oxygen sensitive, but streptolysin S is not. Consequently, streptolysin O only produces hemolysis deep in a blood agar plate, whereas streptolysin S produces hemolysis around surface colonies as well. Both hemolysins are highly toxic for neutrophils and macrophages and streptolysin O is a cardiotoxin. Streptolysin O elicits a neutralizing Ab, designated antistreptolysin O (ASO) but streptolysin S is nonantigenic. *The levels of ASO in serum have proved to be a valuable index of a recent streptococcal infection, particularly with respect to the diagnosis of RF.* These Abs appear in the serum of about 70% of patients and peak at about 3 to 5 weeks after pharyngeal infection.

* There is uncertainty about the basis of the Dick reaction; some evidence indicates that it is not a straightforward toxin-antitoxin regulated event but also involves delayed hypersensitivity.

3. Nicotinamide Adenine Dinucleotidase (NADase)

Nicotinamide adenine dinucleotide (NAD), a respiratory enzyme cofactor, is hydrolyzed by NADase. The enzyme is produced by some streptococci including strains of a number of types such as 3, 4, 6 and 12. The enzyme, which is active only when bound to the cell wall, can kill phagocytes. Whether a phagocyte succumbs undoubtedly depends on the number of streptococci present within the cell.*

4. Streptokinase

Streptokinase is a nontoxic enzyme produced by essentially all strains of *Strep. pyogenes* and by groups C and G organisms as well. Several antigenically distinct streptokinases exist.

By acting on a proactivator of the fibrinolytic system streptokinase brings about the conversion of blood plasminogen to plasmin, a proteolytic enzyme which digests fibrin. Neutralizing Abs to streptokinase become demonstrable in the serum in about 75% of cases of streptococcosis but do not appear to block the spread of infection in tissues.

5. Deoxyribonuclease

Streptococcal deoxyribonuclease (DNase or streptodornase) is a nontoxic enzyme produced by all strains of group A streptococci and by organisms of several other groups as well. Four antigenically distinct kinds of DNases are recognized, A, B, C and D; except for type B, neutralization by specific Ab is irregular. Some strains of *Strep. pyogenes* can produce all 4 serologic types of the enzyme simultaneously. The enzyme contributes to the liquefaction of exudates rich in DNA. In fact, commercial mixtures of streptokinase and streptodornase have been used with limited success for "enzymatic debridement" of wounds and abscesses in order to clear them of fibrin and pus.

6. Hyaluronidase

Streptococcal hyaluronidase is produced in varying amounts by all strains of *Strep. pyogenes,* most notably by strains 4 and 22. Although production of the enzyme *in vitro* is usually difficult to demonstrate, it is evidently produced readily *in vivo* since increasing titers of neutralizing Abs almost always appear in convalescent sera.

7. Proteinase

Streptococcal proteinase, a cathepsin-like enzyme with broad substrate specificity, is produced *in vitro* in varying amounts by certain strains of

* A recent report suggests that streptolysin S rather than NADase may be the leukotoxin studied.

group A streptococci but rarely by strains of the other serologic groups. It is formed autocatalytically from a precursor under reducing conditions.

Low pH (below 6.8) and high temperature (37°C) favor its production. Whether proteinase is produced *in vivo* and to what extent is not known.

8. Other Products

Several additional extracellular factors alleged to represent distinct molecular entities have been reported. Their importance in pathogenesis is controversial. They are lymphocyte mitogen, nephrotoxin, cardiohepatic toxin and a cell sensitizing factor (SF) which sensitizes red cells to agglutination and lysis by serum.

E. Culture

The cultural requirements of *Strep. pyogenes* are similar to those of *D. pneumoniae* (Chapter 10). The organism produces an abundance of lactic acid which lowers the pH of culture media and tends to limit growth. Rich, well-buffered media, particularly those containing blood or serum are favored. Some strains require CO_2 for primary isolation.

F. Resistance to Physical and Chemical Agents

Streptococcus pyogenes is "average" in its resistance to most physical and chemical agents. It is moderately resistant to drying but is destroyed by pasteurization and is readily killed by the common disinfectants. The organism is susceptible to a wide variety of chemotherapeutic agents. Resistance develops readily to sulfonamides and certain antibiotics but, fortunately, not to penicillin, the therapeutic drug of choice.

G. Experimental Models

It is only on rare occasions that *Strep. pyogenes* causes natural disease in wild animals, such as voles and field mice, but when inoculated many strains are pathogenic for the laboratory mouse, guinea pig and rabbit. Virulence may be enhanced by animal passage and in the case of the mouse is frequently attended by an increase in M protein and capsule size. The mouse is commonly used for virulence tests, but unfortunately mouse virulence does not necessarily parallel M protein production or human virulence. The pathogenesis of the sequelae of streptococcal infections in man is poorly understood despite an enormous literature on the subject. No animal models have been developed that closely simulate RF or acute poststreptococcal glomerulonephritis in man.

H. Infections in Man

Streptococcus pyogenes maintains itself in nature as a carried organism in the URT of man, its only constant natural host. The carrier rate in healthy subjects is usually less than 10%, but varies with season and other circumstances, being higher in winter than in summer and highest when URT infections are most prevalent in a population. During epidemics of streptococcal pharyngitis the organisms are heavily encapsulated and rich in M protein; as epidemics decline the M protein content of infecting organisms declines.

The organism has high invasive powers and exhibits a strong tendency to spread via lymphatics. It has great versatility as a secondary invader, particularly in the case of viral infections, and can be a serious secondary invader in smallpox, influenza, and measles. The two most common sites of infection are the nasopharynx and the skin.

1. Pharyngitis

Streptococcus pyogenes is the most common cause of bacterial sore throat (pharyngitis). It is usually contracted from a carrier or an infected subject via droplet infection, direct contact or fomites. "Strep throat" is most frequent between the ages of 5 to 15 years; in most instances the infection is mild and benign. Despite the protection afforded by maternal Ab infections can occur in the newborn, especially in the poorly protected umbilical stump. Since innate immunity is not fully protective, the infant becomes highly susceptible to infection after maternally derived anti-M Ab has waned. With each succeeding infection (which averages about one each year during childhood) or carriage experience the individual develops specific immunity to organisms of the type involved; *thus immunity is type specific and cumulative with advancing age.* Contraction of a new infection only occurs providing the individual has not had previous experience with organisms of the type in question or if the organism is of unusually high virulence or immunity has waned. *Reinfections with organisms of the same type are rare,* and when they occur are usually mild or occult, presumably because of the anamnestic response.

The character of the infection changes with age. The first infections in infancy and early childhood lack a well-defined onset and symptoms, show little tendency to localize, are accompanied by relatively mild inflammatory responses and run a protracted course. Even though pharyngitis in infants is mild, often presenting only a rhinorrhea, suppurative lymphadenitis and otitis media sometimes occur.

Infections in older children and adults are mild and in some 20% of cases pass unnoticed. Severe infections show a greater tendency to localize and are characterized by a sudden and intense inflammatory response. They usually heal without suppurative complications. This change in the character of infection with age is thought to occur because with succeeding infections the individual becomes increasingly sensitive (both immediate and delayed types) to somatic Ags common to all group A streptococci, irrespective of type.

When a child develops a streptococcal sore throat, it is usually observed that at least one or more of the other members of the household (sometimes including adults) contract the disease. The more virulent the organism, the greater the chance of spread.

Severe streptococcal pharyngitis and viral pharyngitis are often mistaken one for the other. Severe streptococcal pharyngitis is commonly heralded by the rapid development of a sore throat of varying intensity (usually without significant cough), fever, leukocytosis, headache, malaise, swollen tender cervical lymph nodes, exudate rich in neutrophils, and often abdominal pain, nausea and vomiting.

2. Scarlet Fever

In a limited number of instances of streptococcal pharyngitis an added complication develops, a skin rash, *the hallmark of scarlet fever*. The rash is commonly generalized and after several days is usually followed by desquamation which is especially evident in the palms of the hands and soles of the feet. Whether the patient with a streptococcal infection develops the scarletinal skin rash depends on whether the particular infecting strain is endowed with the capacity to produce one or more of the 3 different erythrogenic toxins and whether the individual is immune to scarlet fever by virtue of possessing specific antitoxic Abs. About 25% of individuals possess such Abs, presumably as the result of carried organisms or previous infection. Specific antitoxin, if present, can prevent the skin rash (scarlet fever) but fails to convey immunity against streptococcal infection, a property limited to anti-M Ab. Erythrogenic toxins are no longer regarded to produce serious injury and, except for the rash, the scarlet fever patient is not clinically in greater jeopardy than the patient with streptococcal pharyngitis without the rash. Immunization with erythrogenic toxin and the use of antitoxin for therapy are no longer advocated and the Schultz-Charlton blanching reaction produced in scarletinal skin by injecting convalescent serum is seldom used for diagnosis.

The decreasing severity of streptococcosis with associated scarlet fever in the last century has been remarkable; whereas the death rate due to streptococcal infections attended by scarlet fever in Great Britain was over 900 per million in 1861–65, it fell to some 29 per million by 1921–25 and now stands near zero. This change may represent in part an example of evolution of host and/or parasite. Today scarlet fever is principally of interest because it is an example of the unique circumstance in which bacteriophages regulate toxin production by a pathogen.

3. Peritonsillar Abscess

The tissues involved in streptococcal pharyngitis are commonly confined largely to the throat mucosa and local lymphoid structures. In severe cases confluent exudates may accumulate and cover the affected area and the organisms may pass to the cervical lymph nodes and produce an abscess. Involvement of peritonsillar tissues with abscess formation (quinsy) or spread to retropharyngeal tissues, with the attending danger of airway obstruction and thrombophlebitis, probably result most often from a mixed infection with *Bacteroides* species and anaerobic streptococci. Infection sometimes spreads through non-lymphoid tissues of the floor of the mouth with associated abscess formation in the neck, a condition called *Ludwig's angina.* Rarely, group A organisms cause "doughnut lesions" on the palate.

4. Spread to Other Organ Systems

Organisms may also spread readily from the pharynx into the paranasal sinuses, to skin to produce *impetigo,* or directly through the eustachian tube to produce middle ear infection (*otitis media*); spread may also extend to the air cells of the mastoid bone to produce *mastoiditis. Meningitis* may result from invasion through the mastoid bone to the meninges.

Rapid spread from any local site to the blood via lymphatics may occur and may lead to metastatic lesions in joints, bones, endocardium, etc.

Streptococcal bronchopneumonia, often with accompanying bacteremia, usually develops as a complication of some other pulmonary disease, particularly influenza. Because of the tendency to spread through lymphatic vessels, even in retrograde fashion, the organisms readily reach the pleura; hence *pleuritis* with copious pleural exudates commonly develops. *Empyema* (pus in the pleural cavity) occurs in about 40% of cases and bacteremia is frequent.

5. Puerperal Fever

Puerperal fever (childbed fever) is a postpartum infection of the uterus which frequently leads to septicemia and death. It is caused by *Strep. pyogenes* in about 80% of cases; most of the remaining cases are caused by anaerobic streptococci, and *Clostridium perfringens* which frequently colonize the vagina. A substantial number of cases of puerperal fever result from mixed infections which complicates therapy. Infection with *Strep. pyogenes* originates from organisms shed from the respiratory tract of the patient in some 25% of cases and from attendants in the remainder of cases. Without treatment the case fatality rate from disease due to anaerobic streptococci is about 35 to 40% and from disease due to *Strep. pyogenes* about 60%.

6. Infections of the Skin

The skin is the second most common site of infection where 2 types of lesions occur, *pyoderma* and *erysipelas.* Spread may sometimes extend to produce paronychia or vaginitis. Skin and wound infections are of longer duration than pharyngeal infections and are more frequently accompanied by local lymph node involvement and bacteremia. For unknown reasons "skin strains" of streptococci, largely limited to the recently discovered higher-numbered types, are more prone to produce skin infection than other strains. Most skin strains isolated from skin lesions during epidemics lack detectable M protein and capsules and fail to produce mucoid colonies. Nevertheless type specific immunity slowly develops and reinfection with the same type is probably rare.

Pyoderma includes the streptococcal form of impetigo contagiosa which is seen frequently in epidemic form among children and infants, especially in underprivileged families and particularly in warm, humid climates during the summer months. Trauma of skin, insect bites and poor hygiene are predisposing factors. Most skin infections arise from endogenous organisms inhabiting healthy skin of the patient, possibly as the result of colonization. Also, flies and other insects often contribute to transmission by serving as vectors of organisms in open lesions. Following skin acquisition the organisms may spread to the URT and scarletinal rash develops on occasion. The typical vesicular, crusted lesions of *impetigo contagiosa* due solely to the streptococcus are distinct from the *bullous lesions of impetigo caused by the staphylococcus.* However, the staphylococcus commonly superinfects the lesions produced by the streptococcus. Nephritis but not RF sometimes follows streptococcal impetigo.

Erysipelas, the second form of skin infection, usually involves the face and on rare occasions results from group C streptococci. The disease shows some tendency to spread from person to person. It is most common in infancy and middle age and for unknown reasons tends to recur at the same site in the same individual over a span of months to years. Facial erysipelas is usually strictly limited to skin of the face and is thought to result from endogenous throat-derived organisms which probably often enter through abrasions in skin about the nostrils and mouth; there is usually a preceding pharyngitis. The onset is sudden with fever and violent chills; the lesions take the form of spreading cellulitis of facial skin characterized by marked erythema and edema and by sharp advancing margins where the lymph channels are packed with organisms. Erysipelas may also develop in other parts of the body by organisms invading through natural abrasions of the skin or surgical wounds. Spontaneous recovery usually occurs after about a week or more, but without treatment there is danger of spread to the blood stream and the meninges.

7. Poststreptococcal Glomerulonephritis

"Bright's disease," a form of acute hemorrhagic glomerulonephritis, was first described by Bright in 1836 as a frequent sequela of scarlet fever. The disease is produced by relatively few types of group A streptococci and only by certain strains within a type.* Outbreaks within families and schools due to a single strain are common and can follow infection in the pharynx, the skin, or elsewhere. During epidemics the attack rate is 10 to 15% and the latent period may extend from a few days to 10 to 20 days or longer.

* A recent outbreak of nephritis alleged to have been due to a group C streptococcus has been reported.

The death rate is highest in adults and has been variously estimated at 5 to 10% or less; most patients who die succumb to acute disease within a year. *The disease commonly follows type 12 infections, which are primarily pharyngeal, and type 49 infections which occur primarily in skin.* The attack rate in different epidemics due to pharyngeal infection with organisms of a single type can vary greatly (0 to 17% with type 12); this suggests that nephritogenic strains exist. Moreover, the disease has been shown to follow either skin or pharyngeal infections with type 49 organisms. A few strains that belong to types 1, 2, 3, 4, 6, 18, 25 and the provisional types 55, 57 and 60 have also been shown to be nephritogenic. The disease is most common in children over 2 years of age but infants are also affected. Hematuria, edema, hypertension and sometimes gastrointestinal and central nervous system symptoms do not appear until about a week after the beginning of infection. Recurrent attacks are rare because of the limited number of existing nephritogenic strains and because exposed individuals often possess type specific immunity to nephritogenic strains due to prior experience with nonnephritogenic strains of the same type.

The cause of poststreptococcal nephritis is not known and there is no convincing evidence that any known streptococcal component plays a key role in its pathogenesis (Chapter 9). Many investigators believe that the condition is an "immune complex disease." The concept that the major offending Ag is M protein is difficult to accept since both nephritogenic and nonnephritogenic strains produce M protein. Others believe that it results from Abs to streptococcal Ags which cross-react with related Ags of the glomerular basement membrane; such Ags may be limited to the "nephritis prone" individual. Studies on serial renal biopsies taken in different stages of the disease have thrown considerable light on its histopathology. Morphologically *the disease resembles experimental immune complex disease* produced with foreign proteins; serum C levels are sometimes low and typical "grainy deposits" alleged to contain globulins. C3 and streptococcal membrane Ag are frequently seen on the endothelial aspect of the glomerular basement membrane and in the mesangial matrix (see *Fundamentals of Immunology*).* The initial glomerular lesions are generalized and involve endothelial and mesangial cells, but resolving lesions are focal in distribution. Although the acute disease usually undergoes spontaneous resolution, some 10 to 20% of patients, especially those with the greatest glomerular damage and depressed renal function, either die within a year or progress to a chronic form of fibroepithelial proliferative disease characterized by extensive epithelial cell proliferation and crescent formation. Whereas the chronic lesions may gradually heal in some cases they persist for years in others and carry an uncertain prognosis.

* Alternatively, deposits may occur on the epithelial aspect of the membrane.

8. Rheumatic Fever

Rheumatic fever is a serious delayed sequela unique to human infections with *Strep. pyogenes*. It continues to be an important cause of heart disease in children; the attack rate has not changed during the past 3 decades. Its pathogenesis remains one of the most challenging unsolved problems in medicine and has given rise to a multitude of hypotheses and a maze of conflicting opinion. It is acute in nature and usually terminates within weeks. *The disease occurs following infections limited largely if not exclusively to the URT* and affects only some 3% (range 0.3 to 20%) of infected individuals, a figure which appears to vary directly with the virulence of the infecting strain and the magnitude of the immune response. The onset is delayed for about 1 to 4 weeks or more after infection (which passes unnoticed in 40 to 60% of patients) and commonly includes signs and symptoms reflecting widespread involvement of the heart and joints. The cardiac lesions are the most sinister and it has been aptly said that the disease "licks the joints but bites the heart." Other symptoms may include fever, malaise, leukocytosis, chorea, epistaxis, subcutaneous nodular lesions, erythema marginatum and sometimes abdominal pain and vomiting. In decades past, aching in the extremities of children due to RF was so common that it was often mistakenly dismissed as "growing pains"! In many cases of RF medical attention is not sought and in others the disease is misdiagnosed; subsequent rheumatic heart disease may remain as the only indication of a preceding attack of RF. Permanent cardiac damage, particularly of the mitral valve, often occurs, which sets the stage for later serious infection of the damaged valves by other microbes. The subcutaneous nodules of RF tend to develop at sites subjected to frequent injury, such as areas over elbows and shins. The characteristic microscopic cardiac lesion of RF is the "Aschoff body" consisting of epithelioid and giant cells surrounded by lymphocytes, plasma cells and occasionally some neutrophils.

Since RF can follow infection with essentially all types of group A streptococci (except possibly certain "skin strains"), repeated attacks commonly occur over a period of years, each due to a streptococcus of a different type.* There is no convincing evidence that an anamnestic response with shortening of the latent period takes place upon succeeding attacks of RF. Mere carriage of organisms without an immune response to streptolysin O does not induce recurrences. The initial infection usually subsides completely and the organisms are often cleared from the throat before the onset of RF. Since streptococci cannot be cultured from the blood or the lesions, the development of RF evidently depends on events that take place subsequent to infection.

Any theory on the pathogenesis of RF must take into account certain truths, namely that the disease 1) is only observed in human beings and

---

* Whether pharyngitis due to "skin strains" can lead to RF is not known.

only follows infection with *Strep. pyogenes,* 2) follows URT infections but seldom if ever follows skin infections, 3) follows infection with strains representing most, if not all, types of *Strep. pyogenes,* 4) is usually accompanied by the development of a high ASO titer and a long-persisting antigroup A polysaccharide titer, 5) develops in a small percentage of individuals within a population (although there is probably a genetic component in susceptibility to RF; this issue remains controversial), 6) does not occur in infants, 7) does not recur in the rheumatic subject after each and every episode of streptococcal pharyngitis.

One favored theory is that RF represents an allergic response to some streptococcal antigen(s), possibly of membrane origin. Presumably its rarity in children under the age of 3 years is because they have not reached full immunocompetence and have not had time to develop hypersensitivity to streptococcal products. The long latent period of a week or more, the abundance of lymphocytes and plasma cells in the lesions, and the close resemblance between RF and known allergic diseases are compatible with the allergic theory. However, the precise events that occur, and the Ags and Abs or immune cells involved have not been identified.

Another favored theory is that the disease is due to cross-reactive Abs which are stimulated by a streptococcal Ag but react with tissue Ag. This is based on the observation that Abs which are reactive with both streptococci and human heart muscles are present in higher titer in the sera of patients who develop RF than in control subjects who do not. However, the possible role which such cross-reactive Abs may play in the development of RF lesions is unknown.

Still another favored theory is that RF lesions result from the combined toxic and allergenic activities of streptococcal "residue" which localizes at the sites where lesions later develop. This concept is given considerable support by recent work showing that killed streptococci injected into the peritoneum of animals can be carried by macrophages to distant sites in the body, where they lodge and produce lesions resembling the "allergic granulomata" of RF. Evidently the lesions result from a toxigenic-allergenic cell-wall residue, probably a rhamnosyl-mucopeptide complex which is highly resistant to phagocytic digestion by macrophages. Whether streptococcal residues may reach and persist within other cells such as fibrocytes, is not known. They have not been found in the Aschoff body.

Heart valve damage (particularly of the mitral valve) resulting directly from RF or from complicating bacterial infection of such damaged valves (usually subacute bacterial endocarditis) is often life threatening (see section on Streptococci of Other Species).

Schönlein-Henoch purpura, an anaphylactoid phenomenon, and the nodular skin lesion, *erythema nodosum,* sometimes follow streptococcal infections.

I. Mechanisms of Pathogenicity (a Recapitulation)

In common with most pathogenic bacteria, the mechanisms which enable *Strep. pyogenes* to invade and injure the host are largely obscure. Since the majority of streptococci are killed within minutes after ingestion by human phagocytes, especially neutrophils, their notable ability to resist phagocytosis by virtue of surface *M protein* and to a lesser degree the capsule is without doubt the major determinant of virulence. Moreover, virulence for man, particularly as it relates to pharyngeal infection, correlates well with M protein production. Other probable factors of virulence directly concerned with the persistence and sometimes the growth of engulfed organisms are leukotoxin which often kills the phagocyte and the cell-wall mucopeptide complex which resists digestion.

Streptococci which infect skin wounds are often nonencapsulated and of low virulence, whereas those which produce pharyngitis are usually encapsulated and of high virulence. The reason for this paradox is not known. Presumably factors other than capsules and M protein are the dominant factors determining virulence of skin strains. The reasons for the marked tendency of streptococci to spread within tissues and to produce injury are not known but could rest, in part at least, on the independent or cooperative activities of one or more of the following substances: DNase, hyaluronidase and the leukotoxic and tissue-toxic components, streptolysin S, streptolysin O, NADase, M protein and the cell-wall mucopeptide complex.

The pathogenesis of sequelae, which is considered in detail in Section H, is obviously different in RF and glomerulonephritis since the 2 diseases rarely occur simultaneously in the same patient. Although their pathogenesis is not understood, it may well rest on a combination of toxic and immunologic effects involving more than one streptococcal component.

J. Mechanisms of Immunity (a Recapitulation)

Immunity to *Strep. pyogenes* is similar to immunity to *D. pneumoniae,* i.e., it depends primarily on the acquisition of type specific opsonins. Whereas innate immunity, through the agency of surface phagocytosis, may often serve to prevent invasion by streptococci of lesser virulence, it is ineffective against large numbers of highly virulent organisms. In contrast acquired immunity is usually fully protective and repeated attacks with organisms of the same type seldom occur unless the initial infection is arrested by chemotherapy. Whether there is any significant degree of cross immunity between types is uncertain. Once induced, anti-M Abs persist for essentially a lifetime, probably as the result of frequent carrier contact; in the face of infection they are undoubtedly rapidly reinforced by the anamnestic response. Evidently acquired immunity is gained in a cumulative manner upon succeeding encounters with streptococci of new types, be they carried organisms or infecting organisms.

Macrophages from infected rabbits have been shown to carry cytophilic Abs specific for C polysaccharide. However, nothing is known about the possible role of macrophages and delayed sensitivity in either immunity or lesion development in human streptococcal disease.

K. Laboratory Diagnosis

Streptococcal pharyngitis is diagnosed on the basis of both clinical and laboratory findings. Other infections (including diphtheria, infectious mononucleosis and particularly infections due to adenovirus) can simulate streptococcal pharyngitis and make its diagnosis difficult. Virus pharyngitis of short duration is frequent, consequently penicillin treatment of misdiagnosed viral pharyngitis is sometimes mistakenly assumed to represent arrest of a streptococcal infection. Since *Strep. pyogenes* is frequently carried in the URT, a negative culture test is even more meaningful than a positive culture and serves to exclude streptococcal pharyngitis in more than half of the suspected cases. Moreover, since 5 to 10% of the population are nasopharyngeal carriers of *Strep. pyogenes, a positive culture only establishes the possibility that the infection is due to Strep. pyogenes.*

The specimen should be collected with a swab passed over the tonsils and pharynx, including exudate if present, and taking care not to touch the tongue, lips or uvula. Anterior nasal cultures are sometimes needed. Because many strains of *Strep. pyogenes* require CO_2 for initial isolation, prompt culture in an atmosphere of 90% air and 10% CO_2 is advised using blood agar (preferably sheep blood) and a combined pour-streak plate method to permit colony counting and to avoid overlooking beta-hemolytic colonies. Incubation is carried out for 18 to 24 hr. at 35°C and the plates are examined for relative numbers of beta-hemolytic streptococci. The catalase test and culture on low concentrations of bacitracin are used to rule out staphylococci (which are catalase positive) and, presumptively, streptococci of other groups, which unlike most group A streptococci are rarely inhibited by low concentrations of bacitracin.*

Since beta-hemolytic streptococci of various groups may be carried in the throat, final group identification with specific antisera is important. This is most effectively accomplished with a direct slide test using specific fluorescein-tagged Ab applied to cultured organisms from broth inoculated 2 to 5 hours previously with swabbed material. The identification of *Strep. pyogenes* in material from skin infections is complicated by the fact that these are often "mixed infections."

Diagnosis of the sequelae, acute glomerulonephritis and RF, rests largely on clinical grounds and, since living organisms are not directly involved,

---

* An occasional group A strain may be nonhemolytic or alpha-hemolytic and bacitracin-resistant.

throat cultures can only detect carriage. Very few patients with sequelae have seen a physician for treatment of a prior sore throat. Titrations of various Abs are of value as indicators of antecedent streptococcal infection which may have escaped clinical notice, and for assessing the immune response. Antistreptolysin O (ASO) titration serves to rule in or deny the possibility of an URT streptococcal infection and has been particularly useful in the diagnosis of RF. Titers above 250 to 300, *especially if they are rising,* are highly suggestive of a recent pharyngeal infection with *Strep. pyogenes.* Titers of ASO do not rise as the result of carriage. Skin infections seldom engender marked rises in ASO and anti-NADase titers but instead stimulate high titers of anti-DNase B and anti-hyaluronidase Abs. Because nonspecific host responses, such as increased sedimentation rate and C-reactive protein, occur in RF, their absence is useful for eliminating the disease as a diagnostic possibility.

L.   Therapy

The objectives of therapy are to cure the infection, avoid complications and sequelae and prevent transmission of infection to others by preventing carriage. Penicillin is the drug of choice but erythromycin can be used if the patient is allergic to penicillin. Since drug resistance develops to the tetracyclines and sulfonamides they should not be used. In some instances additional measures, such as treatment with cephalosporanic acid derivatives and surgical drainage, may be necessary to halt infection. Whereas penicillin given at the onset of pharyngitis or within a few days thereafter reduces the chances of developing RF, the prevention of acute glomerulonephritis demands treatment at the onset of infection. Treatment should be continued for about 2 weeks.

M.   Reservoirs of Infection

Human carriers and infected subjects are the principal sources of infection. Except for the cow, animals are not important reservoirs of *Strep. pyogenes.* Numerous milk-borne epidemics occurred before wide-scale pasteurization of milk was adopted. Usually the milk was contaminated by infected milk handlers but in some instances the teats and udders of the cows became infected from milkers and then served as massive reservoirs of milk contamination. Consumption of food in which group A streptococci have grown can occasionally lead to massive outbreaks of streptococcal pharyngitis.

N.   Control of Disease Transmission
and Prevention of Sequelae

Transmission of infection is favored by close contact and crowded living conditions, by nasal rather than pharyngeal carriers, and by moist droplets rather than dust particles. Chronic asymptomatic anal carriers are also a reservoir of infection. Prevention of disease transmission involves carrier control and the usual hygienic precautions taken with patients with infectious diseases, particularly within hospitals with their highly susceptible patient populations.

The overall carrier rate for *Strep. pyogenes* is usually under 5% in summer; in winter it is about 10% but on occasion may reach 50% or higher, especially during epidemics of URT infection or streptococcal disease. Carriage is frequent after 1 year of age and decreases during late childhood and puberty to reach an average rate of less than 5% in adults. Convalescent carriage, which varies directly with virulence, usually lasts for only a few weeks, during which time the original infecting organisms are eliminated leaving relatively avirulent M protein-deficient, nontypeable organisms as the last survivors. Evidently this change results from the selective effect of the developing immune state on the carried organisms. Penicillin is effective for clearing carriers and its mass use can quickly reduce the carrier rate and halt an epidemic.

Among the most important and irrevocable outcomes of streptococcal infection are the sequelae. Consequently, principal control efforts center on prevention and early arrest of infection.

In the case of known rheumatic subjects, continuing long-term prophylactic treatment with penicillin has been used successfully for preventing repeated attacks of RF. Benzathine penicillin given monthly by the intramuscular route is preferred. In the absence of cardiac involvement treatment should be continued through the college period, but if cardiac symptoms develop treatment should be continued for life.

In the case of non-rheumatic subjects the question as to how far the therapeutic and prophylactic use of penicillin should be carried is a matter of great concern and debate. Even though penicillin given early in streptococcal pharyngitis dampens the specific immune response and leaves the patient susceptible to reinfection with organisms of the same type, most physicians elect to treat all such patients rather than run the risk of complications and sequelae. However, in the case of carriage, which induces immunity without the threat of infection, it is probably best to withhold treatment unless the carrier poses a special danger to others. In the case of the RF subject for whom long continued penicillin treatment is advocated, it should be recognized that such treatment blocks the natural acquisition of overall streptococcal immunity engendered by the organisms of carriage as well as by those of infection. In theory this circumstance reinforces the concept that the RF subject, especially if he has heart involvement, should be treated prophylactically throughout his lifetime.

Assuming that M protein is not directly involved in the pathogenesis of sequelae a logical future approach to prophylaxis in special risk groups would be to immunize them while under the shelter of penicillin prophylaxis using a pool of M proteins representing types of streptococci which are the most common and important known causes of streptococcal disease in the population. Promising trials on immunization with *highly purified M protein* preparations free of other streptococcal Ags are currently under way.

Streptococci of Other Species

Streptococci belonging to other serologic groups pathogenic for man, e.g. those of groups B, C, D, G, and O, are frequently carried by man; however, infections are relatively rare and are usually mild. For example, only about 1.5% of illnesses due to streptococcal infection in children are due to streptococci of groups other than group A. On rare occasion isolates of pathogenic streptococci have been reported which do not belong to any of the known Lancefield groups. Group B organisms which frequent the vaginal tract often cause infections of mothers and offspring during the perinatal period.

Streptococci of groups D and O are especially worthy of attention because they are the most common causative agents of subacute bacterial endocarditis (SBE). The organisms attack heart valves which are defective or have been damaged in various ways; since RF is the most common cause of valve damage, SBE occurs most frequently on valves injured by this disease. The organisms, which are common members of the normal flora, reach the valves from endogenous sources, such as the mouth and gut, via the blood stream to which they continuously gain entrance in small numbers; 3 common representative species are *Strep. salivarius, Strep. mitis* and *Strep. faecalis* (enterococcus). If untreated, SBE is almost always fatal and irreversible damage often occurs before treatment is instituted. Bacteriologic diagnosis and antibiotic resistance testing are very important. Repeated blood cultures are often necessary for diagnosis and therapeutic management. Since the organisms are highly resistant to antibiotics, therapeutic success, which can be achieved in about 90% of cases, demands prolonged and rigorous treatment with suitable antibiotics or combinations of antibiotics. Penicillin and streptomycin are the combination of choice for treating SBE caused by the enteric streptococci.

Enterococci of Group D (*Strep. faecalis*) are a frequent cause of urinary tract infections. Their ability to grow in 6.5% NaCl broth is an aid in distinguishing them from other streptococci.

Anaerobic streptococci are also worthy of special mention because of their frequent participation in mixed infections, especially wound infections, and their high resistance to penicillin.

References

Bland, E. F.: Declining severity of rheumatic fever. New Eng. J. Med. *262*:597, 1960.

6

Ellen, R. P., and Gibbons, R. J.: M protein-associated adherence of *Streptococcus pyogenes* to epithelial surfaces: prerequisite for virulence. Infec. and Immun. *5*:826, 1972.

Fox, E. N., Pachman, L. M., Wittner, M. K., and Dorfman, A.: Primary immunization of infants and children with group A streptococcal M protein. J. Infec-Dis. *120*:598, 1969.

Ferrieri, P., Dajani, A. S., Wannamaker, L. W., and Chapman, S. S.: Natural history of impetigo. I. Site sequence of acquisition and familial patterns of spread of cutaneous streptococci. J. Clin. Invest. *51*:2851, 1972; *ibid*. Etiologic agents and bacterial interactions. 2863, 1972.

Ginsburg, I.: Mechanisms of cell and tissue injury induced by group A streptococci: relation to poststreptococcal sequelae. J. Infect. Dis. *126*:294, 419, 1972.

Glick, A. D., Getnick, R. A., and Cole, R. M.: Electron microscopy of group A streptococci after phagocytosis by human monocytes. Infect. Immun. *4*:772, 1971.

Glick, A. D., Ranhand, J. M., and Cole, R. M.: Degradation of group A streptococcal cell walls by eggwhite lysozyme and human lysosomal enzymes. Infect. Immun. *6*:403, 1972.

Harvey, H. S., and Dunlap, M. B.: Clinical dilemmas in the use of penicillin in streptococcal illness. Amer. J. Dis. Child. *114*:244, 1967.

Holmes, O. W.: *Medical Essays*. Boston, Mass.: Houghton Mifflin Co., 1883.

Kaplan, M. H.: Multiple nature of the cross-reactive relationship between antigens of group A streptococci and mammalian tissue: cross-reacting antigens and neoantigens conference, Wash., D.C., pp. 48-60, Wms. and Wilkins, May 14-15, 1967.

Kuttner, A. G., and Lancefield, R. C.: Unsolved problems of the nonsuppurative complications of group A streptococcal infections. *Infectious Agents and Host Reactions*. ed. Stuart Mudd. Philadelphia: W. B. Saunders Co., 1970.

Lewey, J. E., Salinas-Madrigal, L., Herdson, P. B., Pirani, C. L., and Metcoff, J.: Clinico-pathologic correlations in acute poststreptococcal glomerulonephritis. Medicine *50*:453, 1971.

Ofek, I., Bergner-Rabinowitz, S., and Ginsburg, I.: Oxygen-stable hemolysins of group hemolysis of group A streptococci. VII. The relation of the leukotoxic factor to streptolysin S. J. Infec. Dis. *122*:517, 1970.

Quinn, R. W.: Dick test results 1969-1971. J. Infect. Dis. *126*:136, 1972.

Slaughter, F. G.: Semmelweis the conqueror of childbed fever. New York: Collier, 1950.

Stollerman, G. H.: Streptococcal diseases. *Cecil-Loeb, Textbook of Medicine,* ed. Beeson, P. B. and McDermott, W., 13th ed. Philadelphia: W. B. Saunders Co., 1971.

Stollerman, G. H., Rytel, M., and Ontiz, J.: Accessory plasma cofactor(s) enhanceing opsonization of encapsulated organisms· J. Exp. Med. *117*:1, 1963.

Vosti, K. L., Lindberg, L. H., Kosek, J. C., and Raffel, S.: Experimental streptococcal glomerulonephritis. J. Infect. Dis. *122*:249, 1970.

Wannamaker, L. W.: Differences between streptococcal infections of the throat and of the skin. New Eng. J. Med. *282*:78, 1970.

Wannamaker, L. W., and Matsen, J. M.: *Streptococci and Streptococcal Diseases.* New York, Academic Press, 1972.

Watson, D. W., and Kim, Y. B.: Erythrogenic toxin. T. C. Montie, S. Kadis and S. J. Ajl, ed., *Microbial Toxins* III, New York: Academic Press, 173 1970.

Williams, R. C., and Gibbons, R. J.: Inhibition of bacterial adherence by secretory immunoglobulin A: a mechanism of antigen disposal. Science *177*:697, 1972.

Weiser, R. S., Myrvik, Q. N., and Pearsall, N. N. *Fundamentals of Immunology*. Philadelphia: Lea & Febiger, 1969.

Zabriskie, J. B.: Streptococcal bacteriophages. J. Infect. Dis. *121*:451, 1970.

Zabriskie, J. B.: The role of streptococci in human glomerulonephritis. J. Exp. Med. *134*:180, 1971.

Chapter 12

Staphylococcus

Most normal human beings carry large numbers of staphylococci and related organisms, both in the nose and on the skin. The relatively nonpathogenic, opportunistic *Staphylococcus epidermidis* is almost always found among the normal flora of the skin and mucous membranes of the respiratory and alimentary tracts, whereas the pathogen *Staphylococcus aureus* is a transient, temporary member of the microbial flora. These gram-positive cocci, members of the family *Micrococcaceae,* were given their genus name *Staphylococcus* because they tend to occur in grape-like clusters (Greek *staphule* = cluster of grapes).

Other members of the same family that are also commonly among the normal flora include species of the genus *Micrococcus,* which are similar to staphylococci in a stained smear, and of the genus *Gaffkya,* which characteristically occur in tetrads as well as irregular masses. All members of these two genera are opportunists and will not be considered further here.

Even though *Staph. aureus* is often carried by healthy individuals, under certain circumstances it causes severe infections and can kill its host. Because of its frequent presence on body surfaces, it is in a position to invade whenever defenses are even slightly impaired. Consequently, it is the most common cause of both traumatic and surgical wound infections, and of superficial skin infections. A frequent and characteristic staphylococcal lesion is the boil or furuncle in the skin. However, the organisms may invade and infect virtually any tissue, causing such diverse diseases as osteomyelitis, bacteremia, pneumonia, and enterocolitis. *Staph. aureus* characteristically causes the formation of large quantities of pus, and is foremost among the pyogenic bacteria.

A. Medical Perspectives

Staphylococci have been recognized as a cause of pyogenic infections since the earliest days of microbiology. During the 1870's, Koch, Pasteur, and other pioneer microbiologists described these gram-positive cocci in pus. However, physicians of that era did not consider that they themselves carried these and other pathogens and shed them into their patients' wounds, causing severe and often fatal postsurgical and postpartum infections. Everyone was, however, well aware of the extremely high postsurgical mortality rate due to infection. In fact, at the University of Aberdeen a large sign in the operating room warned patients: "PREPARE TO MEET THY GOD." Alexander Ogston, a young surgeon at Aberdeen, accepted this state of affairs without question until he visited Edinburgh and was persuaded by Lister that wound infections could be prevented, an amazing and almost heretical concept in those days when pus formation was considered to be an essential stage in wound healing. Ogston was so impressed by Lister's teachings that upon returning to Aberdeen, he tore down and burned the sign, instituted successful aseptic techniques in surgery, and went on to make notable contributions to the study of the staphylococcal etiology of wound infections.

Although the use of aseptic techniques greatly reduced the incidence of iatrogenic (physician-induced) infections, staphylococcal infections continued to occur with high frequency, and many of them were fatal in the preantibiotic era. In the 1940's when penicillin first became available, hopes were high that the end of staphylococcal infections was finally in sight. At that time, most staphylococci were susceptible to penicillin, and it was supposed that this kind of infection would soon be totally under control.

Unfortunately, it was not long before penicillin-resistant strains of staphylococci emerged, at first in the hospital environment, and later throughout the community. It soon became apparent that staphylococci had a greater ability to develop resistance to antibiotics than virtually any other pathogen. New antimicrobial agents that are effective against staphylococci are constantly being discovered; however, there is the ever-present threat that resistant strains of the organism will be selected more rapidly than new agents can be developed. Consequently, efforts are being made to achieve a better understanding of these organisms, the pathogenesis of the diseases they produce, and the mechanisms of immunity to them. Nevertheless, it seems likely that staphylococcal infections will continue to be a major medical problem for the foreseeable future.

B. Physical and Chemical Structure

The staphylococci are facultatively anaerobic, gram-positive spheres about 0.8 to 1.0 μm in diameter. In pus, they occur in irregular clusters, pairs or singly, and occasionally in tetrads or in short chains seldom more than 4 cocci in length. The characteristic grouping in grape-like clusters is most marked among organisms grown on agar media, and results from random division in multiple planes, with failure to separate after each division. In common with most gram-positive bacteria, aged or phagocytized organisms tend to become gram-negative. An antiphagocytic polysaccharide capsule is present in some strains.

The cell wall consists of an outer protein-containing layer and the inner characteristic bacterial mucopeptide layer. Although the antigenic structure of *Staph. aureus* is complex, Ags are of little value for identifying the organisms. However, it is probable that some of the external Ags are important in pathogenesis.

The outer layer of the cell wall contains a substance called protein A. This substance resembles streptococcal M protein in that it is present at the cell surface even on encapsulated cells. It has been clearly demonstrated that protein A is antiphagocytic. It has the unique ability to interact with the Fc region of IgG, thereby interfering with opsonization involving cytophilic Abs.

Specific phage receptor sites are present on the surface of *Staph. aureus* cells. Susceptibility patterns, which involve more than 20 phages, are of great value in typing strains for epidemiological studies. Of the 4 main groups identifiable by phage typing, strains of groups I and III are most often responsible for hospital infections with antibiotic-resistant staphylococci.

C. Genetics

Detectable mutations include gain or loss of ability to form pigment or extracellular products, changes in colony form, and changes in phage susceptibility. However, in terms of human disease, the most important genetic changes are those leading to drug resistance.

D. Extracellular Products

Pathogenic staphylococci produce a variety of important extracellular substances, certain of which are described in Table 12-1. Some of the exotoxins are produced most readily in an atmosphere containing a high concentration (30%) of CO_2.

TABLE 12-1

Some Important Extracellular Products of *Staphylococcus aureus**

Product	Activity	Other Properties
Coagulase	Enzyme that clots blood plasma.	
Staphylokinase	Enzyme that degrades fibrin clots.	
Hemolysins (toxins)	All are hemolytic.	
α	Narrow hemolytic spectrum (limited to RBC of few animal species).	Disrupts many different mammalian cells. Dermonecrotizing. Lethal.
β	Phospholipase (Sphingomyelinase C). Narrow hemolytic spectrum.	Lethal.
γ	—	Cytotoxic for other mammalian cells.
δ	Broad hemolytic spectrum.	Disrupts many different mammalian cells.
Leukocidin	Kills leukocytes.	Two interacting proteins; heat-labile.
Enterotoxin	Emetic.	Heat-stable (100°C, 30 min).
Exfoliatin	Exfoliation of infant skin.	Produced only by organisms of phage group II.
Hyaluronidase	Enzyme that degrades hyaluronic acid.	Also called spreading factor.
Lipases	Enzymes that degrade lipids.	
Proteinases	Enzymes that degrade proteins.	
Penicillinase	Enzyme that splits the β-lactam ring of penicillin.	

*All of the products listed are proteins.

E. Culture

Simple media support the growth of staphylococci over a wide range of temperature (15 to 40°C) and pH (4.8 to 9.4). Although *Staph. aureus* is a facultative anaerobe, aerobic culture on blood agar is usually employed for identification. The large, smooth, frequently beta-hemolytic colonies may be golden yellow due to the production of carotenoid pigments; however, pigment formation is variable, being greater at room temperature than at 37°C and greater in aerobic than anaerobic environments. *Staph. epidermidis,* which lacks pigment, forms smooth, white, colonies which are usually non-hemolytic. Because staphylococci synthesize catalase, the hydrogen peroxide they produce under aerobic conditions does not accumulate to become toxic, as in the case of catalase-negative organisms, such as streptococci and pneumococci.

F.   Resistance to Physical and Chemical Agents

Staphylococci are among the most resistant of the nonsporing bacteria and can survive many adverse environmental conditions enroute from host to host. They are highly resistant to light, extremes of temperature, and drying; hence infection can be transmitted by organisms in dust. They survive in dried pus and sputum for days to weeks and can withstand moist heat as high as 60°C for 30 min. Staphylococci are markedly resistant to phenols and many other disinfectants.

The resistance of many strains of *Staph. aureus* to penicillin usually results from their ability to produce penicillinase. This property is commonly transmitted by transduction and involves plasmids (Chaper 4). Other staphylococcal plasmids have been described which carry genes for resistance to various antibiotics.

G.   Experimental Models

Rabbits and mice are most often used for experimental studies of staphylococci; guinea pigs are used less frequently. The cocci are relatively nonpathogenic for laboratory animals under natural conditions, but may be lethal when injected intravenously or intraperitoneally.

Kittens and monkeys are susceptible to the effects of staphylococcal enterotoxins and have been used for their study.

H.   Infections and Disease in Man

Infections with *Staph. aureus* are characterized by localization, suppuration, and tissue necrosis with resultant scarring. The most frequent lesion, the *furuncle,* often serves as a source for hematogenous spread of organisms, resulting in bacteremia, and diseases such as osteomyelitis and pneumonia.

The intermittent carrier rate is estimated to be about 30 to 50%. The fact that individuals can carry and shed pathogenic *Staph. aureus* over prolonged periods indicates that they and most of their contacts have a substantial degree of immunity. It is only when normal defenses are lacking or are compromised that *Staph. aureus* is likely to invade. Thus infection most often occurs at a site of local injury, such as a burn, abrasion, or other wound. Abnormalities which result in systemic immunodepression and predispose to staphylococcal infection include diabetes, leukemia, renal failure, immunosuppressive therapy, and immunodeficiency diseases involving defects in humoral Ab responses. For unknown reasons, a few ostensibly healthy individuals experience repeated episodes of furunculosis over a period of years.

The colonization of staphylococci on integuments is normally restricted by the antibiosis exerted by members of the normal flora. However, following intensive treatment with broad-spectrum antibiotics, many members of the normal flora of the intestine are decreased in number and their antagonism may be lost, allowing extensive colonization of *Staph. aureus*. A dangerous and often fatal pseudomembranous enterocolitis can result, and there is evidence that enterotoxin-producing strains are often responsible.

Acute osteomyelitis caused by *Staph. aureus* is most common in young boys. In this disease, organisms which become blood-borne, usually from a skin lesion localize in bones, preferentially in the metaphysis of growing bones. Local trauma or strain on bone is predisposing.

Staphylococcus aureus is currently a common cause of bacterial endocarditis, and *Staph. epidermidis* is occasionally implicated. Cardiac surgery patients and drug addicts who use contaminated needles are among those at risk of such infections.

Staphylococcal food poisoning is not an infection, but instead an intoxication resulting from ingestion of contaminated food containing preformed toxin. The source of contamination is usually a food handler who is a carrier. The organisms grow rapidly, even at room temperature, and dangerous concentrations of enterotoxin can accumulate in foods within a few hours. Since the toxin is very heat-resistant, heating does not render enterotoxin-containing food safe for consumption. Following ingestion, symptoms of nausea, vomiting and diarrhea become apparent within 1 to 6 hours. The illness is self-limiting and complete recovery usually occurs within a day or two.

I. Mechanisms of Pathogenicity

Many of the toxins and other substances produced by Staph. aureus *(Table 12-1) probably contribute to its pathogenicity.* The precise contributions of these substances to pathogenesis are not known but must certainly vary from one infection to another.

As stated earlier, both the capsule possessed by some strains and protein A are distinctly antiphagocytic. In addition, most strains produce a leukocidin, which apparently acts on the cytoplasmic membranes of many cell types (including human neutrophils and macrophages) to cause cell lysis.

The alpha-toxin (alpha hemolysin) of virulent staphylococci is highly toxic for human macrophages (but not neutrophils), epithelial cells, and many other types of cells. Alpha-toxin is sometimes called necrotizing toxin, because of its marked capacity to produce necrosis when injected into the skin of a rabbit. It is lethal for mice and rabbits when given intravenously.

This or possibly other staphylococcal toxins are lethal for man, as indicated by the Bundaberg disaster of 1928 in which a diphtheria toxin-antitoxin preparation contaminated with staphylococci caused a rapidly fatal toxic reaction in 12 of 21 inoculated children.

Although some of the toxins of staphylococci certainly contribute to the establishment of infection and the disease process, the use of antitoxin or killed vaccines has not been generally effective for protecting against infection, presumably because the organism possesses other important virulence factors not represented in the vaccines.

There is strong support for the concept that hypersensitivity reactions, especially of the delayed type, contribute to local tissue damage in staphylococcal infections. For example, repeated infections induced in the skin of rabbits produce local lesions of increasing severity. This state of increased susceptibility can be passively transferred with lymphoid cells but not with serum, the hallmark of delayed-type hypersensitivity states. Immunoglobulins of the class IgG can combine with protein A and C to form a complex on the bacterial surface. This complex, which is chemotactic and lethal for neutrophils, may also contribute to tissue damage.

Most pathogenic strains of *Staph. aureus* produce coagulase. However, since coagulase-negative mutants appear to be fully as virulent as coagulase-positive strains, coagulase either is not an attribute of pathogenicity or is not an essential one.

A variety of other staphylococcal enzymes function to allow survival of the organisms on integuments and invasion of tissue. For example, lipase and esterase produced by staphylococci permit the organisms to survive the antibacterial action of lipids on the skin.

Enterotoxin, which is formed by about a third of the strains of *Staph. aureus,* is the major factor in the pathogenesis of staphylococcal food poisoning. It is a heat-stable trypsin-resistant protein exotoxin. Although the manner by which the ingested toxin acts is not known, it appears to stimulate centers in the CNS, thereby inducing vomiting. Three antigenic types of enterotoxin have been described and 90% of toxin-producing

TABLE 12-2

Lytic Groups of Staphylococcus Typing Phages Included in the Internationally Agreed Set of Typing Phages

Lytic Group				*Phages*					
I	29	52	52A	79	80				
II	3A	3B	3C	55	71				
III	6	7	42E	47	53	54	75	77	83A
IV	42D								
Not allotted			81	187					

strains belong to the bacteriophage pattern lytic group III (Table 12-2). The production of one type of enterotoxin (type A) has been shown to be induced by a temperate phage, and it is probable that this is the case for all types of staphylococcal enterotoxin.

Recently, it has been shown that some *Staph. aureus* of phage group II produce a toxin responsible for exfoliation of infant skin. The activity of this exotoxin causes the so-called "scalded-skin syndrome" in which the skin peels off in large sheets. The toxin in appropriately named *exfoliatin*.

J. Mechanisms of Immunity

It is apparent that the forces of innate immunity which contribute to protection against *Staph. aureus* are amplified by acquired immunity. Humoral Abs are important in protection, as evidenced by the fact that patients with immunoglobulin deficiencies are especially prone to develop staphylococcal infections. Opsonization probably makes a major contribution to humoral immunity by promoting phagocytosis especially by the neutrophil, a phagocyte essential to antistaphylococcal immunity.

Inability to correlate the titer of humoral Abs, as measured by any particular test, with the degree of existing immunity could result from the heterogeneity of Abs formed against staphylococcal Ags. For example, Abs specific for various surface Ags and toxins (such as leukocidin and alpha-toxin) probably contribute to protection. Titers of any one of these Abs may reflect only a fraction of total immunity.

The abscess, with its barrier of fibrin, phagocytes, and granulation tissue around the area of suppuration, is important in localizing infection. The dangers involved in breaking the barrier around a staphylococcal infection are readily apparent as evidenced by the observation that systemic infections are often preceded by the "squeezing" of a pimple or abscess. Although delayed hypersensitivity reactions may contribute to local tissue injury, they are probably beneficial from an overall standpoint in that they tend to localize the infection and thus discourage life-threatening systemic spread of organisms. This does not exclude the possibility that an exaggerated delayed sensitivity reaction could interfere with immunity.

K. Laboratory Diagnosis

The presence of typical single or clustered gram-positive cocci in pus from lesions, or in blood or other body fluids, is suggestive of staphylococcal infection. Identification of *Staph. aureus* is made by cultural characteristics and demonstration of coagulase production. Blood agar prepared with rabbit blood is recommended for culture because it is a rich medium which best demonstrates the hemolytic properties of the organism. *Coagulase production* and the *ability to ferment mannitol* distinguish most pathogenic strains of staphylococci from nonpathogenic strains. *Catalase production,* a trait of all staphylococci, is a useful characteristic to distinguish staphylococci from the catalase-negative streptococci which may be similar morphologically on stained smears. Selective media containing a high concentration of NaCl (5% to 7.5%) are often used to isolate the *salt-resistant* staphylococci from mixtures of organisms.

Neither antigenic analysis nor phage typing is useful for routine diagnosis. Antibodies to the teichoic acid of *Staph. aureus,* which are present in low titer in most normal adults but increase during long-term infections with the organism, are occasionally used for determining the cause of infections, such as endocarditis.

Staphylococcal food poisoning is commonly diagnosed on the basis of clinical evidence alone. Usually the food involved is heavily contaminated with typical gram-positive cocci which can be seen in direct smears. Cultures yielding large numbers of *Staph. aureus* are confirmatory. Feeding tests on kittens have not proved to be practical for diagnosis.

L. Therapy

Penicillin G is recommended for the treatment of penicillin-susceptible staphylococcal infections; unfortunately most strains produce penicillinase and are therefore resistant to penicillins G and V and to ampicillin. Most of these strains are susceptible to methicillin, cloxacillin, and cephalothin. Obviously, *antibiotic sensitivity testing is essential, since staphylococci may be resistant not only to penicillin but to a variety of other therapeutic agents.*

Prior to the development of antibacterial chemotherapeutic agents, the only effective treatments for staphylococcal infections were surgical drainage of suppurative lesions and correction of underlying predisposing causes. Today, *drainage of lesions* is even more important than formerly because chemotherapeutic agents do not diffuse readily into areas of suppuration nor do they act effectively in such areas. In the case of drugs such as penicillin, which are only effective against growing organisms, therapeutic failure probably rests in part on the fact that many organisms in purulent exudates are not growing. Also, the activity of certain chemotherapeutic agents is destroyed by the products of tissue necrosis.

Even though serotherapy and vaccine treatments have been widely used in the past, they are not of proven value.

M. Reservoirs of Infection

Although certain domestic animals such as cattle and horses may carry and may become infected with *Staph. aureus,* the human carrier (especially the nasal carrier) is essentially the only source of infections in man. The carrier state is usually established in the newborn infant within the first few days of life and becomes intermittent with age.

The factors which determine the carrier state are not known. However, infants which possess maternal IgG Abs but lack or possess only small quantities of Abs of other immunoglobulin classes have a higher carrier rate than adults. This suggests that Abs of classes other than IgG, or the forces of cellular immunity, or both, contribute to immunity in adults. The most dangerous carriers are food handlers and those in frequent contact with susceptible individuals (such as medical attendants in contact with patients). In the hospital environment the most dangerous carriers (because of their frequent contact with patients) are found among the hospital personnel themselves, especially individuals employed in operating rooms, surgical wards and nurseries.

N. Control of Disease Transmission

Control of transmission of staphylococcal disease is currently centered about hospitals and clinics where susceptible individuals are concentrated. Successful control demands great vigilance by the entire personnel of the institution, under the guidance of experts. The measures used include rigorous hygiene, detection of carriers, control of contacts, control of airborne and fomite spread, and tracing sources of infection by means of phage-typing and antibiotic-resistance patterns (Table 12-3). Among the strains of *Staph. aureus* responsible for hospital epidemics, phage type 80/81 has been a frequent offender.

In general, antibiotic treatment of carriers is of limited value. However, it is of use for certain medical personnel who are known to shed virulent organisms and who must remain in contact with patients.

TABLE 12-3

Use of Antibiogram and Bacteriophage Type in Distinguishing Epidemic Strains of Staphylococci[a]

		Staphylococcus	
Patient	*Antibiogram*[b]	*Bacteriophage* *Type*	
1	RRSRR	80/81	
2	RRSRR	80/81	
3	RRSRR	80/81	
4	RRSRR	80/81	
5	RRSRR	54/83	
6	RRSRR	54/83	
7	RSSSR	80/81	
8	RSSSS	80/81	

[a]It is apparent that the first 4 strains have the same characteristics and probably were from the same source.
[b]R-resistant, S-sensitive to the antibiotics penicillin, tetracycline, chloramphenicol, erythromycin, and streptomycin respectively.

Surgical patients, especially those who have received intensive antibiotic therapy, and newborns in hospital nurseries are at particular risk of infection with virulent staphylococci. Currently, a promising procedure for protecting such individuals is being evaluated. It involves inoculating the patient's mucous membranes with the competitive nonvirulent strain 502A, with the objective of establishing the nonvirulent organisms and thereby precluding colonization by virulent staphylococci.

Antiseptic solutions, especially those containing hexachlorophene, are of value in decreasing the numbers of staphylococci carried on the skin. At present there is question as to the safety of continued exposure to hexachlorophene because of its toxicity, but there is no doubt as to its efficacy in decreasing the incidence of staphylococcal infections in the hospital environment.

Control of staphylococcal food poisoning depends principally on proper food handling. Prompt refrigeration of food is essential to prevent growth of staphylococci and consequent production of enterotoxin. Efforts are made to detect carriers among food handlers and to remove them from situations where they could contaminate food. However, adequate refrigeration of food is the most effective control measure and is usually sufficient to prevent outbreaks of the disease. It should be emphasized that large containers of food cannot be cooled adequately because of the time required to decrease the temperature throughout the food mass. Staphylococci can grow and secrete toxin as the food cools; therefore, large quantities of foods that support staphylococcal growth should be prepared immediately before use.

References

Crowder, J. G. and A. White. Teichoic acid antibodies in staphylococcal and non-staphylococcal endocarditis. Ann. Intern. Med. 77:87 (1972).

Elek, S. D. *"Staphylococcus pyogenes* and its Relation to Disease." Livingstone, Edinburgh (1959).

Kapral, F. A. and M. M. Miller. Product of *Staphylococcus aureus* responsible for the scalded-skin syndrome. Infect. Immun. 4:541 (1971).

Melish, M. E., L. A. Glasgow, and M. D. Turner. The staphylococcal scalded-skin syndrome: Isolation and partial characterization of the exfoliative toxin. J. Inf. Dis. 125:129. (1972).

Montie, T. C., S. Kadis and S. J. Ajl (eds.). "Microbial Toxins" Vol. III, Chapters 5-8, Academic Press, New York (1970).

Mudd, S. "Infectious Agents and Host Reactions" Chapter 9, W. B. Saunders Co., Philadelphia (1970).

Surgalla, M. J. and G. M. Dack. Enterotoxin produced by micrococci from cases of enteritis after antibiotic therapy. J. Amer. Med. Assoc. 158:649 (1955).

Wadstrom, T. and R. Mollby. Some biological properties of purified staphylococcal haemolysins. Toxicon 10:511 (1971).

Wentworth, B. B. Bacteriophage typing of staphylococci. Bact. Rev. 27:253 (1963).

Chapter 13

Neisseria

Neisseria meningitidis, 165

Neisseria gonorrhoeae, 175

The genus *Neisseria* comprises a number of nonpathogenic and pathogenic species which parasitize animals and man. Several nonpathogenic species are among the normal flora of the upper respiratory tract (URT) of man including *N. catarrhalis, N. sicca* and *N. subflava.*

Only two species of the genus *Neisseria* are important pathogens of man, *N. meningitidis,* the cause of epidemic cerebrospinal meningitis, and *N. gonorrhoeae,* the cause of gonorrhea. Man is their only natural host.

On rare occasions certain nonpathogenic neisseriae, especially *N. catarrhalis* and *N. subflava,* produce opportunistic infections, including meningitis.

Neisseria meningitidis

A. Medical Perspectives

Few microbes produce a higher mortality than *N. meningitidis* and none kills more quickly; death often occurs within a few hours after the first symptoms appear.

Cerebrospinal meningitis is the most common of the serious infections produced by *N. meningitidis,* and explosive epidemics of the disease have probably occurred for untold centuries. Despite its neurological nature and epidemicity, meningococcal meningitis was not recognized as a clinical entity until Vieusseux presented his classic description of the disease in 1805. The causative organism was first isolated by Weichselbaum in 1887.

Epidemics of meningococcal meningitis occur most frequently under circumstances in which large numbers of individuals, especially from different geographic regions, are brought together under crowded and stressful conditions. For example, major epidemics have occurred repeatedly among recruits in military camps of the USA during this century. Epidemics are especially common and mortality rates are unusually high in certain geographic areas, such as the "meningitis belt" of Northern Africa, where over half a million cases were reported between 1939 and 1962. During epidemics the mortality rate in untreated cases averages 70% and ranges from 20 to 90%. Carriers are important in spread of the disease, and mounting carrier rates to high values often presage the onset of epidemics. Both case and carrier rates are highest in males.

Treatment of meningococcal disease with specific antiserum, which was introduced by Flexner in 1913, reduced the average mortality from 70 to about 50%. The introduction of sulfonamide treatment was a marked advance in therapy and further reduced the mortality to about 10%. Initially sulfonamides were highly effective for eliminating carriers and for mass prophylaxis to arrest epidemics. However, after a time increasing numbers of "carried" and "case" strains of sulfonamide-resistant meningococci arose; in the USA this occurred successively in large numbers of strains of serogroups B and C. Sulfonamide-resistant strains of group A have recently appeared in foreign countries. Moreover a changing pattern of serogroup prevalence has also taken place in the USA since World War II involving a shift from strains of groups A to B to C. The widespread occurrence of sulfa-resistant strains has seriously limited the usefulness of sulfadiazine for therapy and carrier control. For some unknown reason sulfa-resistant strains persist despite the fact that treatment with sulfadiazine has been largely abandoned.

Although penicillin has provided an effective substitute drug for therapy, it is relatively ineffective for eliminating the carrier state, probably because the concentrations of the antibiotic achieved in the tears and mucous secretions which bathe the nasopharynx are too low.

Whereas meningococcal infections continue to be of public health importance, it is unlikely that they will ever be as serious a threat as they have been in the past, and there is high hope that better control may soon be achieved through the use of meningococcal polysaccharide immunizing agents and new drugs for controlling carriers.

B.   *Physical and Chemical Structure*

Neisseria meningitidis is a nonsporing, nonmotile, gram-negative, oblong diplococcus arranged with its long axis parallel to the line of division. The opposing surfaces of the two organisms are flattened and slightly concave which gives the cells a kidney-bean shape; its dimensions are approximately 0.8×0.6 μm.

The organisms contain metachromatic granules and stain readily with the usual stains, albeit in ageing, autolyzing cultures they tend to become swollen and distorted and may fail to stain.

The medically important chemical components of the cell are the endotoxin of the cell wall, the capsular Ag which determines the presently recognized serogroups and an acid-resistant high molecular weight protein which is the basis of the serotypes. Initially 4 serogroups A, B, C and D were described. More recently other serogroups including Bo, 29E, 135 and X, Y and Z have been added. Some strains are nongroupable. Strains of the serogroups Y, 29E and 135 and the nongroupable strains appear to possess lower virulence than strains of groups A, B and C. Group C organisms are subdivided into at least 6 serotypes and group B organisms into 11 serotypes. *Serogrouping* and *serotyping* are currently of little practical value except for epidemiological studies. Organisms of group B have been reported to possess a thermolabile Ag related to certain strains of *E. coli;* meningococci and gonococci share some 8 heat-stable Ags.

Although *in vivo* grown organisms of groups A and C present capsules demonstrable by the capsular swelling test, group D organisms usually lack a demonstrable capsule. Encapsulation is irregular in cultured group B organisms apparently because the capsular substance is readily depolymerized by autoenzymes.

The capsular Ags of groups A and C are polysaccharides with mol wts above 100,000, whereas the specific capsular Ag of group B is a polysaccharide-polypeptide complex which can be freed of peptide by trypsin. Apparently group B polysaccharide is unique in being a sialic acid polymer consisting principally of n-acetyl-neuraminic acid. Whereas polysaccharides of groups A and C purified with cationic detergent are highly immunogenic for man, group B capsular material appears to be a poor immunogen.

The capsules of meningococci are antiphagocytic and the capsule is an important factor in virulence; its antiphagocytic effects are neutralized by specific Ab which serves to opsonize the organism.

Marked chemical and biological heterogeneity exists among various endotoxins and there is some evidence that meningococcal endotoxin may be more complex than the endotoxins of the rod-shaped gram-negative bacteria.

C. Genetics

Repeated subculture of smooth (S) encapsulated strains of *N. meningitidis* on artificial media selects for rough (R) nonencapsulated avirulent mutants which soon dominate in the culture. Inoculation of mice with rough organisms artificially coated with mucin reverses the selective process and virulent organisms can be recovered from the animals.

Meningococci readily develop resistance to drugs, including sulfonamides and streptomycin.

Transformation with DNA can be accomplished. However, genetic variation due to episomes has not been demonstrated.

D. Extracellular Products

A number of extracellular enzymes are produced but no extracellular product is known to be important in pathogenesis. The organism produces an enzyme, indophenyl oxidase, which is the basis of the oxidase test used for detecting colonies of neisseriae. Meningococci produce a heat-labile (65°C for 30 min) enzyme(s) which causes autolysis in ageing cultures. Bacteriocins (meningocins) which permit the identification of numerous subgroups within the serologic groups B and C are valuable tools for epidemiologic studies.

E. Culture

Neisseria meningitidis is fastidious in its nutritional requirements; it grows well on chocolate agar. It is highly sensitive to trace metals and fatty acids present in most culture media. Consequently agents, such as serum or starch, are often added to culture media in order to bind and neutralize these toxic components. Stock strains tend to be nutritionally less fastidious than freshly isolated strains and many of them can grow on synthetic media. The organism prefers aerobic conditions and grows poorly, if at all, under strict anaerobic conditions. Most strains require added CO_2 for primary isolation and proliferate best at pH values of 7.4 to 7.6. The organism grows over a temperature range of 25 to 42°C (optimum 37°C); however on primary isolation it is especially sensitive to sudden reductions in temperature.

For primary isolation a modified Thayer-Martin (T-M) selective medium called "Transgrow medium" is preferred which serves as both a transport and growth medium for both *N. meningitidis* and *N. gonorrhoeae*. It permits transport at ambient temperatures for 2 to 4 days or longer, especially if incubation is carried out overnight before transport. The medium selects against common contaminants including nonpathogenic neisseriae. Following growth on laboratory media, the organisms tend to die rapidly; hence continued maintenance in culture requires frequent transfer or use of a "maintenance medium" such as the medium of Levine and Thomas which allows survival for 1 to 2 months.

On blood agar the colonies are nonhemolytic, elevated, moist, smooth and bluish-gray in color; they range from 1 to 5 mm in diameter. Rough, smooth and mucoid colonial types occur depending on the presence and amount of capsular polysaccharide produced, the rough colonies being formed by organisms lacking capsules.

Like all neisseriae, the colonies of *N. meningitidis* show a positive oxidase reaction with the oxidase reagents dimethyl- or tetramethyl-paraphenylene diamine. The treated colonies first turn pink and then black due to oxidation of the dye. Organisms in treated colonies die after a few minutes.

F.   Resistance to Physical and Chemical Agents

Neisseria meningitidis is notoriously susceptible to destructive physical and chemical agents. It is highly sensitive to disinfectants and many chemotherapeutic drugs and is easily killed by desiccation and heat. It dies within a few days at 0°C but can be preserved at extremely low temperatures.

Although the neisseriae have the major characteristics of most gram-negative bacteria, i.e. carry endotoxin in their cell walls and are susceptible to destruction by Ab and C, they possess a characteristic in common with many gram-positive bacteria, namely susceptibility to penicillin.

G.   Experimental Models

No experimental models closely resembling disease in man have been developed. The 15-day-old chick embryo is perhaps the best model; irrespective of the site of inoculation the organisms produce a bacteremia followed by elective localization in the lungs and CNS. The mouse model is commonly used but is highly artificial; fatal infection can be produced, providing the inoculum is suspended in mucin. Apparently the mucin serves to protect the organisms against phagocytosis until they have had time to synthesize capsular polysaccharide sufficient to afford maximum protection against phagocytosis.

H. Infections and Disease in Man

Although *N. meningitidis* often colonizes the nasopharynx of man, *it seldom, if ever, causes clinically evident nasopharyngeal infection* and rarely causes primary pneumonia.

Between epidemics the carrier rate ranges from 5% or less to about 20%. On a world-wide basis epidemic disease results most frequently from group A organisms. The disease is most common in late winter and early spring; in civilian populations large scale epidemic disease peaks in cycles of about 10 years. Morbidity and mortality rates are highest among infants between the ages of 4 months to 1 year. Mortality rates are also very high in extreme old age.

Infection is usually acquired as the result of recent close association with a healthy carrier and results primarily from droplet infection. Clinical disease appears about 2 to 3 days or more after exposure. Apparently, and for unknown reasons, colonizing organisms occasionally transgress the mucosa of the nasopharynx to reach the bloodstream and/or the CNS to produce disease. Although chilling and fatigue are presumed to predispose to infection, this is uncertain, and the possible mechanisms responsible for invasion are unknown. Patients often give a history of preceding sore throat but whether this ever represents a meningococcal pharyngitis is debatable. It is probably most often due to a virus. Overcrowding, especially in sleeping quarters, contributes importantly to the chances of developing meningococcal infection; whether this rests on the "quantity of exposure" is not known. The possibility that deficiencies in secretory IgA Abs or antecedent or coincident viral infections predispose to meningococcal infection is likewise uncertain. Moreover the precise routes and mechanisms by which the organisms invade the bloodstream and the CNS are obscure. Whereas most investigators believe that in case of anatomic defects infecting organisms can sometimes pass directly from the nasopharynx to the CNS without entering the bloodstream, it is the consensus that in the absence of such defects invasion of organisms from the nasopharynx is commonly initiated via lymphatics and moreover, that the resulting bacteremia, however transient it may be, is the usual source of organisms producing meningitis.

Bacteremia may be acute or may last for weeks to months; it may be progressive or intermittent and complications may or may not develop. The reasons for such wide variations in the course of meningococcal disease are obscure but probably depend to a substantial degree on differences in the development of specific acquired immunity. Since serum levels of group specific Ag appear to reflect both the severity of meningococcemia and the stage and intensity of the immune response, future studies on serum Ag may throw light on this problem. In a small percentage of cases the initial mild bacteremia is rapidly followed by the development of fulminating meningococcemia with attending widespread thromboembolic metastatic lesions.

Fulminating meningococcemia begins abruptly with chills, headache and dizziness and often terminates in early circulatory collapse and death despite treatment. The metastatic lesions show perivascular infiltration with leukocytes and are often hemorrhagic; in the skin they are present as large irregular geometrical purpuric spots which are especially striking (Fig. 13-1) and commonly yield positive smears and cultivable organisms. The tendency to hemorrhage is presumed to be due to meningococcal endotoxin which causes excessive activation of the clotting mechanism with resulting depletion of blood clotting factors (consumption coagulopathy). In severe cases, especially in infants, extensive hemorrhage into the adrenal glands may occur with associated adrenal insufficiency (Waterhouse-Friderichsen syndrome) and death. Hemorrhage into the pituitary may also occur and contribute to early death.

Mild acute or subacute meningococcemia, a frequent type of infection, is highly responsive to chemotherapy. It may have an insidious onset but is usually heralded by the sudden development of irregular or intermittent fever, leukocytosis, chills and malaise. Other initial symptoms may include skin rash, acute mono- or poly-arthritis, nausea and conjunctivitis. The rash may be mild or severe and may resemble the "rose spots" of typhoid fever. Smears of capillary blood may sometimes reveal intracellular gram-negative diplococci, as do smears of exudates from skin lesions. Skin petechiae may form which develop into ulcers. Some patients recover spontaneously after weeks or months, whereas others develop sequelae or complications, such as meningitis.

On rare occasions a chronic form of meningococcemia develops which often leads to purulent synovitis or arthritis. Culture of organisms from the blood is difficult in such patients; if left untreated they may eventually develop other complications, such as meningitis or endocarditis.

Although *meningitis, the most frequent serious meningococcal disease,* is commonly thought to represent a complication of bacteremia, it is certain that the organisms occasionally invade the meninges directly through anatomic defects, such as those produced by head injury. The disease begins with symptoms reflecting meningeal involvement and generalized infection or a combination of both. The histopathology consists of a fibrin-

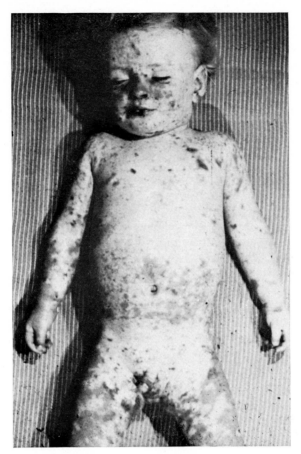

Figure 13-1. Fatal meningococcemia in an infant. (Courtesy Dr. George Ray.)

opurulent type of inflammation which may block the circulation of CSF and compress the brain. Various signs of inflammation of the meninges develop and coma may develop within a few hours. Many complications of meningitis occur, including cerebral thrombosis, brain abscess, transient or permanent paralysis, hydrocephalus and altered cerebration. Relapses are frequent and may occur several times during a period of one to two years. The mortality ranges from 2 to 6% despite chemotherapy.

Differential diagnosis of meningococcal infection should include consideration of a number of diseases such as typhus, typhoid fever, subacute bacterial endocarditis, rheumatic fever, diabetic coma, and uremia.

Although attendants seldom contract infection from patients, it is common practice to regulate the patient's contacts until 48 hours of treatment have passed and to monitor known contacts for evidence of carriage and developing illness. Attempts should be made to eliminate convalescent carriage of organisms before discharging patients. (Section N)

I. Mechanisms of Pathogenicity

Bacteriocin typing and drug resistance studies have established that "epidemic strains" of meningococci exist. Presumably they are more invasive and "toxic" than other strains, but the factors responsible for these attributes have not been fully elucidated. It is unlikely that *N. meningitidis* grows or survives long within phagocytes; hence the organism is considered to represent an extracellular pathogen. *In common with other extracellular pathogens, such as D. pneumoniae, the capsule is an important determinant of virulence and anticapsular antibody affords group-specific protection against infection presumably by acting as an opsonin.*

The basis of the profound toxemia of meningococcal infections is not known. A protein (P substance) which is toxic for animals has been reported but its role in the toxemia of infections in either animals or man has not been established. Endotoxin probably plays an important role in pathogenesis by producing vascular damage, evidently involving mechanisms common to those of the Shwartzman reaction. It has been reported that endotoxin produces lesions in animals similar to those attending natural disease in man and that anti-endotoxin protects animals against lethal doses of either endotoxin or living meningococci.

J. Mechanisms of Immunity

Immunity to meningococci is complex and is only partially understood. Herd resistance is relatively high. The innate resistance of man to meningococcal infection is probably substantial, but the nature of the protection it affords is unknown. In contrast, it is known that acquired immunity is a major force of resistance and that the titer of serum bactericidal activity is strongly correlated with resistance to infection; for example maternal IgG Abs provide substantial humoral immunity to young infants until 4 to 6 months of age when they become more susceptible than at any time during life. It is presumed, but not proved, that the course of infection is largely determined by developing forces of specific acquired immunity. Antibodies with agglutinating, precipitating, complement fixing, opsonic and bactericidal activities arise early (5 to 15 days) in the course of infection. They belong to the immunoglobulin classes IgG, IgM and IgA. Most of them are directed against surface Ags including the *capsular immunogens* which engender specific *serogroup* immunity. The role which *serotype* Abs may play in immunity has not been elucidated; however in the case of group B organisms they totally account for the bactericidal Abs in serum.

Antibody-containing sera afford specific protection to both mice and men. However, all of the various Abs and Ab activities which may convey protection to either mouse or man are not known.

It is tempting to assume that secretory IgA may contribute to immunity to nasopharyngeal carriage but this is pure speculation. Carriage to nongroupable strains of meningococci stimulates cross-reactive bactericidal Abs against numerous but not all meningococci of other groups. The nature of the cross-reactive Ag(s) involved is not known. In this regard it is of interest that children are frequent carriers of the relatively avirulent nongroupable strains and thus acquire broad cross-reactive immunity to meningococci. Whereas some individuals may remain chronic carriers of meningococci for years, the carrier state is usually temporary, presumably because of the early development of acquired immunity to the carried organisms. After 2 weeks of carriage most individuals are resistant to infection by the organisms they carry, a circumstance resembling the development of specific immunity to carried pneumococci. Protective Abs can be demonstrated in the sera of 80% of healthy individuals. They are probably initiated, broadened and reinforced throughout life by intermittent exposure to carried organisms. It is thought that immunity acquired by carriage does not selectively promote a shift in carriage from typable to nontypable organisms as in the case of the streptococcus.

Whether anti-endotoxins afford substantial protection against invasion by meningococci or injury resulting from infection is not known. In any event anti-endotoxin has not been found useful for therapy despite favorable results in animals.

K.   Laboratory Diagnosis

The procedures for bacteriological laboratory diagnosis of meningococcal infections include examination and culture of spinal fluid, joint fluid, blood and nasopharyngeal secretions as indicated.

In routine bacteriological diagnosis it is common practice to culture 10 ml of fresh blood in 10 volumes of an appropriate liquid medium, such as tryptose phosphate broth, and to spread 0.1 ml of blood on a plate of chocolate agar or Thayer-Martin selective medium. In cases of fulminating septicemia and sometimes in lesser states of septicemia the organisms can be demonstrated in the buffy coat with the Gram stain. Repeated blood culture may be needed on occasion. Incubation is carried out under 10% CO_2 and the broth is observed and examined for growth of gram-negative diplococci during a week of incubation. The oxidase test is applied to colonies on plates. Oxidase-positive colonies of characteristic morphology are picked promptly and organisms are identified by fermentation tests and agglutination tests with known antisera. *Neisseria meningitidis* can be distinguished from *N. gonorrhoeae* and other common species of neisseriae by the fermentation of different sugars and the ability or lack of ability to grow on nutrient agar and at the temperature of 22°C.

Fresh specimens of spinal fluid are examined by capsular swelling tests and precipitin tests with known antisera and by culture and direct staining for typical gram-negative diplococci. Since organisms are abundant in spinal fluid, direct smears of spinal fluid sediment will often reveal them both free and within phagocytes. The organisms tend to occur in large numbers within some individual phagocytes but not others. Cultures are often positive before leukocytes appear in spinal fluid and reduction in the glucose content of the fluid occurs. Organisms which frequent the respiratory tract and which may be mistaken for *N. meningitidis* are *N. catarrhalis, N. sicca* and members of the genera *Moraxella* and *Veillonella.*

Positive bacteriological findings on blood and spinal fluid are highly significant indicators of meningococcal disease but positive nasopharyngeal cultures only indicate carriage of the organism. In some instances examination and culture of other specimens, such as aspirates of skin lesions and joints, are indicated.

L. Therapy

Although it is often desirable to determine the susceptibility of an infecting organism to an antimicrobial drug before initiating therapy, *early treatment of acute meningococcal disease is so crucial that the presence of typical organisms on smear justifies the initiation of chemotherapy before cultural and sensitivity tests are completed.* Certain drugs do not pass the normal blood-brain barrier readily. The concept that this precludes their therapeutic value in meningococcal meningitis is not true because the blood-brain barrier tends to be broken in inflammation. Consequently during about the first 3 days of effective treatment the barrier remains moderately permeable to drugs which would not pass the normal barrier in appreciable amounts. Sulfadiazine readily reaches the spinal fluid but because of the ubiquity of sulfa-resistant strains is no longer the drug of choice. Instead, penicillin G in massive doses is used even though it has limited capacity to pass the normal blood-brain barrier. Sometimes a combination of sulfadiazine and penicillin G is used, especially if the infection is severe and the organism is not sulfa-resistant. *Drug treatment should be initiated promptly* and if adrenal insufficiency or intravascular coagulation is suspected appropriate special supportive treatment should be added. Recurring symptoms of infection should be monitored for the possible occurrence of superinfection with another organism, as well as for changes in drug resistance of the infecting meningococcus.

M. Reservoirs of Infection

Man is the only known reservoir of meningococcal infection.

N. Control of Disease Transmission

As stated earlier meningococcal infection is usually acquired by recent close association with healthy carriers rather than contact with patients.

Because carrier rates and morbidity rates of endemic meningococcal disease are low, preventive measures directed at either carriers or patients are relatively ineffective for controlling interepidemic infection. This is in contrast to epidemic disease which appears to rest on both a high percentage of susceptibles in the population to the type of meningococcus involved and a high incidence of carriers of "virulent" organisms. Under these circumstances regulation of carriers is a highly effective preventive measure.

Chemoprophylaxis among close contacts of carriers continues to be a recommended practice. However, because of the current prevalence of sulfonamide-resistant strains, chemoprophylaxis must often be carried out with other drugs, the most promising of which is minocycline. Rifampin is of temporary and limited value because of the rapid emergence of rifampin-resistant strains.

Immunization with purified high molecular weight capsular polysaccharides of groups A and C is under field trial and gives good promise of being effective in reducing the carrier rate and protecting against infection. If the immune response to these polysaccharides mimics the response of man to pneumococcal polysaccharide the induced immunity should be durable. Effective immunogens would be of great value for preventing epidemics under circumstances where the chances that an epidemic will develop are high.

Neisseria gonorrhoeae

A. Medical Perspectives

Although gonorrhea undoubtedly occurred among early civilizations, it was not clearly described until the 13th century when Guielmus de Saliceto recognized the disease as a distinct clinical entity of venereal origin.*

For centuries gonorrhea was considered to be an early stage of syphilis, an opinion which was erroneously reinforced by the famous experiment of John Hunter, who in 1767 acquired syphilis by inoculating himself with exudate from a patient who allegedly had gonorrhea, but who evidently had *both syphilis and gonorrhea*. It was not until the work of Hill (1790), Bell (1792) and Ricord (1831-1860) that syphilis and gonorrhea were clearly defined as distinct diseases. Neisser discovered the causative organism of gonorrhea in 1879 and Loeffler cultured it in 1882. Until recent decades bacteriologic diagnosis was usually made by smear alone and

* The term "gonorrhea" was first used by Galen in the first century to designate another disease.

therapy was of little or no value. The marked effectiveness of sulfonamide therapy introduced in 1935 was short-lived because of the rapid emergence of resistant strains, and it was not until 1943 that penicillin was shown to be a highly valuable therapeutic agent.

However, in spite of effective chemotherapy and improved methods for diagnosis, the disease is probably more prevalent today than at any time in history. Again, as is so often true, the opportunities for controlling a disease with a highly effective chemotherapeutic or prophylactic agent have come to naught; in the present instance because of changing social mores, complacency, ignorance and public indifference. Indeed it has become almost axiomatic that the development of a highly effective chemotherapeutic agent which can commonly cure a disease and cope with its life-threatening complications leads to lack of interest on the part of research workers and lack of concern on the part of the medical profession and the public. Today gonorrhea is a world-wide pandemic disease of staggering proportions; over 25% of cases are among teenagers and the highest incidence is in the 20 to 24 year age group. The threat it poses destroys what little solace might be taken in the fact that gonorrhea is seldom life-threatening; the mounting number of cases with serious complications presents a major public health problem.

The incidence of the disease is difficult to assess because the actual number of cases is at least 5 to 10 times the number reported. It is estimated that private physicians report only 10% of the cases they treat. Also, the disease is usually self-limiting and many cases go undiagnosed. In recent years the annual increase in incidence has exceeded 12% in the USA. It is probable that in 1971 the number of new cases was between 2,000,000 and 6,000,000 in the USA and over 65,000,000 in the world at large. There are many reasons for the continued rise in the incidence of gonorrhea, some related to the inherent nature of the disease, such as the short incubation period, lack of adequate immunity to reinfection and inadequate methods for detecting carriers, and others related to social attitudes and sexual behavior including the 7 P's: promiscuity, perversion (sexual), pornography, permissiveness, "pot," "pads," and "the pill." The disease is currently out of control and, for the present at least, has outstripped the opportunities for containing it, even with the best case finding methods and treatments available. It appears that short of a sharp reversal in social attitudes and sexual behavior the disease will be controlled only by new approaches, such as better methods for detecting carriers and the development of a vaccine.

B. *Physical and Chemical Structure*

Neisseria gonorrhoeae is similar to *N. meningitidis* with respect to morphology and staining properties. Irregular "giant forms" are frequently

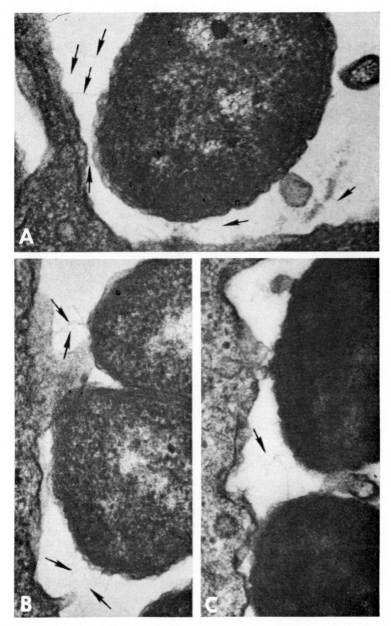

Figure 13-2. Pilated T-2 gonococci are numerous in association with amnion cells both after exposure to the cells in suspensions (A) or as monolayers (B and C). Pili can be seen extending from the gonococci (arrows) toward the plasma membranes of amnion cells in these thick sections. In some instances (A and B) several pili course from each organism to the amnion cell surface. × 80,000 (A and B) and × 60,000 (C). (From Swanson, J.: J. Exp. Med. *137*:578, 1973.)

present in ageing cultures and a decrease in stainability occurs *in vivo* within a few hours after initiation of penicillin therapy. The gonococcus possesses pili (Fig. 13-2). Although the organism contains numerous surface and cytoplasmic Ags they have not been critically analyzed and their relation to structure and virulence is largely unknown. The organism possesses a cell wall endotoxin, and a specific surface polysaccharide Ag (K-like Ag) which is related to meningococcal capsular Ags A and B. The K-like Ag never lends the appearance of a detectable capsule and rapidly diminishes on subculture, a change which is associated with conversion from smooth (S) to rough (R) colonial growth. Subculture also results in the loss of pili and virulence (Section C). Pilus protein is species specific but whether the pili of different strains of gonococci are antigenically distinct is not known.

The organism possesses other Ags related to Ags of organisms of the genus *Pasteurella* and common to the genus *Neisseria* including a somatic polysaccharide. Wall-less L forms can be produced by growing the organisms in the presence of penicillin. Such forms have been found in synovial fluid in untreated gonococcal arthritis.

When large numbers of either living or heat-killed gonococci are injected into animals toxic death results, presumably due to endotoxin.

C. Genetics

Four colonial types of *N. gonorrhoeae* have been described. The small-colony virulent types 1 and 2 are piliated; they predominate in the exudates of acute infections and appear in primary culture on suitable media. On repeated subculture on liquid media they soon convert to avirulent nonpiliated types 3 and 4 which are poor in surface K-like Ag. Type 1 can only be maintained in culture by cultivation on special media. Although pili are associated with virulence and may be a key to virulence, they are probably not the sole determinant of virulence. Autoagglutinability varies among colonial types and appears to depend in large part on the presence of peculiar regions on the surface of the organism which promote adherence to adjacent organisms (zonal adherence).

Although *N. gonorrhoeae* readily develops resistance to the sulfonamides, resistance to penicillin has developed to a lesser degree; at present no strains are encountered which are not clinically susceptible to penicillin. Penicillin resistance may be due to small-step mutations. Strains resistant to other antibiotics, including streptomycin, have been encountered and multiple-drug resistance has emerged, the basis of which has not been elucidated; it is unlikely that episomes are involved. Whether changes in drug resistance are accompanied by changes in virulence remains unknown.

D. Extracellular Products

Extracellular products produced by the gonococcus include a weak hemolysin and an oxidase which is important in the oxidase test. Bacteriocins (gonocins) have been found which may prove to be valuable in epidemiologic work for strain identification.

E. Culture

The growth requirements of the gonococcus are very similar to those of the meningococcus. It grows best under aerobic conditions at 35°C to 36°C over a pH range of 7.2 to 7.6. Some strains do not grow at 37.5°C and growth ceases below 30°C or above 38.5°C; this temperature sensitivity was the basis of artificial fever therapy attempted several decades ago. After 48 hours of incubation on Thayer-Martin (TM) medium or "Transgrow medium" at 36°C to 37°C small oxidase-positive colonies appear as raised, translucent, finely granular mucoid structures about 5 mm in diameter. Glucose is the only sugar fermented; acid and gas are produced. The organism dies out on culture media within 3 to 4 days but can be preserved for weeks by covering the cultured organisms with paraffin oil. Preservation for years can be accomplished by storage at −70°C.

F. Resistance to Physical and Chemical Agents

The gonococcus is highly susceptible to most chemicals including the common disinfectants. Its high suceptibility to silver nitrate is the basis of the practice of preventing ophthalmia neonatorum by placing drops of a 1 to 2% silver nitrate solution in the eyes of newborn infants. The organism is usually killed by sunlight and drying within 1 to 2 hours. For susceptibility to chemotherapeutic agents see Sections C and L.

G. Experimental Models

Good experimental models of gonorrhea in man are greatly needed; it is only recently that disease closely simulating human gonorrhea has been produced in the very expensive model, the chimpanzee. Consequently most of the research on pathogenesis has been accomplished by the use of human volunteers. Infection can be produced in the chick embryo, in the anterior chamber of the rabbit's eye, and in mice injected intraperitoneally with mucin-coated organisms. The use of immunosuppressed animals as models has not been tried extensively.

H. Infections and Disease in Man

Gonorrhea is the *most frequently reported infectious disease* in the USA. About 30% of cases develop serious complications, and chronic disease lasting many years is not uncommon. Infections are principally of venereal origin and the lesions are usually confined to the urogenital tract. In past decades the disease appeared to be more common among males than among females. However, this pattern is now reversed, possibly because of contraceptive pills which raise the pH of the vagina toward neutrality and thus favor growth of the organism. The incubation period is usually 2 to 8 days (range 1 to 30 days).

In the male the onset is almost always symptomatic and abrupt and is characterized by frequent painful urination and a yellowish mucopurulent discharge from the urethra, which usually prompts the individual to seek medical attention. *Neisseria gonorrhoeae* has a predilection for parasitizing columnar and transitional (but not squamous) epithelia. The organisms transgress the epithelial layer by passing between adjacent cells and probably through cells as well. Within the subepithelial tissues they grow extracellularly for a short time and engender an acute inflammatory lesion characterized by heavy infiltration with neutrophils, lymphocytes, plasma cells and mast cells. Fever does not develop so long as the infection is limited to the urethra. Spread of the disease, which is by direct extension via lymphatic vessels, often results in *prostatitis, epididymitis* and sometimes sterility. *Most cases undergo spontaneous cure without serious complications.* Occasionally secondary invaders, such as *Staph. aureus,* supplant the gonococcus and prolong the urethritis. In some cases columnar epithelium may be destroyed and replaced by stratified squamous epithelium; sloughing epithelium and the *formation of scar tissue may cause obstruction* or narrowing of ducts. This tendency to obstruct ducts often results in *retention cysts or abscesses.* Strictures of the urethra may lead to urinary tract infection with other organisms. Other less frequent complications are discussed below. In about half of the cases of prostatitis, spread to the rectum and resulting proctitis occurs. In a small percentage of cases the individual may remain infectious for months to years due to asymptomatic chronic disease.

In the female primary infection usually involves the urethra, cervical glands, Skene's glands or Bartholin's glands. The infection spreads to the rectum in about half of the cases. It may involve the fallopian tubes and lead to acute *purulent salpingitis* or *chronic salpingitis* which predisposes to ectopic pregnancy, obliterative fibrosis and sterility. *Gonorrhea in the female (either chronic or acute) is mild or asymptomatic in about 75% of cases* and usually involves the cervix. Consequently discovery of the female "carrier" is most often the result of a search for sources of infection to account for disease detected in the male.

Chronic disease (often undiagnosed) *with vague pelvic and abdominal symptoms and serious complications occurs in about 15% of infected females.* Occasionally spread occurs to produce perihepatitis (Fitz-Hugh-Curtis syndrome).

In some cases of gonorrhea, principally those with a chronic pelvic focus, the organisms *invade the bloodstream* and often reach and produce lesions in the tendon sheaths, joints, heart valves and skin but rarely the meninges. In some cases they may produce widespread lesions in many organs and septic death.

Sexual perversion presents different patterns of disease, proctitis being common in males. Oral-genital practices may lead to pharyngitis and parotiditis as well as genital lesions; pharyngeal carriage has been reported.

Gonococcal bacteremia is usually accompanied by chills, fever and malaise and in about 50% of the cases small *dermal infarcts* due to septic emboli are seen. These infarcts usually occur in the extremities and often show gonococci on smear but seldom contain cultivable organisms. The majority of patients with severe bacteremia, accompanied by chills, fever and skin lesions, complain of *polyarthritis* and/or *tendosynovitis* of the wrist or ankle. Less than 50% of patients with arthritis yield positive blood cultures. It is extremely difficult to culture the organism from the synovial cavity, not only because synovial fluid may be sparse or absent but because the organisms may exist as L-forms at this site or may be limited to the joint capsule or membrane. The clinical picture of gonococcal arthritis without positive bacteriological findings can be mistaken for rheumatic fever; however such patients will respond to trial penicillin therapy within 2 to 3 days if the infection is indeed due to the gonococcus.

Endocarditis, a life-threatening complication, may not only result from bacteremia but may cause it to persist. Consequently if heart murmurs are heard, adequate and prolonged chemotherapy is in order. The rare cases of gonococcal *meningitis* that occur are often mistaken for meningococcal disease and treated as such. The newborn may contract infection of the eyes (*ophthalmia neonatorum*) during passage through the infected birth canal. Before laws were enacted requiring prophylaxis with silver nitrate for all newborn infants (Credé treatment) the disease caused 12% of all blindness but now affects only 0.1 to 0.2% of all newborns and is easily controlled by antibiotic therapy. Gonococcal *conjunctivitis* or *iridocyclitis* sometimes occurs in adults, particularly in patients with gonococcal arthritis and is a tragic complication if not treated promptly since it can rapidly lead to corneal ulceration, perforation and blindness. *Gonococcal vulvovaginitis* sometimes occurs in prepubescent females, usually as the result of intimate contact with infected adults or, on rare occasion, from moist fomites.

I. Mechanisms of Pathogenicity

The mechanisms concerned in the pathogenesis of gonococcal disease have not been elucidated. Virulent *in vivo* grown organisms are resistant to specific antiserum and C because they possess some unknown surface

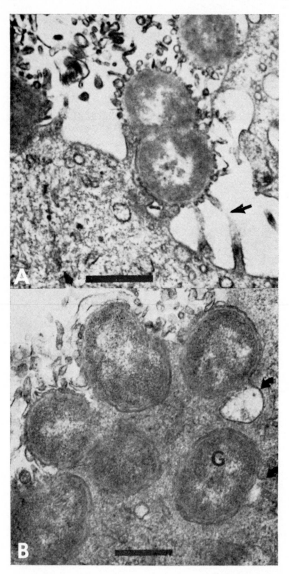

Figure 13-3. Adherence and embedding of gonococci into the epithelial cells of the urethra. A. Processes from a urethral epithelial cell appear to be twisted over and attached to an adjacent gonococcus (arrow). The bar represents 500 nm. B. Electron micrograph showing gonococci deeply embedded in a urethral epithelial cell. Note the membrane of the host cells (arrows) around the gonococcus (G). The bar represents 500 nm. × 36,000 (A) and × 30,750 (B). (Ward, M. E. and Watt, P. J., J. Infect. Dis. *126*:603-604, 1972.)

material (possibly K-like Ag) which presumably covers up Ags important in C killing. Apparently the bacterial surface also possesses substances of unknown nature which are antiphagocytic. The gonococcus is not known to produce any toxin, other than endotoxin, that might injure tissue or kill phagocytes. Although the fate of the organism within phagocytes is controversial, the probability is that it does not grow but instead is killed. There is no evidence that nonantibody humoral factors oppose the organism. The observation that a few neutrophils in an exudate tend to be loaded with gonococci, whereas others are free of organisms is alleged to result from chance phagocytosis of a clump of organisms rather than from intracellular growth.

Recent evidence indicates that gonococci can adhere to and become embedded in the secretory surface of the epithelial cells of the urethra. Occasionally the organisms are seen in the cytoplasm encased within membrane-bound structures (Fig. 13-3). Whether this results from phagocytosis or endoencystment and what the fate of these intracellular organisms may be is unknown. The bacterial surface component responsible for adherence is not known but could be associated with pili or the special regions on the bacterial surface responsible for the phenomenon of "zonal adherence." Apparently the gonococcus may assume the role of an intracellular as well as an extracellular parasite with all of its implications, e.g. inapparent infection, carriage and escape from the usual forces of defense, namely antimicrobial humoral factors and professional phagocytes.

Subculture on the usual media results in loss of virulence, which is associated with loss of pili; surface Ags, resistance to phagocytosis by professional phagocytes, and resistance to killing by Ab and C. Although the only certain correlate of virulence is the presence of pili on the cell, other key determinants of virulence probably exist.

Whereas endotoxin may contribute to pathogenesis because of its inherent toxicity it is not a key factor of virulence since it is present equally in both virulent and avirulent gonococci.

Obviously there is urgent need for research directed to the questions of virulence factors and the relations between the organism and phagocytes. Since it is possible that virulence factors are synthesized only *in vivo,* it may be necessary to use *in vivo* grown organisms for such studies. Important unanswered questions are: whether leukotoxins are produced, whether and to what extent the organisms grow within either phagocytes or other cells and what the nature of the surface materials are that cause adherence and prevent phagocytosis and Ab-C killing.

J.   Mechanisms of Immunity

Innate immunity to gonorrhea does not prevent primary infection in any instance; all human beings appear to be essentially equally susceptible. Although it is often stated that acquired immunity does not arise in gonorrhea, this is obviously not true since most cases of the disease undergo spontaneous recovery. However the contention that immunity is weak cannot be denied since chronic disease is common. Immunity to gonorrhea is complex, and concepts of its nature will demand revision as more knowledge is gained about the role of the organism as an intracellular parasite. It is probable that specific acquired immunity involves opsonins and moreover that it is type specific. However, there is little evidence to support this thesis. Observations which are compatible with it are: (1) that such a pattern characterizes other pathogens such as the meningococcus, pneumococcus, streptococcus and *H. influenzae,* (2) that humoral Abs which might act as antitoxins or as bacteriocidins in concert with C appear to be excluded, (3) that there is nothing to suggest that macrophages and the forces of specific cellular immunity are involved, (4) that volunteers who possess antigonococcal Abs show increased resistance to experimental inoculation with the organism (possibly restricted to strains of the type responsible for Abs), (5) that nonantibody factors of immunity against the gonococcus have not been demonstrated, and (6) that reinfection is common. These last observations could result because many type-specific strains may exist and/or that the immune response is weak. The marked susceptibility to reinfection was amply documented many years ago in the diary of the famous author James Boswell, "a compulsive patron of prostitutes," who recorded some 19 attacks of gonorrhea between 1760 and 1790. Evidently he paid dearly for his sexual exploits and promiscuity for the records indicate that he finally died from complications of the disease.

For unknown reasons the humoral Ab response in gonorrhea seems to be poor regardless of whether the infection remains localized or becomes disseminated. All sorts of Abs against all sorts of Ags have been studied, but the immunoglobulin nature and specificity of the Abs that may afford protection remain unknown. Three aspects of immunity may be considered, namely immune forces which may operate against invasion of the epithelial barrier, against organisms within epithelial cells and against extracellular organisms. Antibodies specific for pili are present in patients with gonorrhea but their possible protective function has not been determined. Assuming that pili or other surface components may be antiphagocytic or may serve to promote adherence and colonization on columnar epithelium and thus permit invasion, it would be of particular interest to know whether Abs specific for pili would serve as opsonins or, in case of secretory IgA Abs, would block adherence of organisms to epithelium.

There is great need for intensive research on the nature and mechanisms of immunity in gonorrhea. Special attention should be given to the question of whether acquired immunity is type specific and whether it can be passively transferred with cells and/or serum. The possible role of nonantibody factors of acquired immunity in gonorrhea should also be explored.

New knowledge on immunity could help solve 2 great needs, an effective vaccine and a more suitable method for detecting carriers.

K. *Laboratory Diagnosis*

Fresh exudate from acute lesions having a clinical history of gonorrhea commonly yields positive smears for typical gram-negative diplococci. The organisms are largely intracellular and tend to be present in large numbers in some phagocytes in the smear but not others. *A presumptive diagnosis by smear is fairly reliable in case of the male but not the female; in the latter case it should be confirmed* by culture. False positive microscopic tests, due principally to organisms of the Mima-Herellea group, can usually be avoided by care and the use of proper techniques.

Bacteriologic diagnosis of self-treated cases and of chronic gonorrhea, especially in the female, often fails because the organisms are few in number and are extremely difficult to find even by culture. When only a single specimen is examined the diagnosis may be missed in 20 to 40% of cases. Repeated examination of specimens taken over a period of days or weeks from the glands of Skene and Bartholin and from the cervix and rectum greatly reduces the number of missed cases. Trials on the use of suppository tampons for collecting specimens promise to improve the success of culture.

Specimens should be promptly inoculated after collection, preferably on Thayer-Martin or Transgrow medium and incubated under 10% CO_2 at 35°C to 36°C. In order to prevent spreading growth of contaminating *Proteus* sp. 5 μg/ml of trimethoprim may be added to Transgrow medium. Blood, synovial fluid and spinal fluid should preferably be cultured for a week in a thin layer of ascitic fluid broth under 10% CO_2. Although detection of oxidase-positive colonies of typical morphology on T-M medium affords a presumptive diagnosis of gonorrhea, final identification rests on sugar fermentation tests and/or tests with specific antisera. Effective mass control of gonorrhea demands rapid but accurate bacteriologic diagnosis. Whereas the direct fluorescent Ab (FA) method applied to fresh exudate usually succeeds with acute exudates, the "delayed" FA method in which the specimen is cultured for 16 to 20 hours before applying FA is even more successful than routine culture and is useful in cases of chronic disease.

The immune response in gonorrhea is weak and no useful diagnostic skin test or serological tests have been developed. However, a new test for anti-pilus Ab in serum promises to be useful for detecting carriers.

Simple but accurate methods for detecting asymptomatic infection are sorely needed for carrier detection; serologic and various other immunologic tests such as the macrophage migration-inhibition test and skin tests should be explored further.

L. *Therapy*

The drug of choice in most cases of gonorrhea is penicillin. Whereas most strains were formerly sensitive to about 0.01 units/ml of penicillin, it is common now to find strains for which the MIC (minimum inhibitory concentration) is 2 to 4 units/ml. Consequently, the recommended "one-shot" dose of penicillin for females is now 4.8 million units of procaine penicillin, with probenecid to prolong effectiveness. Parenteral administration is usually best because it assures that the patient receives the full dosage of the drug.

Erythromycin, tetracycline, or kanamycin may be used to treat patients who are allergic to penicillin. Many strains of gonococci have developed resistance to sulfonamides and some to erythromycin or tetracycline. Spectinomycin is a new aminoglycoside that can be used to treat patients who are allergic to penicillin, or patients infected with gonococci possessing a high degree of resistance to penicillin.

Since organisms within cells and abscesses are not readily reached by many chemotherapeutic agents, unusually high doses must often be given to be effective. Also cases of proctitis and pharyngitis may be refractory because of penicillinase produced by other bacteria present in the area of infection. Whether multiple-drug resistance, which is on the increase, will ever progress to the point where drugs will no longer be therapeutically valuable cannot be forecast. Cure is evaluated by weekly cultures continued for 2 to 3 weeks after terminating treatment.

Since some 3% of patients with venereal disease have both gonorrhea and syphilis, penicillin treatment often aborts coexisting cases of early syphilis. Needless to say, all patients with gonorrhea should be subjected to serologic tests for syphilis before treatment and periodically for 6 months thereafter.

M. Reservoirs of Infection

Man is the only reservoir of the gonococcus. The organism is most commonly harbored in the genitalia and rectum. The incidence of disease and carriers is high among prostitutes, averaging some 20%. *Long term carriage is frequent in both women and men.** Whereas patients sometimes contract the disease from the acutely infected mate, infection most commonly results from contact with the asymptomatic chronic carrier who is often unaware of ever having been infected; currently approximately 2 million such carriers exist in the USA. This circumstance was well documented by Boswell who contracted the disease from a "safe" girl friend who believed herself innocent because she had had no lover for 6 months before becoming intimate with Boswell. Lacking the benefit of today's knowledge, Boswell doubted her fidelity; he wrote: "There is scarcely a possibility that she could be innocent of this crime of horrid imposition, and yet her positive asserverations have really stunned me." Since approximately 1% of all females have asymptomatic gonorrhea, it is obvious that the female carrier constitutes the major reservoir of disease transmission; the relative importance of the asymptomatic male remains to be determined.

* The former concept that chronic carriage is largely confined to females who commonly acquire infection from symptomatically-infected males is erroneous.

N. Control of Disease Transmission

The fallacious assumption that a highly effective therapeutic agent can be used to effectively control an infectious disease irrespective of the nature of its transmission and the human elements involved is well illustrated in the case of gonorrhea. No suitably effective practical measures for preventing gonorrhea in the exposed individual have been developed despite the numerous gadgets, ointments, chemical irrigants, etc. that have been tried over the centuries. Various vaccines have been tried without success. Condoms probably afford the best protection. Penicillin, if given in adequate dosage at or near the time of exposure, is an effective prophylactic and should be employed for all individuals known to have had sexual contact with an active case of the disease. Treatment of the patient and his contacts should be continued until cure is effected since sexual relations are apt to continue despite advice to the contrary.

Efficient case finding is a critical but delicate matter which should be reserved for experts. In theory if a good case-finding team is at hand, the rapid identification and prompt treatment of all of the sexual contacts that the patient has had within a week before infection, regardless of whether they present symptoms, should go a long way toward controlling the disease. Of course, contacts of contacts should also be considered since some of the original contacts may have reached the infective stage within a week.

References

Artenstein, M. S., Schneider, H. and Tingley, M. D. Meningococcal infections. I. Prevalence of serogroups causing disease in U. S. Army personnel in 1964-1970. WHO Bull. *45*:275, 1971.

Brown, W. J., Lucus, C. T. and Kuhn, U. S. G. Gonorrhea in the chimpanzee. Brit. J. Vener. Dis. *48*:177, 1972.

Finland, M. Revival of antibacterial immunization: meningococcal vaccines prove promising (Editorial). J. Inf. Dis. *121*:445, 1970.

Frasch, C. E. and Chapman, S. S. Classification of *Neisseria meningitidis* group B into distinct serotypes. IV. Preliminary chemical studies on the nature of the serotype antigen. Inf. and Immun. *6*:674, 1972.

Gotschlich, E. C., Goldschneider, I. and Arnstein, M. S. Human immunity to the meningococcus. V. The effect of immunization with meningococcal group C polysaccharide on the carrier state. J. Exp. Med. *129*:1385, 1969.

Guttler, R. B., Counts, G. W., Avent, C. K. and Beaty, H. N. Effect of rifampin and minocycline on meningococcal carrier rates. J. Inf. Dis. *124*:199, 1971.

Handsfield, H. N., Lipman, T. O., Harnisch, J. P., Tronca, E., and Holmes, K. K.: Asymptomatic gonorrhea in men. New England J. Med. *290*:117, 1974.

Hoffman, T. A. and Edwards, E. A. Group-specific polysaccharide antigen and humoral antibody response in disease due to *Neisseria meningitidis*. J. Inf. Dis. *126*:636, 1972.

Martin, J. E. and Lester, A. Transgrow, a medium for transport and growth of *Neisseria gonorrhoeae* and *Neisseria meningitidis*. Health Service and Mental Health Administration Health Reports *86*:30, 1971.

Ober, W. B. Boswell's Gonorrhea. Bull. N. Y. Acad. Sci. *45*:587, 1969.

Reller, L. B., MacGregor, R. R. and Beaty, H. N. Bactericidal antibody after colonization with *Neisseria meningitidis*. J. Inf. Dis. *127*:56, 1973.

Slaterus, K. W. Serological typing of meningococci by means of microprecipitation. Antonie Van Leuwenhoek J. Microbiol. Serol. 27:305, 1961.

Swanson, J., Kraus, S. J. and Gotschlich, E. C. Studies on gonococcal growth patterns. I. Pili and zones of adhesion: their relation to gonococcal growth patterns. J. Exp. Med. 134:886, 1971.

Ward, M. E., Watt, P. J. and Glynn, A. A. Gonococci in urethral exudates possess a virulence factor lost on subculture. Nature 227:382, 1970.

Ward, M. E. and Watt, P. J. Adherence of Neisseria gonorrhoeae to urethral mucosal cells. J. Inf. Dis. 126:601, 1972.

Chapter 14

Corynebacterium

The genus *Corynebacterium* of the family *Corynebacteriaceae* contains many species parasitic to animals and to man but the only pathogen of major importance for man is *Corynebacterium diphtheriae,* the cause of diphtheria. The virulent form of the organism is notable for the powerful exotoxin it secretes, which serves as the principal agent responsible for its pathogenicity, virulence and immunogenicity. *Corynebacterium diphtheriae is maintained in man, its only natural host, by a small but relatively constant population of chronic carriers who commonly harbor the organism in the nose or nasopharynx.* Certain nonpathogenic corynebacteria (often referred to as "diphtheroids") are commonly found on the mucous membranes of the upper respiratory tract (URT), urogenital tract and eyes. On occasion certain of them may assume the role of opportunists. Two nonpathogens, which are notable because they often confuse the diagnosis of diphtheria, are *C. hofmannii,* a frequent inhabitant of the URT, and *C. xerosis,* which is often present on the conjunctivae. As might be expected, several species of *Corynebacterium* are pathogenic for animals. The focus in this chapter will be on *C. diphtheriae* and the infections it produces.

A. Medical Perspectives

No serious bacterial disease of man is more thoroughly understood and controlled than diphtheria, largely because the disease is a simple toxemia uncomplicated by invasion of organisms beyond the local lesions they produce on external integuments and because artificial immunization produces strong immunity which commonly persists for months to years.

Diphtheria, a world-wide disease, was first accurately described as a clinical entity by Bretonneau of Tours in 1821. However, clear references to the disease are found among the earliest writings of civilized man. The Greeks recognized diphtheria as a disease of the throat and tonsils, which often suffocates its victims; the Spanish called it "garrotillo" (after a tourniquet-like method for strangling criminals), the Italians "gullet disease" and the English "throat distemper" or "morbus suffocans." Bretonneau recognized the *false membrane* as being highly characteristic of the infection and consequently named the disease *diphtheritis* after the Greek word *"diphthera"* meaning leather, skin or membrane. He observed that diphtheria is communicable and proposed that it is caused by a specific germ. However, the causative organism was not observed until 1883 (Klebs) and fully established as the causative agent until 1884 (Loeffler). Based on his observation that, although the growth of organisms in infected guinea pigs was limited to the site of inoculation, damage occurred in distant organs; Loeffler (1884) reasoned that the organism must produce a toxin. The truth of this postulate and the role of antitoxin in immunity was established when Roux and Yersin (1888) discovered the toxin in culture filtrates and Frankel, von Behring and Kitasato (1890) discovered that the sera of immunized animals contained a neutralizing substance (antibody) which protected against the toxin.

Prior to the advent of antitoxin therapy and mass immunization, diphtheria was a dreaded disease which regularly took a huge toll of lives, especially infants and young children among whom morbidity and mortality are highest. Even in advanced countries it was the single leading cause of death among children. Sometimes whole families were wiped out. For example, during an epidemic in the Atlantic Coast States in 1735-1740 some 20% of all children under 15 years of age died of the disease.

In the decades before immunization procedures were introduced, periodic pandemics occurred, which sometimes swept the world. For example, in Spain the year 1613 is known as the "year of the garrotillo," and a world-wide pandemic originated in France in 1850 which began its decline in 1885 but did not terminate until about 1941. The mortality rate tends to be high during pandemics, but its relation to the cause of pandemics is not known. The cause(s) of pandemics is an enigma but could be related to evolutionary changes in the organism and the host population (Section N).

Advances, including the introduction of antitoxin treatment in 1891, the Schick test for measuring immunity in 1913, and immunization with the toxin-antitoxin complex (von Behring, 1913) markedly improved the control of diphtheria; however, it was not until after the highly effective immunogen, diphtheria toxoid, was developed by Ramon in 1923 that the important contribution of mass immunization to control the disease was fully realized (Section N). Since then *immunization of children in advanced countries has become routine, and diphtheria seldom occurs.* Moreover, antitoxin treatment of the disease reduces the average mortality from about 18 to 5%.

Sporadic outbreaks of diphtheria still occur in the USA, involving a few hundred cases and fewer than 100 deaths annually, including an increasing number in adults. Nevertheless, there is little reason to expect that the disease will become a major health problem again so long as mass immunization of children is continued and good epidemiology is practiced. Until better world control of diphtheria is effected, it is probable that the disease will never be completely eradicated from any large population for an extended period of time. Consequently, *relaxation or abandonment of any of the current public health practices would lead to serious epidemics.* The future outlook for control of diphtheria in the world at large is far less promising than it should be, and in certain underdeveloped countries the disease remains a major medical problem.

B. Physical and Chemical Structure

Corynebacterium diphtheriae is a slender, highly pleomorphic, gram-positive, nonsporing, nonencapsulated, nonmotile, rod-shaped organism which varies from 2 to 6 μm in length and from 0.5 to 1.0 μm in diameter. The organisms are often clubshaped and sometimes pointed; they tend to appear in clumps arranged in angular aggregates resembling Chinese letters. When stained with Loeffler's alkaline blue or toluidine blue, cytoplasmic granules of polymerized polyphosphates stain metachromatically and present a reddish hue. This staining behavior lends a characteristic beaded appearance to the organisms.

No features of chemical structure are of known medical importance. Surface polysaccharides and proteins have been found and antigenic types described; however, they bear no relation to virulence, which depends principally on the amount of toxin produced.

C. Genetics

When cultured on selective-differential media containing potassium tellurite, 3 principal colonial types are seen. They were initially termed "gravis," "intermedius," and "mitis" to designate differences in the severity of disease produced (Section E); however, the relationship between virulence and type is not constant.

A more interesting aspect of the genetics of *C. diphtheriae* was introduced by the remarkable and biologically important discovery of Freeman in 1951 that *toxin production, and consequently virulence of C. diphtheriae, can be induced in nontoxinogenic strains by exposure to temperate bacteriophage,* a process called *lysogenic conversion.* Similar relations between toxinogenicity and lysogeny have since been discovered in other species of bacteria. Apparently all toxin-producing strairs of *C. diphtheriae* carry the latent virus "prophage β" and all potentially toxinogenic strains of avirulent *C. diphtheriae* are susceptible to β phage. Other phage-susceptible species, *C. ulcerans* and *C. ovis,* carried by horses and sheep, can infect man.

Strains of *C. diphtheriae* which have been ridded of prophage β and toxinogenicity by exposure to ultraviolet light can be reconverted to the lysogenic state and toxinogenicity by exposure to β phage or certain of its mutants. Evidently toxin production is specific for β phage or certain of its mutants since lysogeny produced with other phages does not result in toxinogenicity.

In lysogenic conversion, the entering DNA of the phage becomes integrated with the bacterial genome and toxin production is evidently under the direct control of prophage β. How frequently nontoxinogenic strains may be converted to toxinogenic strains or vice versa under natural conditions is not known. However, it is possible that chance lysogeny of potentially high toxin producing strains could be responsible for the initiation of epidemics. Strains differing in virulence and toxinogenicity occur, presumably due to attributes of the organisms not coded for by β phage.

Although it is conceivable that a phage mutation could occur which would lead to the production of a new and chemically different toxin, this has not been observed and, to date, the toxins produced by all strains of *C. diphtheriae, C. ovis* and *C. ulcerans* appear to be antigenically identical.

The manner by which viral DNA induces toxin production is not known; however, toxin production is favored by certain growth conditions, especially submerged culture in alkaline liquid media (pH 7.8 to 8.0) containing a certain low level of iron ranging near the value of 100 μg/ml. Toxin production is greater the longer the period between phage induction and cell lysis; apparently low levels of iron prolong the induction-lysis period and thus promote increased toxin production. The slow-growing Park and Williams strain 8 (PW8) of *C. diphtheriae,* which can grow at lower concentrations of iron than other strains, is the most potent toxin-producer isolated to date, producing toxin *in vitro* equal to about 5% of its dry weight. Despite its high *in vitro* toxinogenicity the PW8 strain is avirulent for animals. This implies that toxin is not the only determinant of virulence or that it is not produced *in vivo* by this strain of *C. diphtheriae.* Whether the *in vivo* iron concentration is unsuitable for toxin production by PW8 or whether avirulence rests on inability to colonize or some other basis is not known.

D. Extracellular Products

The only extracellular product of recognized medical importance is diphtheria toxin, a slow-acting exotoxin that inhibits protein synthesis (Section I). It is lethal for susceptible animals in quantities of 100 μg/kg. Diphtheria toxin is a heat-labile protein consisting of a single polypeptide chain having a molecular weight of about 63,000. Proteolytic digestion of "intact toxin" yields "nicked toxin," which is a complex composed of two polypeptide fragments, A (mol wt 24000) and B (mol wt 39000), linked by at least one disulfide bridge. When dissociated with thiols only Fragment A is found to be enzymatically active. Whereas Fragment A is highly stable to heat, acid and alkali, Fragment B is easily denatured. Toxicity demands the whole molecule which cannot be reconstituted from Fragments A and B. The first step in toxin activation is the nicking of toxin and the final step, the dissociation of nicked toxin. The conditions in the animal body at the cellular level apparently favor the nicking of toxin and the dissociation of nicked toxin; consequently, *intact toxin* is toxic on injection.

Animal models for quantitative measurement of toxin and antitoxin have been developed. *The minimum lethal dose* (MLD) of toxin is the smallest amount which will kill a 250 gram guinea pig within 4 to 5 days. Twelve MLD's injected by accident have been observed to kill a child. Antitoxin is measured by its capacity to protect animals against either the local or the systemic effects of toxin. Currently the measurement of toxin and anti-toxin is done by use of the international standard antitoxin stored at Copenhagen, Denmark.

In vitro precipitin (flocculation) tests are not suitable for measuring either toxin or antitoxin since toxin can spontaneously denature to form toxoid without losing its capacity to bind Ab; moreover the precipitating and neutralizing capacities of Abs do not correlate in different preparations.

E. Culture

Corynebacterium diphtheriae is an aerobe and grows poorly if at all under anaerobic conditions; it has simple nutritional needs and grows over wide ranges of temperature (15 to 40°C) and pH (7.2 to 8.0).

For many years Loeffler's coagulated serum medium was the medium used for laboratory diagnosis; however, potassium tellurite is an additional medium of great value since it inhibits most contaminating bacteria while allowing recognizable colonies of *C. diphtheriae* to develop. The color of the colonies on tellurite medium, which ranges from gray to black, is due to reduction of the tellurite to tellurium, a property shared by few of the other bacteria which may be present in the respiratory tract. The 3 major colonial types, gravis, intermedius, and mitis, can be separated on the basis of colony size, color and form. The gravis strains produce large, flat, rough dull-gray to black colonies, whereas the mitis strains produce small, smooth, convex colonies with glossy-black centers and crenated edges. Diphtheroid colonies are shiny gray-black with grayish-white edges.

Corynebacterium diphtheriae can be distinguished from *C. ulcerans* and from two common nonpathogenic diphtheroid species, *C. xerosis* and *C. hofmannii,* by colonial appearance on tellurite medium and by biochemical reactions. Distinction between avirulent and virulent strains of *C. diphtheriae* demands virulence tests of toxin production (Section G) because avirulent, nontoxinogenic strains occur which are otherwise indistinguishable from virulent *C. diphtheriae.*

F.   Resistance to Physical and Chemical Agents

Corynebacterium diphtheriae is "average" in its resistance to physical and chemical agents. It is readily destroyed by most of the common disinfectants and by heating sufficient to destroy vegetative bacterial cells. The organism is sensitive to erythromycin, penicillin and several other antibiotics. It is highly resistant to drying and may remain alive and infective for days to weeks in dust.

G.   Experimental Models

Laboratory animals vary widely in their susceptibility to infection with *C. diphtheriae* and to diphtheria toxin; the monkey, rabbit, guinea pig and pigeon being highly susceptible and the rat and mouse highly resistant. It is of singular interest that varied susceptibilities of different species of animals to diphtheria toxin correlate with the susceptibility of their respective cultured cells to the toxin *in vitro.*

Disease resembling diphtheria in man can be produced in animals by introducing the organism into the respiratory tract or skin. For example, if a large dose of virulent *C. diphtheriae* is injected intracutaneously or subcutaneously into a guinea pig, the organism will remain localized but the animal will die within 12 hours to several days (depending on dosage) due to the systemic effects of liberated toxin. Within a few hours the injection site becomes tender, edematous and hemorrhagic; degenerative changes occur in heart, liver and kidneys and the adrenals show intense congestion, which is usually accompanied by hemorrhage. Low doses of toxin produce late paralysis.

Death following the injection of either the organisms or the toxin can be prevented by prior administration of specific antitoxin. *The demonstrated protective action of antitoxin in animals challenged by injecting live organisms constitutes the "animal virulence test."* Insight into the mechanisms by which toxin produces cell injury has been gained by studies on the action of toxin on cell cultures (Section I).

H. Infections in Man

Man is the principal reservoir of *C. diphtheriae* and infection is commonly acquired from a patient, a person with subclinical infection, or a carrier, via respiratory droplet passage or direct contact. Less frequently transmission may result from insect bites (skin infection), contaminated milk, fomites or dust. Diphtheritic lesions of skin or of other sites may occasionally serve as sources of respiratory tract infection.

Following an incubation period of 2 to 7 days, pharyngeal infection is usually heralded by a headache and a sore throat of slight to moderate intensity *but notably devoid of the erythema and pain characteristic of streptococcal pharyngitis. Prostration* is a singular finding and tends to be out of all proportion to the early low grade fever which is usually present. *Differential diagnosis should, most notably, include streptococcal infection, Vincent's disease, infectious mononucleosis, mycotic infection, agranulocytic angina and adenovirus infection with exudate.*

The general course of the disease varies greatly depending on microbial virulence, host resistance and whether respiratory tract obstruction occurs; the mortality in untreated cases varies markedly among different epidemics and has ranged from about 12 to 30% or more. Presumably the highest mortalities are due to organisms that produce the greatest amounts of toxin *in vivo.* Late symptoms of injury of cranial and peripheral nerves often develop. Whereas in severe cases death may occur within 24 to 48 hours, *in other cases the patient may live for several weeks to finally die of cardiac damage.* In individuals who have previously developed antitoxin, the disease tends to be mild and is frequently not recognized because of the anamnestic response. *Presumably the anamnestic response alone in the initial absence of antitoxin can abort the development of disease when the infecting organism is of low virulence.*

Evidently the organisms first reach and colonize the surface of the mucosa of the throat before lesions appear. It is presumed that the small amount of toxin initially produced soon kills underlying epithelial cells and induces a local inflammatory exudate in which further growth of organisms is favored. With time the initial small yellowish-white lesions, which are usually on the tonsil, coalesce and may spread laterally to include wide areas over the tonsils, posterior pharynx and nares, uvula, soft palate, larynx and trachea. Infection may occasionally spread through the eustachian tube to the middle ear. The tough grayish-white *"pseudomembrane"* which forms, consists of necrotic epithelium embedded in a fibrinous exudate rich in red cells and leukocytes. When hemorrhage occurs the membrane may darken and if it is forcefully dislodged points of hemorrhage appear and a new layer of exudate forms. Membranes which eventually loosen and separate naturally may cause *respiratory tract obstruction.*

The cervical lymph nodes become swollen and tender and in severe cases massive edema of the neck may develop (bull-neck). It is notable that the *growth of the organisms tends to be largely restricted to the mucosal layer* and any spread of live organisms to the draining lymph nodes and blood, which may occasionally occur, is commonly either an early or terminal event. The reason(s) for such strict localization and failure of the organism to invade deep tissues and produce distant lesions is not known.

There are two principal causes of death, one the systemic effects of toxin and the other, local obstruction of the respiratory airway. The most life-threatening effects of the systemic toxemia are cardiac damage and depression of respiration. Cardiac failure results from necrosis of the myocardium or peripheral circulatory collapse. Myocarditis usually becomes manifest after the 2nd week and death may result during the next 2 months or later. Paralysis of the soft palate due to cranial nerve involvement usually appears after the 3rd week and leads to the characteristic regurgitation of fluid through the nose during attempts to swallow. Late complications, including paralysis of oculomotor, facial, pharyngeal, laryngeal, diaphragmatic, intercostal and peripheral muscles, may occur.

The second major cause of death, obstruction of the respiratory airway, is due to either excessive edema or a detached pseudomembrane. Membranes deep in the throat or trachea (laryngeal diphtheria) pose the greatest threat. *Obstruction by a detached membrane is a fortuitous event and can occur with great suddenness; it cannot be forecast on the basis of clinical examination,* a point which cannot be overemphasized since emergency intubation or tracheotomy can often be lifesaving.

Patients who recover from diphtheria, including those who show symptoms of neurotoxic injury, usually show no permanent effects of the disease. Clinical recovery is not attended by prompt elimination of the organisms, and the convalescent carrier state, which may persist for 1 to 2 months or longer, constitutes a reservoir of infection for others (Section N).

Extrarespiratory infections may occur in sites such as the ear, conjunctivae, vagina, anterior nares, umbilicus and skin wounds. *Skin diphtheria is largely confined to the tropics and subtropics* where it occurs with considerable frequency, and constitutes a major reservoir of infection. The rare case of extrarespiratory infection that occurs in Northern USA (less than 1% of all *C. diphtheriae* infections) is often misdiagnosed. Such infections usually begin at a site of minor injury and develop as a chronic spreading "punched-out" ulcer covered by a gray membrane. Although skin diphtheria is not as life-threatening as pharyngeal diphtheria, presumably because toxin is produced at a slower rate in skin or reaches the circulation less readily, *ulcers may persist for months and the disease often leads to peripheral neuritis* (missed cases of mild respiratory infections may likewise lead to late peripheral neuritis).

The pathogenesis of skin infections is not fully understood, and there is no good correlation between serum antitoxin levels and resistance to skin infection. Instead *resistance to skin infection apparently results from the natural acquisition of immunity unrelated to antitoxic immunity. Also skin infections often involve nontoxinogenic rather than toxinogenic strains.* The peak incidence of skin diphtheria in Southern USA occurs in late summer and early fall, evidently because skin diphtheria is commonly associated with infected insect bites, many of which involve mixed infections with staphylococci and/or streptococci.

Apparently antitoxic immunity is less effective in opposing infection by *C. diphtheriae* in skin wounds and skin lesions of various sorts than in the throat.

The role which skin infections with toxinogenic and nontoxinogenic strains play in herd immunity and the epidemiology of respiratory tract diphtheria is not known.

Taken together, the above observations exemplify the subtleties of host-parasite relationships and invite the speculation that early in the evolution of parasitism by *C. diphtheriae* the organism may have been a non-toxinogenic opportunist parasitizing insect-bitten primitive man and that later the fortuitous development of toxinogenicity by lysogenic conversion endowed the organism with enhanced powers of invasiveness and pathogenicity, especially in the respiratory tract.

I. Mechanisms of Pathogenicity

In the intact animal certain cells and tissues appear to be more susceptible than others, particularly peripheral nerves, pericardium, diaphragm, heart muscle, liver and kidneys. As stated in Section D, chemical studies involving cell cultures and animals have indicated that the toxicity of the native diphtheria toxin molecule depends on the enzymatic nicking of toxin *in vivo* and upon contributions of both Fragments A and B. Fragment A is able to catalyze ADP ribosylation of free Transferase II thus inhibiting protein synthesis by blocking transfer of amino acids from tRNA to the growing peptide chain.* Evidently procaryotic cells resist the toxin because their G factor substitutes for the role played by Transferase II in eucaryotic

---

* Transferase II (transfer factor II) has recently been renamed elongation factor 2 (EF2).

cells. Presumably either Fragment A with the help of Fragment B or the whole "nicked toxin" molecule crosses the cell membrane and makes contact with Transferase II in the cytoplasm. This evidently requires time since antitoxin can block the action of toxin on cultured cells if added as late as 30 min to 1 hour after adding toxin, but not later. It has been proposed that the events leading to toxicity involve a two-step process, the first step being the rapid fixation of toxin to binding sites on the cell surface via the hydrophobic B portion of the molecule and the second step a combination of cell membrane activities, including peptidase action, and the reduction of disulfide bonds which leads to the release of Fragment A into the cell interior where it can cause injury. Thus variations in susceptibility of various mammalian cells may depend on whether they have suitable binding sites for toxin, and membrane activities which allow fragmentation and penetration of toxin into the cells. Apparently only 200 to 300 toxin molecules are required to kill a cultured cell. Whereas a shutdown in protein synthesis by cells takes place in 1½ to 3 hours, morphologic evidence of injury does not appear until several hours later. *Recently it has been reported that cells rich in interferon are highly resistant to diphtheria toxin, presumably because interferon blocks the binding of toxin to the cell membrane.* For considerations of pathogenicity at the organ and systemic levels see Section H.

Apparently nontoxinogenic strains may sometimes produce mild respiratory tract disease often with membrane formation but without systemic toxemia. The injury produced is presumed to be due to a cell-wall toxin resembling endotoxin. Whether actual membrane formation in such cases may result from mixed infections is controversial.

Corynebacterium ulcerans produces a nonfilterable skin necrotizing toxin; some strains produce classical toxin as well.

J. Immunity

The dominant factor responsible for acquired immunity to respiratory diphtheria is antitoxin; however the relative roles played by Abs of various classes of immunoglobulins are not known. Much of the Ab may be nonprecipitating. Evidently the power of the organism to invade the respiratory mucosa and to injure depends largely on toxin, for only toxinogenic strains are known to readily produce systemic disease, and antitoxin immunity is protective. However total immunity to toxinogenic strains undoubtedly involves both antibacterial and antitoxic immunity and is never complete. The nature of antibacterial immunity is unknown.

The nature of immunity to skin diphtheria is less certain than the nature of immunity to respiratory tract diphtheria (Section H). Since skin infection occurs in an existing wound and usually involves other organisms *the factors which determine susceptibility and resistance to skin diphtheria are probably multiple and complex.*

Antitoxic immunity is powerful in preventing infection and disease but the extent to which it may discourage carriage of virulent organisms is uncertain. Little is known about the carriage of avirulent organisms in either immunized or nonimmunized populations or what, if any, influence they may have on carriage or infection by virulent organisms. In some studies the carriage rate of avirulent organisms has been found to be substantial, especially among strains of the mitis type. Healthy subjects exposed to carriers usually acquire carriage which terminates within a few days or weeks.

Although high herd immunity induced by mass immunization with diphtheria toxoid is accompanied by a low carrier rate of virulent organisms, it is uncertain whether such low carrier rates are due principally to antitoxic immunity per se or to a lesser chance of acquiring carriage because of a lowered incidence of disease and paucity of carriers in the population. Whereas virulent organisms can be carried in the face of antitoxic immunity, long term carriage is rare. It is obvious that *the nature of immunity regulating carriage of either virulent or avirulent organisms is uncertain. Indeed the factors which oppose carriage may be more concerned with forces of "antibacterial" immunity and the antagonism afforded by the normal flora of the respiratory tract than with acquired immunity to toxin.*

Because immunity to respiratory tract diphtheria is due largely to antitoxin, susceptibility to the local effects of a small dose of toxin injected into the skin (the Schick test) provides a rough measure of immunity and is occasionally used for this purpose.

The *nonimmune individual who is not allergic to the toxin* will give a *true Schick-positive reaction* by responding to the Schick test dose of toxin (1/50 MLD for the guinea pig) with a late spreading inflammatory reaction of long duration, which is characterized by erythema, swelling and tenderness. The reaction usually appears by about 24 hours and peaks on the 5th to 7th day. In contrast *the immune individual who is not allergic to the toxin* will give a *"true Schick negative"* test by failing to react to the toxin. The average threshold level of antitoxin in serum that determines whether an individual will be Schick positive or negative is about 0.03 units/ml.

The Schick test is complicated by the fact that some individuals, especially among older children and adults, may possess a delayed type of hypersensitivity to the toxin (immediate sensitivity is extremely rare). Consequently the Schick test is conducted by *injecting highly purified toxin* intradermally into the volar surface of one forearm and a *control toxoid preparation* into the opposite forearm.* In case the individual is *both*

---

*The use of highly purified toxoid preparations has largely eliminated allergic reactions due to contaminating antigens.

immune and allergic, allergic inflammation will develop at both sites within 12 to 18 hours but, because the true toxin reaction is lacking, will fade within 48 to 72 hours. This is the so-called *"pseudoreaction."* In the occasional individual who is *nonimmune but allergic* to the toxin the early allergic reaction present at both sites will fade by 48 to 72 hours leaving a persisting toxin reaction (*Schick reaction*) at the toxin site. This is called the *"combined reaction."* Allergic reactions to toxin are rare in young children but increase in incidence with age and are lower in toxoid-immunized populations than in populations not artificially immunized, presumably as the result of a higher carrier rate and more frequent inapparent infections in nonimmunized populations. *The Schick test often incites the production of antitoxin, especially if the anamnestic response is involved.*

Although the Schick test is only an approximate measure of existing immunity, it is an even less accurate measure of susceptibility to the actual disease since it does not fully allow for the anamnestic response, which in the face of infection can be profound, or exposure to highly virulent organisms, which can overwhelm some Schick-negative individuals. However, *in general, individuals who are Schick-negative are immune to diphtheria and those who are Schick-positive are susceptible* and need immunization. Since administration of the usual immunizing dose of toxoid can cause violent reactions in allergic individuals, adults and older children to be immunized should first be tested for sensitivity to toxoid. The usual, albeit not infallible procedure, is to administer the *Moloney test* with 0.1 ml of a 1:10 dilution of toxoid, and then to proceed cautiously with immunization, depending on the nature of the local response. *In allergic individuals 3 weekly injections using the Moloney test dose of toxoid will usually serve to reawaken a good immunity.* Although Moloney-negative individuals can be given the full immunizing dose of toxoid, it is safer to give repeated small doses of toxoid.

K. Laboratory Diagnosis

In diphtheria the difference between recovery and death often hinges on the promptness of administering antiserum; delays involving hours or even minutes may be crucial. No rapid and reliable routine method for laboratory diagnosis has been developed to date. Consequently it is current practice to diagnose the disease on clinical grounds alone, which is most difficult in mild cases, and to use the laboratory only to judge the accuracy of clinical diagnosis in retrospect.

Material used for laboratory diagnosis should be collected directly from the lesions by the physician before any therapy is begun and promptly transported to the laboratory for staining and culture. A smear, stained with dilute fuchsin, should be made and examined to rule out the possibility of Vincent's disease, and a tellurite plate, a blood agar plate and a Loeffler's slant should be inoculated and incubated at 37°C. No attempt should be made to identify *C. diphtheriae* by examining smears made from material taken directly from the lesions because the results are frequently erroneous and misleading. The cultures should be observed after 15 to 24 hours at 37°C and, if negative, again at 48 hours. The blood plate should be examined for beta hemolytic streptococci, the tellurite plate for colonies typical of *C. diphtheriae* and Loeffler's medium for organisms with morphology typical of *C. diphtheriae*. Special procedures for rapid diagnosis, including the fluorescent Ab technique on direct smears, and toxin detection in saliva have been proposed but have not been found to be suitable for routine laboratory use.

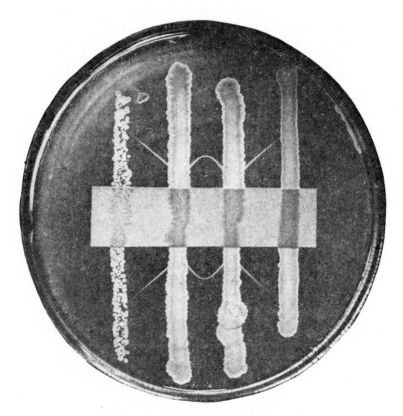

Figure 14-1. Gel diffusion test for toxin-producing *Corynebacterium diphtheriae*. The organism are streaked at right angles to a paper strip impregnated with diphtheria antitoxin. The outer two strains are avirulent, whereas the two inner strains are virulent. Note the precipitin arcs indicating lines of identity. A known virulent strain can be placed next to a suspected virulent strain to establish identity of a toxin-producing isolate (E. O. King, M. Frobisher and E. I. Parsons. Am. J. Pub. Health *39*:1314, 1949).

Final identification of virulent *C. diphtheriae* demands a virulence test for toxinogenicity which is done with a pure culture derived from a tellurite colony. In some laboratories animal virulence tests have been replaced by the simpler *in vitro* double-diffusion precipitation-in-gel test of toxinogenicity devised by Elek, which serves to specifically identify toxin-producing organisms growing on agar into which specific antitoxin is allowed to diffuse (Figure 14-1). The test is only reliable when done with care using suitable antiserum, control strains and base medium. A new virulence test is a toxigenicity test on cultured HeLa cells.

L. Therapy

If clinical evidence indicates that there is any reasonable chance that the patient has diphtheria, material for culture should be collected promptly and antitoxin treatment initiated as soon as skin and ophthalmic tests for serum sensitivity can be completed (about 30 minutes).

Administering antiserum to an occasional nonsensitive patient who may not have diphtheria only entails the risk of developing serum sickness which is generally self-limiting, and not permanently harmful. The lethal activities of the toxin are so irrevocable that *no patient should be denied antiserum if there is any likelihood that the disease is diphtheria.*

Since toxin is quickly bound by tissues and soon rendered unavailable for neutralization by Ab, *the success of therapy demands early treatment* with an *adequate dose of antitoxin* (Table 14-1). Antitoxin treatment begun on the first day is highly effective but after the 4th day is of little or no value. The mortality among untreated patients varies greatly in different epidemics ranging from about 12 to 50%. Among all treated cases the average mortality is about 5%. Antitoxin, consisting of concentrated gamma globulins from immune serum, is usually administered intramuscularly but never subcutaneously as a single dose (100 U to 500 U/lb body weight)

TABLE 14-1

The Influence of Delay in Antitoxin Administration on Mortality in Diphtheria

	Antitoxin Given On	Cases	Case Fatality (%)
	1st day of disease	225	0
	2nd day of disease	1,441	4.2
	3rd day of disease	1,600	11.1
	4th day of disease	1,276	17.3
	5th day of disease and upward	1,645	18.7

Russell, W. T.: The epidemiology of diphtheria during the last forty years. Med. Res. Council, Special Report. London No. 247, 1943.

in order to ensure maximum immediate neutralization of toxin.* Another objective is to provide an excess of free Ab which will persist for many days beyond the time when a clinical cure is effected. A second injection of antiserum may occasionally be needed. Patients who are sensitive to the antitoxic serum pose a special problem and must be either placed on "desensitization treatment," which consists of giving the antiserum cautiously in small increasing increments, a procedure which carries considerable risk of anaphylaxis, or given antisera produced in some other animal, such as the goat, sheep, rabbit, or man (such antisera are often not available). Antibiotics such as erythromycin, penicillin and the tetracyclines have no therapeutic value against preformed toxins but tend to discourage continued toxin formation and complications due to other pathogens. In addition, antibiotic therapy tends to render the patient noninfectious for others by hastening the elimination of *C. diphtheriae* from the primary lesions and arresting convalescent carriage which otherwise often persists for 1 to 2 months or longer. Convalescent carriers pose a public health problem and should remain in isolation until carriage is terminated (Section N). *The exercise of vigilance to prevent or relieve respiratory tract obstruction is another matter of first order importance in therapy and cannot be emphasized too strongly.*

Future prospects for improving therapy are difficult to envision unless research on the mechanisms of toxin action should reveal some biochemical means for blocking injury by toxin after it has become fixed to cells.

M.   Reservoirs of Infection

The principal reservoirs of infection are human carriers and patients with the disease. On rare occasions animals have served as reservoirs; for example, unpasteurized milk from cows with teat lesions incited by hand milkers who were carriers has caused epidemics. Public health practices in advanced countries are highly effective for limiting and controlling reservoirs of infection and usually succeed in arresting epidemics.

N.   Control of Disease Transmission

An understanding of the epidemiology of diphtheria in different populations demands consideration of numerous factors including the carrier rate, passive immunity in the newborn, opportunities for the acquisition of active immunity both naturally and artificially, opportunities for maintaining active immunity by artificial booster immunization or carrier contact and other possible factors.

Experience has shown that most infectious diseases are only effectively prevented when immunization procedures are introduced which strongly

*One unit of antitoxin neutralizes about 100 MLD of toxin.

immunize a large majority of the population; in the case of diphtheria when 70% or more of the total population is immune, the chain of disease transmission is severely weakened, and its spread becomes limited and manageable.

Prevention of diphtheria in the USA currently rests principally on mass immunization of children, carrier regulation, and isolation of active cases. In addition, possible contacts are given booster immunization and sometimes short-term prophylaxis with antibiotics.

Populations in which mass immunization is not practiced are typified by high carrier rates of virulent organisms (about 5%), a high proportion of immune adolescents and adults, and frequent and sizable epidemics confined principally to children (Chapter 9). *Populations in which mass immunization is practiced* are typified by low carrier rates (a small fraction of 1%), a low proportion of immune adolescents and adults and infrequent small epidemics, often among adolescents and adults.

In *"nonimmunized" populations* immunity is often incited naturally by carried organisms, especially by strains of low virulence, and is maintained in the majority of adults by frequent contact with carried organisms. Consequently many newborn infants in such populations (probably 90% or more) are well protected by maternally derived Ab. Moreover, because of the high carrier rate an appreciable number of such infants become actively immunized by carrier contact while they still possess a degree of protection due to maternal Ab. Those infants with maternally derived Ab who do not experience contact with carried organisms lose their passively acquired immunity after a few months and become highly susceptible to diphtheria. They constitute a large susceptible segment in such populations upon which epidemics feed.

In populations in which mass immunization of young children is practiced essentially all individuals remain immune for several years and sometimes through puberty into adulthood, and the case and carrier rates are low. Because of the low carrier rate, the booster effect of carrier contact on the maintenance of immunity among adults is largely lost. However, epidemics among adolescents and adults are infrequent in such populations because the reservoirs of infection, the carriers and cases of disease, are low. Since many mothers in such populations do not have appreciable serum levels of antitoxin most infants lack passive immunity and need early immunization with toxoid.

Ideally immunization should not only be instituted early in infancy (about 3 months of age) but should be continued into childhood and even adulthood with booster doses of toxoid given at appropriate intervals. Otherwise even the capacity to respond anamnestically may ultimately wane to the point where its effectiveness in the face of infection is largely lost. Substantial immunity is maintained for about 3 to 5 years after immunization. Immunity is not absolute and individual responses vary greatly.

Because continuing immunization into adulthood is not commonly performed, and herd immunity among adults and adolescents is low in advanced countries *it is important to detect and control carriers and to take emergency prophylactic measures in the case of outbreaks of the disease.* This should include quarantine of patients, booster immunization and administration of antitoxin or preferably antibiotics to possible contacts. Cases of active disease should be isolated through convalescence until carriage of the organisms is eliminated; nasal carriage persists longer than throat carriage. Whenever chronic carriers of virulent organisms are discovered in a population, efforts should be made to eliminate carriage. Certain antibiotics, especially erythromycin, are useful for this purpose. Incubationary carriers are rarely detected and constitute especially dangerous reservoirs of infection. A better understanding of the role of phage on virulence conversion in nature and of the factors which determine the carrier state is needed in order to devise more effective methods for detecting and eliminating the carrier state.

Immunization of children is commonly accomplished with highly purified toxoid precipitated with alum or adsorbed to aluminum phosphate gel as adjuvant. The immunizing dose consists of 10 to 20 LF units in a 0.5 to 1.0 ml volume. The material is usually combined with pertussis vaccine and tetanus toxoid to form a pool of Ags. Immunization is begun at 3 months of age. Two doses of the Ag given one month apart followed by the first booster dose at 1 year of age and the second at the beginning of school usually provide adequate protection until adolescence. Schick testing a few individuals before and after immunization serves as check on the adequacy of immunization. In mass-immunized populations allergy to toxin is infrequent in young children and Schick testing prior to immunization is not practiced. In adults allergy to toxin is more frequent and, as indicated in Section J, immunization of adults should be carried out on an individual basis after Moloney testing.

References

Barksdale, L.: *Corynebacterium diphtheriae* and its relatives. Bact. Rev. *34*:378, 1970.

Belsey, M. A., Sinclair, M., Roder, M. R. and Leblanc, D. R.: *Corynebacterium diphtheriae* skin infections in Alabama and Louisiana. New Eng. J. Med. *280*:135, 1969.

Brooks, G. F., Bennett, J. V. and Feldman, R. A.: Diphtheria in the United States, 1959-1970. J. Inf. Dis. *129*:172, 1974.

Collier, R. J. and Kandel, J.: Structure and activity of diphtheria toxin. I. Thiodependent dissociation of a fraction of toxin into enzymatically active and inactive fragments. J. Biol. Chem. *246*:1496, 1971.

Drazin, R., Kandel, J. and Collier, R. J.: Structure and activity of diphtheria toxin II. Attack by trypsin at a specific site within the intact toxin molecule. J. Biol. Chem. *246*:1504, 1971.

Freeman, V. J.: Studies on the virulence of bacteriophage-infected strains of *Corynebacterium diphtheriae*. J. Bact. *61*:675, 1951.

Gill, D. M. and Dinius, L. L.: Observations on the structure of diphtheria toxin. J. Biol. Chem. *246*:1485, 1971.

Gill, D. M.: Structure-activity relationships in diphtheria toxin. J. Biol. Chem. *246*: 1492, 1971.

Gill, D. M., Pappenheimer, A. M. and Uchida, T.: Diphtheria toxin, protein synthesis, and the cell. Fed. Proc. *32*:1508, 1973.

Groman, N. B.: Evidence for the active role of bacteriophage in the conversion of nontoxigenic *Corynebacterium diphtheriae* to toxin production. J. Bact. *69*: 9, 1955.

Wilson, G. S. and Miles, A. A.: *Topley and Wilson's Principles of Bacteriology and Immunity*. Vol. II 5th Ed., Williams and Wilkins, Baltimore, 1964.

Chapter 15

Bacillus

Members of the genus *Bacillus* are sporeforming rods of the family *Bacillaceae* which grow best under aerobic conditions. Most species are saprophytic inhabitants of soil, water and decaying organic matter. Very few are highly pathogenic for animals and only one, *Bacillus anthracis,* the cause of anthrax (Charbon, Milzbrand), is a pathogen for man. On rare occasions, nonpathogenic species, such as *Bacillus cereus* and *Bacillus subtilis,* produce opportunistic infections in man and animals.

A. Medical Perspectives

Anthrax played an important role in the early development of medical bacteriology (Chapter 1). It was employed as a model by such investigators as Davine, Koch and Pasteur; Koch used *B. anthracis* to perfect his pure culture technique and to prove his famous postulates on the etiology of infectious diseases, and Pasteur demonstrated the worth of his attenuated anthrax vaccine in a public field trial which brought him world acclaim.

Herbivores, ranging from goats to wild elephants, are common primary hosts of *B. anthracis;* infection is most frequent *in cattle* and occurs in "anthrax regions" where the soil serves as the reservoir of infection. Diseased herbivores and their products and remains serve as the principal sources of infection for carnivores and omnivores, including man. Being a sporeformer, the organism can remain alive and infectious on dried material for decades, including all sorts of animal products that have not been properly sterilized or disinfected. Anthrax has been the bane of domesticated bovines for centuries. It was probably among the "7 plagues of Egypt" at the time of the Pharaohs and *remains a threat to the livestock industry in areas where pastures with suitable soils have become contaminated.*

Recent studies have thrown new light on the natural history of *B. anthracis* and lend strong support to the concept that the organism is a *soil saprophyte* which, in its pathogenetic role, should be considered to be an opportunistic pathogen and *facultative parasite.* Infection of herbivores commonly results from spores. However, the relative importance of different routes of infection is uncertain and varies, depending on whether the animals are stable fed or pastured. In grazing animals, infection probably occurs most frequently through breaks in the skin (many of which are inflicted by biting insects) which are exposed to soil, dust, or water contaminated with spores. Infection probably occurs less often by ingestion or inhalation of contaminated forage foodstuffs and dust. Carriage of the organism does not occur and transmission by blood-sucking insects is infrequent. Direct animal-to-animal transmission among herbivores is uncommon and *the organism is not capable of perpetuating itself in nature solely within animal hosts.* Although it has long been known that "anthrax regions" are established by contamination of the soil by diseased animals and their excreta and products, the manner by which the organism persists in such regions has been difficult to elucidate. Fields have been known to harbor the organism for 50 to 100 years under circumstances in which the chances of recontamination were highly unlikely. It was first proposed that spores may be able to survive in soil for decades without germinating and that long spore survival plus periodic recontamination by diseased animals may account for prolonged persistence of the organism in soil. *Instead, it now appears that prolonged persistence in soil depends on irregular periodic cycles of spore germination, vegetative growth and resporulation as determined by the microenvironment.* Prolonged persistence of the organism occurs only in soils having pH values near neutrality or above, particularly calcareous soils, and demands spore-vegetative cell-spore recycling. Recycling occurs under restricted conditions of temperature, moisture, pH and available organic matter. Such conditions are only met periodically in "incubator areas" which are often only small locales within a field. Water-killed grasses and decaying vegetation overlaid by silt deposits favor the growth of *B. anthracis.* Ponds, ephemeral streams, etc. provide ideal incubator areas when flood-drought cycles occur to cause growth and killing of vegetation and when minimum daily temperatures above 60°F obtain to promote spore formation. Humidity above 80% and temperatures above 70°F favor spore formation. Consequently, within an "anthrax region" the production of crops of spores adequate to incite anthrax outbreaks tends to occur focally and sporadically, sometimes years apart. *It is highly probable that once the organism becomes established in the soil of a favorable region it seldom if ever fails to persist indefinitely as a saprophyte unless incubator areas are eliminated by natural events or altered land management, such as soil drainage and tillage.* Obviously it is important to maintain constant vigilance to avoid the establishment of new "anthrax regions" since, once established, they may remain indefinitely as a cardinal sin of pollution against both man and beast.

Anthrax, which has been endemic in Africa, Asia and Europe for centuries, was spread to distant lands with the advance of Western civilization. Anthrax regions in the USA are distributed principally in areas of old Spanish and French settlements of the South and Southwest, along the routes of the early cattle drives from Texas to Montana and in the neighborhood of tanneries in the New England States.

Although good sanitary practices and vaccination have brought anthrax in developed countries under good control, large numbers of domesticated and wild animals and thousands (20,000 to 100,000) of human beings are afflicted each year in the world at large. Anthrax remains one of the major livestock diseases in the world and threatens to increase unless better control practices are adopted. It is currently a danger to the animals on the big game preserves of Africa where adding oral vaccines to the waterholes is being considered.

Anthrax is declining in the USA. During the period 1945 to 1952, 2,785 outbreaks and 14,708 deaths occurred among livestock. Small outbreaks continue to occur almost annually, with livestock losses ranging from tens to hundreds. However, recent human infections number only in the tens. *If all individuals at high risk were to be appropriately immunized with the new improved vaccines available, the incidence of human anthrax in the USA should drop to near the vanishing point.*

B. Physical and Chemical Structure

Bacillus anthracis is a large sporeforming gram-positive nonmotile, encapsulated rod averaging about 1.5 × 6 μm in size. Whereas cultured organisms grow in long chains and form central spores, organisms in infected hosts occur singly and in short chains and are devoid of spores. The capsule, a polypeptide composed of D-glutamic acid, is antiphagocytic and is one of the key materials in virulence, the other being a toxin. The formation of both toxin and capsules is favored by the presence of CO_2 and media rich in serum. Other components of the cell are not of medical importance.

C. Genetics

Mutants of B. anthracis vary in their nutritional requirements, ability to form spores, colony morphology, virulence and resistance to drugs, bacteriophage and lysozyme. Repeated subculture tends to select for avirulence. Sporulation bears no relation to virulence because nonsporing mutants and sporeformers are equally virulent when injected into animals.

D. Extracellular Products

Among the numerous extracellular substances produced, a toxigenic system composed of 3 proteins or lipoproteins designated factors I, II and III is apparently responsible for the toxic manifestations of anthrax. Whereas no one factor alone is toxic, combinations of factors I + II, II + III or I + II + III are toxic, the last combination being the most toxic.* The injected toxin-complex causes edema and necrosis in the rabbit's skin and death in most species of animals when given intravenously. The toxin injures phagocytes and "enhances virulence" when injected simultaneously with the organisms. Factor II, which is alleged to be the most immunogenic, is often referred to as the "protective antigen." However, the other factors are also protective immunogens.

E. Culture

Bacillus anthracis is aerobic and facultatively anaerobic. It grows best at a pH range of 7.0 to 7.4 over a temperature range of 12 to 45°C (optimum 35°C). The organism can be grown on simple media. Colonies are small, opaque, grayish-white and tough. They have fringed edges due to hair-like loops consisting of long, parallel chains of cells. The colonies of encapsulated strains are smooth and those of nonencapsulated strains are rough. Spores are only formed in old aerobic cultures. The organism is proteolytic and fermentative.

F. Resistance to Physical and Chemical Agents

Whereas vegetative forms of B. anthracis possess the usual resistance of nonsporing bacteria, the spores are highly resistant to drying, heat (boiling 10 minutes) and most disinfectants (oxidizing agents are the most lethal). The organism is susceptible to a number of antibiotics (Section L).

G. Experimental Models

Only an exceptional animal species is completely resistant to injected B. anthracis, the frog being one; epidemics involving many species have

* The toxin-complex is often designated simply as toxin.

occurred in zoos. Whereas the white rat is markedly resistant, the mouse and guinea pig are highly susceptible. An unexplained reverse relationship exists between resistance to infection and to toxin, resistant species being more susceptible to toxin than susceptible species.

Herbivores, such as sheep and cattle, have been used as experimental models. Ingested spores survive stomach acid and pass through the intestinal epithelium to germinate and multiply in the submucosa and draining lymph nodes. In about 80% of cases (range 75 to 100%) the organisms reach the blood to produce septicemia and toxin-death, often within a few hours or even minutes after symptoms are first noticed (apoplectic anthrax). Indeed, except for possible cases of primary meningitis, death in both animals and man infected with *B. anthracis* is almost invariably a consequence of septicemia and the action of the toxin. Some strains or breeds of animals, belonging to species that are highly susceptible to natural infection, such as the long-fleeced algerian sheep, are unusually resistant to infection.

H. Infections in Man

Anthrax is usually established in man by spores present in animal products and seldom by direct host-to-host passage of vegetative cells, such as by blood-sucking insects. Infection commonly results from spores entering through skin abrasions (95% of cases in the USA); on occasion spores enter through the respiratory tract by inhalation of dusts from hair, hides, ivory, bone meal, feces or wool (woolsorter's disease). In some regions of the world the organisms may enter the alimentary tract following ingestion of raw or inadequately heated meat, milk or blood products. The disease is most frequent among herdsmen, veterinarians, butchers and industrial workers who handle animal products (industrial anthrax).

The *localized lesion* of *cutaneous anthrax,* the *malignant pustule,* is usually solitary; it is characteristically painless, necrotizing, seropurulent, ulcerous and hemorrhagic leading to a *black eschar,* the basis of the term "anthrax" which is derived from the Greek word "anthrakos," meaning coal. It is surrounded by an area of intense nonpitting edema due to a gelatinous exudate in the tissue. The lesion heals spontaneously in about 80% of subjects without appreciable local lymphadenopathy. In about 20% the draining lymph nodes become so extensively involved that septicemia and death due to the toxin result within a few days.

Pulmonary anthrax is almost always fatal because septicemia leading to early toxin-death (24 hrs) usually sets in before effective therapy can be instituted. Nonproductive cough and vague pulmonary symptoms commonly prompt the mistaken diagnosis of "viral pneumonitis," unless anthrax is suspected. Apparently the inhaled spores do not remain in the alveoli but, instead, are transported by alveolar macrophages to the lymph

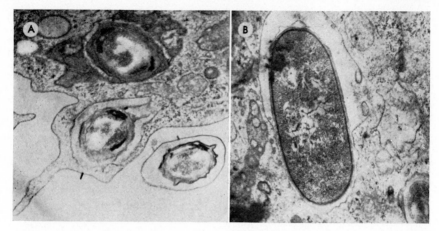

Figure 15-1. Sections of alveolar macrophages containing (*A*) phagocytized anthrax spores, 17,000 ×. (*B*) Anthrax spore that germinated in the phagosome, 27,200 ×. (From Shafa, F., Moberly, B. J., and Gerhardt, P.: J. Infect. Dis. *116*: 401, 1966. The University of Chicago Press.)

nodes where they germinate and usually overwhelm lymph node defenses to incite a septicemia. Spores germinate within macrophages *in vitro* and presumably *in vivo* as well (Fig. 15-1). The resulting vegetative cells escape and multiply extracellularly. Hemorrhagic mediastinitis is a common complication. Pleurisy associated with precordial distress and with organisms in the pleural fluid occurs on occasion and can serve as a useful diagnostic clue.

Meningitis or pneumonia secondary to mediastinal lymph node involvement is very rare. Subclinical infections may sometimes occur, as indicated by specific Ab responses, but chronic infection or carriage of the organisms in either animals or man has not been documented.

I. Mechanisms of Pathogenicity

Spores of B. anthracis *are engulfed by macrophages but are not destroyed.* The spores germinate to yield vegetative cells that escape and multiply extracellularly. Following skin infection a few vegetative organisms probably always reach the draining lymph nodes but only occasionally (20% of cases) escape to the blood in sufficient numbers to cause septicemia and death. In systemic disease the organisms are usually confined largely to lymph and blood channels and rarely enter the CNS. At death the bacilli may reach such enormous numbers in animals of certain species that blood capillaries, especially of the viscera, can become literally occluded with them.

The toxic basis of death in septicemia was not appreciated until the discovery of anthrax toxin in 1954. The mechanisms responsible for systemic toxicity are poorly understood. Evidently injury is irreversible because *late destruction of bacilli with antibiotics does not prevent toxin death*. Toxin seems clearly to have primary toxicity for the CNS, leukocytes and certain cultured cells. However, there is little evidence to indicate what cell types may be attacked to account for the edema, hemorrhage and necrosis of the local lesion, the malignant pustule, or the hemoconcentration, extreme anoxia, respiratory failure and renal failure of systemic shock.

Virulence is due to the combined effects of the toxin and the capsule; whereas both are antiphagocytic, the toxin has the additional pathogenetic activity of being toxic for other cells as well as phagocytes.

J. Mechanisms of Immunity

The forces of immunity presented by different animal species appear to vary greatly. Compared to animals, man is moderately resistant. In susceptible animals and man the destruction of *B. anthracis* probably depends largely on the activities of neutrophils. It is questionable whether cellular immunity or nonantibody anthracidal substances present in serum play a significant role in either innate or acquired immunity. Antigenic virulence factors of most bacteria are effective immunogens and, in theory, acquired immunity to anthrax should involve the combined effects of antitoxic and anticapsular Abs. However, protection by anticapsular Ab has only been demonstrated in the mouse. The capsular polypeptide acts as a hapten. The role of antitoxin in protecting against infection is easily demonstrated; it evidently acts on toxin in two ways, namely, by blocking its antiphagocytic effects and by blocking its "toxic effects." The fact that natural infection and certain live vaccines induce greater and more durable immunity than toxin preparations suggests that important immunogens other than toxin exist.

The best animal vaccines are spore preparations made from lowly virulent, nonencapsulated, toxinogenic strains plus alum-precipitated toxin administered with or without antiserum. Although an effective alum-precipitated, pooled toxin is available for use in man, better vaccines will doubtlessly be developed in the future as knowledge about immunogens and the nature of anthrax immunity advances. A better means of assessing anthrax immunity in man and more information on the possible role of anticapsular Abs in immunity are needed.

K. Laboratory Diagnosis

Blood should be examined by smear and culture in all subjects in whom anthrax is suspected. Wright-stained smears of exudates from early, but not from late, cutaneous lesions usually show an abundance of typical encapsulated organisms, whereas sputum from patients with pulmonary anthrax (which, locally, is largely restricted to pulmonary lymph nodes) seldom yields positive smears or cultures. In septicemia, Wright-stained smears of centrifuged sediment of blood cleared of red cells with 3% acetic acid often reveal the organism. Specimens should be cultured on a selective medium that will suppress contaminants; suspected outgrowth should always be checked for pathogenicity in guinea pigs or mice since other organisms, especially *B. cereus,* closely resemble *B. anthracis.* Other identification procedures include the string-of-pearl type of growth on nutrient agar containing 0.05 unit penicillin per ml, lysis by γ phage and fluorescent Ab techniques applied to direct smears from lesions or cultured organisms.

L. Therapy

In cutaneous anthrax, treatment with animal antisera, which is moderately successful, has been replaced by highly effective drugs, especially penicillin and the tetracyclines. In pulmonary anthrax, drug therapy and supportive measures are usually initiated too late to be of value.

M. Reservoirs of Infection

Whereas the only constant and permanent reservoir of infection of herbivores is soil, the only reservoir for man is the infected animal or its excreta or products.

N. Control of Disease Transmission

Anthrax is a reportable disease in both man and animals. Control of the disease in animals by vaccination and sanitary practices is the first and major step for preventing infection in man. Vehicles that may contribute to infection in animals and man and to contamination of soil are: fertilizers, animal feeds, animal products, offal and wastes, industrial wastes, fodders, hay, insects, carrion birds and wild animals. Insects that have fed on sick or dead animals are a special hazard to man. Also in recent years many cases of human anthrax have been traced to bone meal. Control measures include restrictions on the importation, movement, handling and processing of vehicles and animals from anthrax areas and disposal of infected animals by burning or deep burial in lime pits. It must be kept in mind that vegetative cells which escape from the infected animal via excreta, blood and exudates readily form spores. Unique examples of breaks in surveillance that have led to human epidemics are: a large outbreak during World War I due to imports of contaminated hair used to make shaving brushes and a recent small outbreak among factory workers engaged in cutting and polishing ivory.

Alum-precipitated toxin-vaccines and occasionally chemoprophylaxis are useful measures for protecting individuals in high-risk occupations, such as veterinarians. In anthrax regions, vaccination must be repeated annually to be effective.

References

Lincoln, R. E., and Fish, D. C.: Anthrax toxins. In *Microbial Toxins*. Vol. III. T. C. Monte, S. Kadis and S. J. Ajl, eds. New York: Academic Press, 1970, p. 361.

Shafa, F., Moberly, B. J., and Gerhardt, P.: Cytological features of anthrax spores phagocytized *in vitro* by rabbit alveolar macrophages. J. Infect. Dis. *116*:401, 1966.

Van Ness, G. B.: Ecology of anthrax: anthrax undergoes a propagation phase in soil before it infects livestock. Science *172*:1303, 1971.

Wilson, G. S., and Miles, A. A.: *Topley and Wilson's Principles of Bacteriology and Immunity*. 5th ed. Baltimore: Williams & Wilkins, 1964.

Chapter 16

Clostridium

Tetanus, 218

Gas Gangrene, Anaerobic Cellulitis and *Cl. perfringens* Food Poisoning, 224

Botulism, 228

The genus *Clostridium* includes the anaerobic members of the family *Bacillaceae;* it comprises a large number of species of gram-positive spore-forming rods. Although most species lead only a saprophytic existence, some exist as both saprophytes and parasites. Many species can assume the role of *opportunistic pathogens* for man. Clostridia are present in soil, dust, sewage and mud and some species are often abundant in animal and human feces and sometimes in the female genital tract. A special attribute of the clostridia is that, in common with all members of the family *Bacillaceae,* the spores which they form are extremely resistant to physical and chemical agents and can survive in nature for long periods of time. Unlike the more susceptible vegetative cell they are highly resistant to many common disinfectants and some spores can survive 100°C. Consequently, the sterilization procedure of autoclaving at 120°C for 15 minutes or more is expressly designed to kill spores.

The pathogenic clostridia are characterized by their capacity to synthesize and secrete highly potent exotoxins which are important in the pathogenesis of the 5 diseases of man that they produce, namely, *tetanus, gas gangrene, anaerobic cellulitis, Cl. perfringens food poisoning and botulism.* Although the clostridia are widely distributed in nature, infections due to these organisms are comparatively rare. Lacerated external wounds, large or small, particularly puncture wounds contaminated with foreign materials such as soil, dust, feces, bits of clothing and fragments of glass, that often contain spores, favor the development of clostridial infections by providing anaerobic and other conditions that allow spore germination and bacillary multiplication. Injuries involving the intestines or uterus also frequently provide sites of clostridial infection.

It should be emphasized that irrespective of the cause, e.g., chemical or physical injury or lack of blood supply, any area of dead or dying tissue to which clostridial spores may gain access is a potential site of clostridial infection. Since the organisms cannot tolerate the aerobic environment of live tissue with an intact blood supply, they can only extend the initial lesions by secreting toxins that kill surrounding tissues, which they can then invade. Except for specific antitoxins, host defenses have little opportunity to act against organisms in the zone of infection. Phagocytes cannot migrate far from vital vascularized tissue to reach organisms in the zone of devitalized tissue, especially organisms contaminating foreign bodies. These facts emphasize the importance of prompt and thorough debridement and drainage of wounds, with removal of all devitalized tissue and foreign materials. The above considerations also make it obvious that the virulence factors of clostridia must rest with their extracellular products and that the defenses of the host must rest largely with antitoxic Abs. The fact that aerobes growing in a wound can promote the growth of anaerobes by creating anaerobic conditions also emphasizes the necessity of directing therapy at control of these organisms as well as the anaerobes themselves.

All of the medically important clostridia are obligate anaerobes which can be cultivated in meat infusion broth media containing a reducing agent, such as thioglycollic acid, or on agar plates incubated in an anaerobic jar (90% N_2 plus 10% CO_2). As a general rule they produce malodorous organic amines derived from their enzymatic action on proteins and peptides. Chopped meat and milk media are commonly used for obtaining primary cultures. A few clostridia are partially aerotolerant and will grow feebly in the presence of low tensions of O_2.

An abbreviated classification scheme of the medically important clostridia is presented in Table 16-1.

Tetanus

A. Medical Perspectives

Tetanus, a horrifying clinical disease, was recognized by the early Greeks and old drawings depict the lumbar spasm of tetanus.

The infectious nature of *tetanus* or *lockjaw* was not proven until 1884 when Carlo and Rattone produced tetanus in rabbits. Kitasato isolated the causative agent *Cl. tetani* in pure culture in 1889. In 1890, Von Behring and Kitasato succeeded in immunizing animals by injecting small amounts of toxin and Ramon developed the highly effective immunogen, tetanus toxoid, in 1923. Prior to the development of antitoxin, and especially toxoid, tetanus was a major medical problem, particular during wars and in other high-risk situations. Tetanus, gas gangrene and other wound infec-

TABLE 16-1
A Classification of the Medically Important Clostridia

Position of Spores	Both Proteolytic and Saccharolytic Properties		Proteolytic but No Saccharolytic Properties	Saccharolytic but No Proteolytic Properties	Neither Proteolytic nor Saccharolytic Properties
	Proteolytic Predominating	*Saccharolytic Predominating*			
Central or subterminal	Cl. sporogenes Cl. histolyticum Cl. bifermentans Cl. sordellii Cl. botulinum A, B, F	Cl. perfringens A to E Cl. septicum Cl. chauvoei Cl. novyi A to D Cl. botulinum C, D, E	—	Cl. fallax Cl. multifermentans	—
Oval and terminal	—	—	—	Cl. tertium	Cl. cochlearium
Spherical and terminal	—	—	Cl. tetani	Cl. tetanomorphum Cl. sphenoides	—

Adapted from Willis, A. Trevor: *Clostridia of Wound Infection.* London: Butterworths & Co. Ltd., 1969.

tions have taken a frightful toll of lives during wars; it is said that during the Civil War in the USA many more soldiers died of wound infections (largely tetanus and gas gangrene) than died in battle. Tetanus antiserum given the wounded saved many lives during World War I and mass immunization with toxoid during World War II reduced deaths from tetanus to essentially zero in the allied military forces! At the present time the estimated annual case rate of tetanus in the world at large exceeds 350,000 and the number of deaths 160,000. Currently in the USA the annual number of deaths from tetanus is less than 200, largely because of immunologic control. Tetanus is readily prevented by immunization, which represents one of the triumphs of immunology. *Since therapy is often of little or no benefit, every effort should be made to promote routine immunization with tetanus toxoid, including proper booster injections for those at high risk.* With adequate attention to active immunization and prophylactic passive immunization with antiserum, tetanus does not pose a future medical problem of any magnitude in the USA.

B.   Physical and Chemical Structure

Clostridium tetani is a relatively slender gram-positive rod about 3 to 5 μm in length and 0.3 to 0.7 μm in diameter. The young vegetative cells have peritrichous flagella. They develop swollen spores that are located terminally giving the cells the appearance of drumsticks or rackets (Fig. 16-1). The mature spores, which are spherical, do not stain readily with the Gram stain. Accordingly, developing spores appear as nonstainable refractile inclusions within the cell.

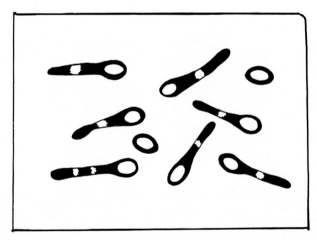

Figure 16-1. A diagrammatic representation of the racket appearance of *Clostridium tetani* undergoing sporulation. Note the spherical spores that are mature and free of any vegetative cytoplasm. The clear areas in the vegetative part of the cell are vacuoles.

C. Genetics and Variability

Antigenic variability of somatic and flagellar Ags occurs. However, all strains of *Cl. tetani* produce only one antigenic type of tetanus toxin.

D. Extracellular Products

All virulent strains of *Cl. tetani* produce tetanus toxin which is a powerful heat-labile (5 min at 65°C) neurotoxin (tetanospasmin) liberated from the organisms by diffusion as well as by autolysis. One milligram will kill 50 to 75 million mice. It has been estimated that 0.13 μg is a lethal dose for man. The toxin is a crystallizable protein of about 60,000 mol wt. It spreads from the local site of infection along motor nerves and via the blood.

The toxin acts in the inhibitory synapses of nerves by blocking the normal function of the inhibitory transmitter. *Tetanolysin, another toxin, is distinct from "tetanus toxin";* it causes lysis of erythrocytes and kills neutrophils.

E. Culture

Clostridium tetani grows only under the strictest of anaerobic conditions. For further information on culture see chapter introduction.

F. Resistance to Physical and Chemical Agents

See chapter introduction.

G. Experimental Models

There are no routine animal models for tetanus although laboratory animals are susceptible to tetanus toxin.

H. Infections in Man

Clostridium tetani is an opportunistic pathogen which initiates infection by chance. It is important to emphasize that even trivial puncture wounds, especially if "dirty," are potential sites of tetanus infection; for example, tetanus can occur at injection sites in drug addicts and at the site of an insect bite. *Neonatal tetanus* (tetanus neonatorum) occurs when the severed umbilical cord stump (a debilitated tissue) becomes infected soon after birth. It is a major cause of infant mortality in underdeveloped countries; it is most effectively controlled in these regions by immunizing prospective mothers. *Since the organism does not invade healthy tissue having an adequate blood supply, tetanus infection remains localized in the wound area. The clinical symptoms are the result of the action of tetanus toxin which diffuses from the site of infection to reach the blood stream.* High concentrations of toxin exist at the local site and continue to diffuse and reach the blood stream for some time after growth of the organisms has been arrested by antimicrobial therapy. In general the severity of tetanus is inversely proportional to the incubation period, which may vary from several days to many weeks, and to the onset period (interval between the first sign and generalized spasm). If the incubation period is less than 9 days and the onset period is less than 48 hours, the attack will probably be severe. Tetanus is characterized by violent, painful convulsive contractions of voluntary muscles, usually beginning in the muscles near the infected wound (local tetanus) and the masseter muscles, followed by progressive involvement of other voluntary muscles throughout the body. Once observed the symptoms of severe tetanus are never forgotton; the rigid facial muscles create a sneering countenance and the painful contraction of voluntary muscles, especially of the legs and back, may be so violent that vertebrae are fractured. The patient assumes a rigid position with arched back, the weight being borne on head and heels (opisthotonos) (Fig. 16-2). Fever, sweating and cardiovascular symptoms, which are usually present during the peak of severe illness, apparently result from overactivity of the sympathetic nervous system. Death usually results from spasms affecting the muscular apparatus involved in respiration. In a nonfatal case of tetanus the symptoms progress to a point and then gradually regress.

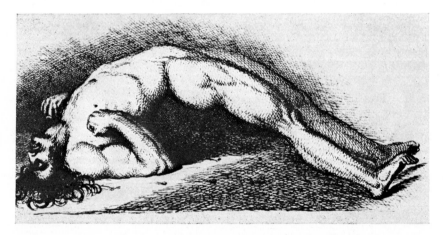

Figure 16-2. Tetanus in a British soldier wounded in the battle of Corunna in 1809. Note the rigid position of opisthotonos and the "sardonic smile" of lockjaw involving spastic paralysis of muscles which persist in working against one another despite intense pain and exhaustion. Reproduced from a drawing by the Scottish surgeon Sir Charles Bell published in 1832 in his book *The Anatomy and Philosophy of Expression.*

I. Mechanisms of Pathogenicity

The toxin has a strong affinity for certain nerve tissues and once combined cannot be neutralized by antitoxin. It alters nerve function but no cytotoxicity or local lesions have been found. Ultimately the toxin is inactivated somehow because *patients who recover from tetanus have no apparent residual neurologic defects*. The action of tetanolysin, the cytotoxin, does not contribute importantly to pathogenesis.

J. Mechanisms of Immunity

Tetanus toxin can be neutralized by specific Ab providing the Ab can react with the toxin before it reaches its target.

K. Laboratory Diagnosis

The diagnosis of *tetanus* rests on clinical grounds; as a rule the fully developed disease is not confused with other diseases. The organism is sometimes difficult to isolate and its mere presence in a wound does not confirm or establish the existence of tetanus. Consequently wound culture is not done routinely.

L. Therapy

There is no successful specific treatment for *tetanus*. Proper nursing care should include the placing of a padded tongue depressor between the teeth to prevent biting of the tongue, and removal of URT secretions by suction and postural drainage. Sedatives and muscle relaxants are very important to prevent tetanic seizures. A centrally acting muscle relaxant such as diazepam and a sedative such as sodium thiopental form a useful combination. *Large doses of penicillin, tetracycline or some other effective antibiotic should be administered to all patients with tetanus.* Antibiotics not only act directly on *Cl. tetani* but restrict the growth of contaminating aerobes which help to maintain anaerobic conditions favoring *Cl. tetani*. Active immunization with tetanus toxoid should also be started at the onset of therapy. Since antimicrobial chemotherapy does not interfere with the diffusion of preformed toxin from the site of infection, antiserum should be administered although it may seem to be of little or no value. Human tetanus-immune globulin is preferred over horse serum antitoxin. Careful debridement of the wound and the establishment of adequate drainage under the protective cover of antitoxin is highly important. Tracheostomy with nasogastric-tube feeding, to prevent inhalation of pharyngeal contents and to permit artificial respiration, is another valuable therapeutic measure in severely ill patients. A combination of curare and intermittent positive pressure ventilation through a cuffed tracheostomy tube and anti-coagulants may be indicated in the most severe cases. Patients with mild tetanus usually survive, but in those with more severe disease the best treatment only reduces the mortality from about 45% to 20%.

M. Reservoirs of Infection

Clostridial spores are widespread in nature and are particularly prevalent in soil and feces.

N. Prevention of Disease

Mass immunization with tetanus toxoid is the first and most effective step for preventing tetanus. Ideally, active immunization with alum precipitated toxoid should be performed during the first year of life, and a booster dose of toxoid should be given at the age of 15 to 19 years and each decade thereafter. Preventive measures following injuries which predispose to tetanus include wound debridement, drainage, administration of antitoxin, a booster dose of toxoid and early chemoprophylaxis with drugs, such as penicillin or tetracyclines. *In all instances in which there is any reasonable chance that tetanus may develop a booster dose(s) of toxoid should be given. Antibiotics alone are ineffective if given later than about 4 to 6 hours after injury.* If foreign antiserum to which the patient is sensitive is given, it may be rapidly rendered ineffective by immune elimination; there is also the problem of anaphylaxis and serum sickness.

Gas Gangrene, Anaerobic Cellulitis and Cl. perfringens Food Poisoning

Gas gangrene and anaerobic cellulitis are often mixed infections involving more than one of a number of species of clostridia. If untreated they are highly fatal diseases. Whereas gas gangrene involves infection of voluntary or uterine muscle with severe local and systemic effects, anaerobic cellulitis, a less serious disease, involves subcutaneous tissue with effects which are more severe locally than systemically.

Since *Cl. perfringens* is the most common and important species involved in the diseases covered in this section, it is given the most attention.

A. Medical Perspectives

Gas gangrene is chiefly a disease of warfare although a significant number of civilian cases occur. The disease has always been an important medical problem and although improvements in prophylaxis and therapy have been made it will undoubtedly continue to be of substantial concern for the foreseeable future.

B. Physical and Chemical Structure

Clostridium perfringens is an encapsulated, nonmotile, gram-positive rod that occurs singly and in pairs. Unlike *Cl. tetani* the spores occur in the subterminal position.

C. Genetics and Variability

Clostridium perfringens is classified into 5 serologic types based on the toxins it produces. Other species of clostridia involved in gas gangrene also produce many and varied toxins. Variants of *Cl. perfringens* that produce low levels of some of the toxins can be isolated.

D. Extracellular Products

Clostridium perfringens, type A, the most frequent and important agent of gas gangrene in man, produces a wide array of extracellular toxins that possess varying degrees of necrotizing and hemolytic activity. The most important toxin is the α toxin which is lecithinase C. Other products include collagenase, proteinase, hyaluronidase and deoxyribonuclease. Certain "food poisoning" type A strains produce a heat-labile enterotoxin; they usually produce only small amounts of α toxin. The other clostridial species also produce many different toxins which probably play important roles in the pathogenesis of anaerobic cellulitis.

E. Culture

Clostridium perfringens, type A, can be identified by culture on agar plates containing egg yolk. Lecithinase C (α toxin) causes a precipitate to form around the colonies because it destroys the emulsifying action of lecithin. Specific Ab to α toxin can be incorporated in the agar to neutralize this effect and thus identify the toxin. Double zones of hemolysis, an inner zone of complete hemolysis and an outer zone of partial hemolysis, give a characteristic "target" appearance to *Cl. perfringens* colonies on blood agar.

F. Resistance to Physical and Chemical Agents

For information on this topic see chapter introduction.

G. Experimental Models

Guinea pigs, pigeons and rabbits are the most susceptible animals to experimentally induced *gas gangrene*. They usually die within 12 to 48 hours. At death the injection site is purplish red and the adjacent muscles and subcutaneous tissues crepitate when pressed due to bubbles of gas in the tissues. *Clostridium perfringens* can be typed by protecting infected mice with specific antitoxins.

H.   Infections and Disease in Man

Clostridium perfringens, Cl. oedematiens (Cl. novyi) and *Cl. septicum* are the most frequently recognized etiologic agents of gas gangrene; however, other species of clostridia have been isolated from gangrenous lesions. Although the latters' etiologic roles in the disease are uncertain, it is possible that by synergistic action they may sometimes contribute substantially to pathogenesis. Mixed infections with clostridia or with clostridia and certain pyogenic organisms are common. Only about 5% of patients with wounds and devitalized tissues potentially suited for the development of gas gangrene develop the disease. Clostridial infections of the uterus account for a large proportion of gas gangrene seen in a civilian practice; they are primarily the result of criminal abortions. With new abortion laws now in effect, it is probable that such infections will soon be rare.

The incubation period in gas gangrene may be as short as 4 to 6 hrs and as long as 72 hrs or more. Intense edema and pain develop in the wound. Moderate fever, early delirium and extreme prostration occur. Leukocytosis and thrombocytopenia are common findings and massive hemolysis leading to anemia and renal failure may be observed within 24 hours after onset.

If gas gangrene infection is of sufficient magnitude, enough toxin will be produced to incite a progressive cycle of tissue destruction and extension of the infection. The organisms ferment tissue carbohydrate and protein components leading to the accumulation of bubbles of hydrogen gas between muscle fascia and in other tissues, which can be detected by crepitation under pressure. Excessive gas promotes extension of the lesion by dissecting tissue and exerting pressure effects that interfere with the blood supply. Without treatment the death rate is essentially 100%.

Food poisoning caused by *Cl. perfringens* type A is more common than was formerly realized. It is due to ingestion of contaminated food containing preformed *Cl. perfringens* enterotoxin which causes hypersecretion by the small intestine. This type of food poisoning is similar to staphylococcal food poisoning. The incubation period is less than 18 hours. *Enteritis necroticans* is a rare but severe intestinal disease caused by type F strains of *Cl. perfringens* and is usually diagnosed only during surgery or at necropsy.

I.   Mechanisms of Pathogenicity

Gas gangrene is a progressive infection because the various toxins destroy tissue, thus creating an expanding anaerobic environment in which the organisms can spread. The primary lesion may extend to involve an entire extremity. Massive edema coupled with gas production within the tissues, toxemia and hemolytic anemia account for the pathologic picture. Alpha toxin probably plays the dominant role in the destruction of tissue.

J. Mechanisms of Immunity

The only known acquired defense against gas gangrene results from Abs specific for extracellular toxins. Antibodies are probably incapable of neutralizing toxin that has fixed to cells. Passive immunization is probably of some benefit when antitoxin is given early, in conjunction with the other modes of treatment.

K. Laboratory Diagnosis

The diagnosis of *gas gangrene, clostridial cellulitis* or other clostridial infections such as *postabortal sepsis* rests largely on clinical findings. Bacteremia seldom occurs in *gas gangrene* but is common in postabortal sepsis. Since clostridia are present in small numbers in most external wounds, their isolation is of little significance in diagnosis of wound infections unless a quantitative approach is used. Gram-positive bacilli can sometimes be found in abundance in smears from biopsied muscle and identified by the fluorescent Ab method.

L. Therapy

Early diagnosis of gas gangrene and prompt application of proper therapeutic regimens are very important if success is to be achieved. The success of treatment is often tenuous and a few patients die even when treated by all the modes of therapy, namely, surgical debridement, antibiotics, antitoxins, hyperbaric oxygen and, in extreme cases, the old procedure, amputation. Amputation may sometimes succeed when other methods fail.

The most important approach for treating gas gangrene and less severe clostridial wound infections involves immediate extensive surgical debridement and open drainage. The administration of hyperbaric oxygen to create aerobic conditions in the wound provides another form of therapy which can produce prompt improvement in the patient. Penicillin is the antibiotic of choice. Polyvalent antitoxin appears to have very limited value and has been discontinued as a method of treatment in many medical centers.

M. Reservoirs of Infection

Clostridial spores are ubiquitous in nature and are particularly prevalent in soil and feces. Infection occurs on occasion due to lack of aseptic practices such as the use of unsterilized surgical instruments.

N.   Prevention of Disease

Gas gangrene can only be prevented by guarding against traumatic injuries and instituting proper prophylactic procedures for patients at risk, such as wound debridement, drainage and chemoprophylaxis. Because of the large number of species of organisms and toxins involved, immunization with toxoids is not considered to be practical even among persons at high risk.

Anaerobic cellulitis is usually a mixed infection with more than one clostridial species, often including species such as *Cl. bifermentans, Cl. fallax* and *Cl. histolyticum;* it is a limited infection and does not involve muscles. The disease may represent an infection that has become stabilized as the result of host control of the infection which in turn limits the amounts of necrotizing toxins produced.

Botulism

Botulism is a rare, but severe and often fatal, type of intoxication caused by eating food containing toxin produced by growth of the causative organism *Cl. botulinum.*

The disease is more common in animals than in man. For example, large outbreaks have been reported in cattle, poultry and ranch-raised mink. One of the principal concerns of wildlife management groups has been the massive outbreaks of botulism among waterfowl that feed in shallow waters rendered anaerobic at certain times by the high oxygen demand of aquatic flora.

A.   Medical Perspectives

The first case of human *botulism* described (van Ermengem, 1896) was caused by pickled ham contaminated with *Cl. botulinum.* Most of the cases of botulism in the USA result from eating home-canned vegetables and some fruits, whereas in Europe most cases are due to eating smoked, salted or spiced fish and meats. A total of 1,669 cases and 948 deaths due to botulism was recorded in the USA between 1899 and 1967; during the past decade an average of about 20 cases/year was reported.

The threat of botulism will continue in the future because heat-sterilization methods are always subject to errors. It is seldom that even a few months pass without the threat of botulism from large batches of improperly sterilized commercially canned foods.

B.   Physical and Chemical Structure

Clostridium botulinum is a motile gram-positive rod that occurs singly or in short chains. Swollen spores generally appear in a subterminal position.

C. Genetics

Clostridium botulinum comprises several types of organisms, each of which produces at least 1 of 6 serologically distinct forms of the exotoxin. The production of toxins C and D has been shown to depend on lysogeny by certain bacteriophages and some strains of *Cl. botulinum* have been shown to produce both A and F toxins.

D. Extracellular Products

Clostridium botulinum produces a powerful neurotoxin. It is a classical exotoxin which is destroyed by boiling (100°C) for 10 min, but not by gastric juices; hence it passes the stomach to reach the small intestine where it is absorbed. The 6 known serologically distinct toxins and the respective types of organisms that produce them are designated A, B, C, D, E, and F. Less than 1 μg of a toxic polypeptide derivative (mol wt 150,000) is lethal for man and 1 mg will kill 20,000,000 mice.

E. Culture

It is important to stress the fact that growth of *Cl. botulinum* does not occur at pH values below 4.5. Consequently those home-canned foods which are highly acidic do not cause botulism.

For additional information on culture see chapter introduction.

F. Resistance to Physical and Chemical Agents

Canning techniques in which boiling water is used under ambient conditions (cold pack method) are not adequate for killing spores of *Cl. botulinum* which can withstand 100°C for 3 to 5 hours. This accounts for the high incidence of outbreaks following consumption of home-canned food.

G. Experimental Models

Laboratory animals are highly susceptible to botulinum toxin and are useful for detecting and identifying the toxin in food; the type of toxin in a food can be determined by demonstrating specific protection with a known antitoxin. Mice are commonly used for this purpose.

H. Disease in Man

It should be emphasized that botulism is not an infectious disease but, instead, is a severe intoxication resulting from the ingestion of improperly preserved food containing preformed toxin. Cases due to types A, B and E are the most common; those due to F are rare. The E toxin is most often associated with improperly preserved fish.

After absorption in the intestine the toxin reaches susceptible neurons by way of lymphatics and the blood circulation. Symptoms usually begin within 12 to 36 hours after ingestion of food containing the toxin, but may appear as early as a few hours or as late as 8 days. The shorter the incubation time the more severe the disease. Cranial nerve terminals are affected earliest and most severely. Symmetric descending weakness or paralysis occurs, but sensory and mental functions are not impaired. Hearing may be altered and vision is impaired, probably because of involvement of extraocular muscles. Diplopia develops and nystagmus and fixed dilated pupils may be present. No fever develops, but the mouth tends to become dry and painful. Double vision is followed by difficulty in swallowing and bulbar paralysis. Death usually results from respiratory failure, cardiac arrest, aspiration pneumonia or a combination of these events. The fatality rate is high, but varies with the type of toxin ingested; 75% of patients ingesting type A toxin succumb, whereas only a 20% mortality occurs following ingestion of type B toxin. Recovery from botulism is slow but is usually complete without permanent damage.

I.   Mechanisms of Pathogenicity

Botulinal toxin is absorbed by mucous membranes throughout the gastrointestinal tract and ultimately blocks transmission in cholinergic nerve fibers. Toxins have decreasing affinity for nerve tissue in the order A > E > B; as a result, type A toxin can only be detected in the blood for a few days after ingestion, whereas type B toxin persists for as long as 3 weeks. The toxin apparently interrupts neural impulses close to the point of final branching of terminal nerve fibrils short of the motor end-plate and prevents release of acetylcholine.

J.   Mechanisms of Immunity

Immunity against botulism rests on neutralization of the toxin by antitoxic Ab and can be induced by either active or passive immunization. Antitoxin can neutralize free toxin but is ineffective against toxin that has been fixed to tissue.

K.   Laboratory Diagnosis

The diagnosis of botulism rests primarily on clinical findings. If the suspected food is available, helpful confirmatory evidence of botulism may be gained by injecting mice with extracts or saline emulsions. If the toxin is present the mice will die within 24 hours but can be protected by type specific antiserum. Fresh serum from the patient with botulism is also toxic for mice; the toxin can be identified by mouse protection tests with A, B, E and F antitoxins.

L.   Therapy

Since death from *botulism* is a consequence of respiratory failure, *early tracheostomy and the use of a mechanical respirator are of utmost importance.* In addition, trivalent type A-B-E antitoxin should be administered promptly by the iv route.* Type E or bivalent type A-B antitoxin can be used if the causative type is known. Since the antisera are produced in horses, appropriate skin tests for horse serum sensitivity must be conducted prior to administration of antitoxin. Antiserum administration should never be delayed while waiting for laboratory results. Present evidence indicates that mortality is significantly decreased by proper administration of specific antitoxin in combination with supportive therapy. *Prophylactic administration of antitoxins is important and effective in those subjects who have eaten toxin-containing food but whose symptoms of botulism have not become apparent. The first case of botulism, in a group of individuals who have eaten contaminated food, becomes an important index case demanding that prompt measures be taken to protect the remaining exposed subjects.*

M.   Reservoirs of Contamination

The spores of *Cl. botulinum* are widespread in nature throughout the world and are found in many soils and muds. Since the organisms are so ubiquitous, all raw foods may be considered to be potentially contaminated. The different types of *Cl. botulinum* have distinctive geographic distribution patterns. Whereas type A is the most common type in North America, type B predominates in Europe. Type A organisms predominate in the soils of Western USA but type B organisms predominate in Central and Eastern USA. The type E organism has been isolated from salmon on the West Coast and from fish of the Great Lakes. Type F *Cl. botulinum* has been found in salmon and marine sediments of the West Coast and in crabs from the York River of Virginia.

N.   Prevention of Disease

If food to be preserved is contaminated with botulinum spores, the environment in the food mass is anaerobic, and the pH is near neutrality or above, any spores which may survive the heat treatment may germinate, grow, and produce toxin.

The gas produced in canned food may or may not cause the can to bulge and a detectable foul odor may be evident. *Suspected food should never be tasted since only a short sojourn of a trace of food in the mouth, even if rejected, may allow absorption of enough toxin to be lethal.*

* Botulinal antitoxins are available at the USPHS Center for Disease Control, Atlanta, Georgia, and the Lederle Laboratories, Pearl River, New York.

Botulism can be effectively prevented by properly canning and preserving foods. As an additional precaution, all home-canned foods that could support the production of botulinal toxin should be boiled for at least 10 minutes before consumption. Antiserum together with other prophylactic measures, including induced vomiting, gastric lavage and purgation, should be used whenever there is reasonable chance that toxin-containing food has been ingested. Although active immunization with pentavalent toxoid is effective, it is only employed for high-risk individuals, e.g., laboratory workers who handle the toxin. The toxoid has been used successfully for protecting animals against botulism.

References

Ajl, S. J., Kadis, S., and Montie, T. C.: *Microbial Toxins.* Vols. I, IIA, III. New York: Academic Press, 1970 and 1971.

Craig, J. M., and Pilcher, K. S.: Clostridium botulinum type F isolated from salmon from the Columbia River. Science *153*:311, 1966.

Eklund, M. W., Poysky, F. T., and Reed, S. M.: Bacteriophage and the toxigenicity of *Clostridium botulinum* type D. Nature (New Biol.) *235*:16, 1972.

Hitchcock, C. R., Haglin, J. J., and Arner, O.: Treatment of clostridial infections with hyperbaric oxygen. Surgery *63*:759, 1967.

Hoeprich, P. D.: *Infectious Diseases.* New York: Harper & Row, 1972.

Koenig, M. G., Drutz, D. J., Mushlin, A. I., Schaffner, W., and Rogers, D. E.: Type B botulism in man. Am. J. Med. *42*:208, 1967.

Williams-Walls, N. J.: Type E botulism isolated from fish and crabs. Science *162*: 375, 1968.

Willis, A. Trevor: *Clostridia of Wound Infection.* London: Butterworth & Co., Ltd., 1969.

Chapter 17

Escherichia coli and Related Enteric Bacteria

The normal human adult excretes in the feces approximately 100 billion *Escherichia coli* organisms daily, along with lesser numbers of other gram-negative rods of the family *Enterobacteriaceae*. The members of this family are widespread in nature and range from obligate parasites to saprophytes with low parasitic potential (Table 17-1). They include the genera *Salmonella* and *Shigella,* whose members are commonly pathogenic. Most of the other members of this family are normally nonpathogenic but can act as opportunistic pathogens. It is this group of opportunistic enterobacteria that will be considered in this chapter.

Escherichia coli and some of its close relatives are commonly referred to as "coliforms." Included in the coliform group are members of the genera *Enterobacter, Klebsiella, Serratia, Hafnia, Citrobacter,* and *Arizona.* In

TABLE 17-1

Genera and Species of the Medically Important Members of the Family *Enterobacteriaceae*

Tribe	Genera and Species
Eschericheae	Escherichia coli Shigella dysenteriae Shigella flexneri Shigella boydii Shigella sonnei
Edwardsielleae	Edwardsiella tarda
Salmonelleae	Salmonella choleraesuis Salmonella typhi Salmonella enteritidis Arizona hinshawii Citrobacter freundii
Klebsielleae	Klebsiella pneumoniae Klebsiella ozaenae Klebsiella rhinoscleromatis Enterobacter cloacae Enterobacter aerogenes Enterobacter hafniae Enterobacter liquefaciens Serratia marcescens
Proteeae	Proteus vulgaris Proteus mirabilis Proteus morganii Proteus rettgeri Providencia alcalifaciens Providencia stuartii

Modified from: Edwards, P. R., and Ewing, W. H.: *Identification of Enterobacteriaceae,* 3rd ed. Minneapolis: Burgess Publishing Co., 1972.

addition to the coliforms, most of which ferment lactose, the relatively non-pathogenic enteric rods include non-lactose-fermenting organisms of the genera *Proteus* and *Providencia*.

The prototype species of the coliforms, E. coli, *has probably been studied more intensively than any other microbe. It is important as an indicator of fecal contamination* (for example, in water supplies) because it is abundant in feces, durable in external environments and easily detected. Other highly pathogenic bacteria that are spread by fecal contamination, such as *Salmonella typhi,* are less durable in the external environment and usually comprise only a small fraction of the total number of organisms excreted by an infected individual; because of small numbers they frequently cannot be detected in water containing them; nevertheless this water would be unsafe for human consumption.

The first of the following sections centers on *E. coli* and some general properties of the coliforms. This is followed by separate discussions of the

TABLE 17-2

Properties of the Coliforms and Related Enterobacteria

Genus	Lactose Fermentation	Motility	Other Useful Characteristics
The coliform group			
Escherichia	+	+	Metallic sheen on eosin-methylene-blue media; flat colonies
Enterobacter (Aerobacter)	+	±	Raised colonies; lack sheen on eosin-methylene-blue media
Klebsiella	+	−	Mucoid colonies due to capsules
"Paracolon bacilli"	− or slowly +	+	
Serratia	+	+	
Citrobacter	+	+	
Arizona	variable	+	
Proteus	−	+	Some species exhibit swarming motility on solid media; rapidly degrade urea to yield ammonia
Providencia	−	+	Urea not degraded

+ = most strains positive.
− = most strains negative.
± = some strains positive.

genera *Klebsiella* and *Proteus,* and brief mention of a similar genus, *Alcaligenes,* that belongs to a different family. Table 17-2 summarizes some important properties of these organisms.

Escherichia coli

A. Medical Perspectives

Despite the fact that *E. coli* is not highly pathogenic, it is of great medical importance because of the frequency and potentially serious nature of the infections that it causes. The organism normally lives in the intestine without causing apparent harm. However, because of its presence in feces, it often reaches, and incites disease in, other areas of the body, especially the urinary tract and peritoneum. In the decades before the advent of modern surgery and antimicrobial chemotherapy, many died of *E. coli* infections such as peritonitis attending rupture of the appendix and perforations of the intestine. Even today, such infections with this organism are often difficult to manage because of rapidly changing patterns of drug resistance; hence they continue to be important causes of illness.

The increasing use of immunosuppressive therapy and antibiotics for a variety of conditions has led to an increased incidence of all kinds of opportunistic infections, including those caused by enteric bacteria. Such infections will undoubtedly remain a major medical problem in the future. In addition, it has been shown that some strains of coliforms are relatively virulent because they produce enterotoxins and that certain strains can cause epidemic enteritis, especially in infants. Thus, *E. coli* and its relatives have commanded increasing respect for their pathogenic capabilities as more is learned about them.

B. Physical and Chemical Structure

All members of the family *Enterobacteriaceae* have a similar antigenic structure (Fig. 17-1). They are gram-negative, nonsporing rods, measuring about 1.0 to 2.0 $\times$ 0.5 μm. Motile organisms of this family possess peritrichous flagella. The flagellar protein (H Ag) is serologically distinct in various strains, even within a single species. If a K Ag (capsular or envelope polysaccharide or protein) is present, it may mask the structural somatic (O) lipopolysaccharide Ag that is an integral part of the cell wall. In *E. coli* the K Ags are grouped into 3 categories: L, A and B. Serotypes of *E. coli* are determined by the various combinations of O, K and H antigens. For example, the strain designated O119:B14:H6 has somatic Ag 119, capsular Ag B14 and type 6 flagellar Ag.

Electron microscopy reveals an abundance of pili scattered over the cell surface of many strains of enterobacteria (Fig. 2-3). Some of these

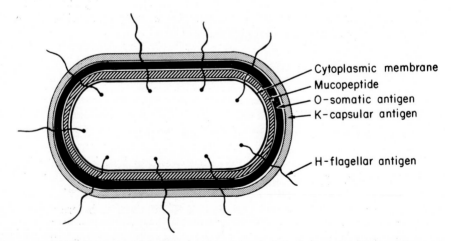

Figure 17-1.   Diagram depicting the antigenic components of enterobacteria.

organelles are sex pili that function in conjugation (Chapter 4), and some serve as attachment sites for specific bacterial viruses. It has been suggested that the common or "hold fast" pili may serve for attachment of bacteria to host cells (Chapter 2).

C. Genetics

Much of what is known about microbial genetics was learned from studies of E. coli. By using transduction and conjugation as tools, the "chromosome" of *E. coli* has been partially mapped. References concerning the genetics of this group of organisms are included at the end of this chapter.

Of particular medical importance is the ability of the enterobacteria to rapidly acquire multiple drug resistance through exchange of episomes or plasmids, such as resistance transfer factors (Chapter 4).

Episomes also control toxinogenicity and the production of bacteriocins (Chapter 2) by these bacteria. For example, colicins, which are bacteriocins formed by certain strains of *E. coli,* kill other strains selectively. Hence they can be used for strain typing, a procedure of value in epidemiologic studies.

The relationships between the enterobacteria are complex and there is often a thin dividing line between genera. These organisms are highly variable and cannot always be neatly categorized. Genes are readily transferred between different species within a genus and even between different genera. Therefore, it is not surprising to find that the taxonomy of the *Enterobacteriaceae* is constantly being changed.

D. Extracellular Products

Although enterobacteria produce a wide variety of enzymes, little is known about the roles of secreted enzymes in the pathogenesis of enterobacterial infections. It is thought that the bacteriocins produced are important in regulating the normal flora by antibiosis.

Certain strains of *E. coli* isolated from human beings and animals produce enterotoxins. Both heat-stable and heat-labile forms of enterotoxin have been described; however, it is postulated that these represent different forms of the same toxin. The heat-stable enterotoxin contains protein, but there is evidence suggesting that the active protein may be part of the same carbohydrate-lipid-protein complex that contains the glycolipid responsible for endotoxin activity. It is of interest that the cholera-like symptoms produced by the heat-labile protein are prevented by antitoxin made against pure cholera enterotoxin.

E. Culture

Escherichia coli has simple cultural requirements. It can grow on a defined glucose-salts medium and thrives on many richer media, such as blood agar and eosin-methylene-blue medium. It is facultatively anaerobic and readily ferments glucose, lactose and certain other sugars, producing both acid and gas. All of the coliform group have similar growth requirements. Biochemical and serologic tests are used to identify the various organisms.

F.   Resistance to Physical and Chemical Agents

The usual physical and chemical agents employed for disinfection are generally effective against the enteric rods; also, these organisms are readily killed by pasteurization and by chlorination. They can live for weeks to months at room temperature or below, and can survive for long periods in soil, water, or other suitable environments.

The enterobacteria are susceptible to a number of antibiotics, but resistant strains tend to emerge rapidly in the face of antibiotic therapy.

G.   Experimental Models

Rabbits and other laboratory animals are used to produce experimental urinary tract (UT) infections with the coliforms. Swine have been employed extensively to study the effects of *E. coli* enterotoxin. The mouse model has been used to demonstrate virulence of *E. coli*. Certain strains that are prevalent in UT infections are virulent for young mice when injected intracerebrally, whereas others, such as those causing enteritis in infants, are avirulent for mice.

H.   Infections in Man

The coliforms are the most common cause of UT infections, the majority of which result from invasion by endogenous normal flora along an ascending route. Organisms enter the UT by natural means or may be introduced on catheters or other instruments. *Their persistence in the UT is favored by anesthesia, paralysis, or any other agency that interrupts the normal voiding reflex, or by anatomic abnormalities that permit retention of urine.*

Urine is an excellent culture medium and readily supports the growth of *E. coli* and many of the other bacteria that gain entrance into the bladder. The resulting cystitis may be self-limiting, or the infection may ascend further to reach the kidneys and cause pyelonephritis. The *E. coli* O serotypes most frequently found in UT infections are 1, 2, 4, 6, 7, 25, 50 and 75.

Urinary tract infections are much more common in females than in males for various reasons; for example, in the female the alimentary and UT orifices are proximal to each other, the urethra is short, and the infecting organisms may be mechanically introduced into the urethra during sexual intercourse. Urinary tract infections occur in persons of all ages and stand among the most frequent infections of the female. They may be acute, intermittent or chronic, symptomatic or asymptomatic and can lead to permanent renal damage with all of its consequences; therefore, they are currently the subject of intensive research.

It is convenient to classify UT infections into 4 categories: uncomplicated and complicated acute infections and asymptomatic and chronic bacteriuria. *Uncomplicated acute infections* are characterized by production of the usual symptoms of cystitis (dysuria, pain on voiding) or pyelitis (flank pain, chills and fever) in patients without a history of prior UT infection. In these patients, endogenous *E. coli* is almost always the etiologic agent. *Complicated acute infections* occur in persons with anatomic abnormalities of the UT, and tend to recur until the abnormality is corrected. In contrast to uncomplicated acute infections, which occur most often in women of childbearing age, complicated acute disease is seen most often in young men. In both conditions, however, *E. coli* is most often the etiologic agent. *Asymptomatic bacteriuria* occurs mostly in women without clear-cut UT disease; however, a careful history usually reveals that these patients have had some symptoms of UT infection in the past. The organisms isolated from them are often *E. coli,* but other species of enterobacteria are also frequently found. Asymptomatic bacteriuria is detected in about 5% of women in early pregnancy; unless treated, approximately 40% of these women develop acute symptomatic UT infections later in pregnancy or in the postpartum period. *Chronic bacteriuria* is most frequent in the elderly, the members of both sexes being equally affected. These individuals have repeated episodes of symptomatic infection, usually due to structural abnormalities, such as scarring or strictures, in the UT. Infections of the UT must be distinguished from contamination of collected urine by quantitative urine culture (Section K).

Endogenous coliforms can often be isolated from the infected appendix removed by operation during attacks of appendicitis, from the infected peritoneum, or from any sort of abscess in areas exposed to fecal contamination, e.g., decubitus ulcers. Although these are often "mixed infections," *E. coli* usually predominates and is a major offender.

Enteropathic *E. coli,* comprising a few strains of the organism, is the cause of epidemics of *infantile diarrhea* in nurseries; serotypes 055, 0111 and 0127 are implicated most often. It is of singular interest that these serotypes rarely, if ever, cause UT infections. Other serotypes of *E. coli* have been reported to cause outbreaks of diarrhea in preschool children as well as in the newborn.

Recent evidence suggests that certain enterotoxin-producing strains of *E. coli* are responsible for outbreaks of a cholera-like disease. It is claimed that the production and action of the enterotoxins of *E. coli* and *Vibrio cholerae* are similar (Chapter 20); however, *E. coli* enterotoxin appears to be less potent than cholera toxin.

Some data suggest that a change of environment permits the establishment of a new gut flora with a predominance of *E. coli* serotypes common in the new environment. *Mild diarrheal illness* may occur during the interval when the newly acquired serotypes are becoming established as part of the normal flora. This could explain many cases of the common "traveler's complaint."

Secondary infections in tissues already injured by other bacteria are often caused by the coliforms. The coliforms are also the principal cause of meningitis during the first few weeks of life, especially in infants with meningocele or other predisposing conditions.

I.   Mechanisms of Pathogenicity

The mechanisms of pathogenicity of *E. coli* and similar organisms are poorly understood. Endotoxins probably contribute to the production of disease, as discussed in Chapter 9. The polysaccharide K Ags of some strains may also be important in inhibiting Ab-C killing and phagocytosis by masking other Ags. Although certain O serotypes are definitely associated with particular diseases, such as UT infections and infantile diarrhea, there is no evidence to indicate that the O Ag is itself a virulence factor.

Studies on the pathogenesis of *E. coli*-induced diarrhea and colitis have led to the conclusion that strains of *E. coli* can cause intestinal disease by either of at least 2 mechanisms: some strains produce enterotoxin, resulting in a diarrheal syndrome resembling cholera, and other strains, which are capable of penetrating epithelial cells, produce a dysentery similar to shigellosis.

J.   Mechanisms of Immunity

Immunity to the coliforms is also poorly understood. Natural "barriers" are important in preventing infection. For example, *under normal circumstances,* E. coli *seldom infects the urinary tract, in spite of frequent exposure of the urethra to the organism;* small numbers undoubtedly enter the tract from time to time by way of the urethra, but sphincters controlling urinary flow and other mechanisms prevent most of them from reaching the bladder and the few that do are either killed or flushed out by the urinary flow before they can become established.

Humoral Abs against H, O and K Ags are often produced during *E. coli* infections, but the roles that they may play in protecting against subsequent infection are not known. Persistent or recurring kidney infections with *E. coli* often lead to substantial titers of humoral Abs against somatic O antigen of the infecting strain; in contrast, during bladder infections, humoral Ab titers seldom rise above the normal range. Therefore, serum Ab titers against O antigens are a useful diagnostic aid in differentiating pyelonephritis from cystitis, but have no demonstrable relation to effective immunity.

When serum Ab titers are high, small amounts of anti-O Ab are demonstrable in the urine of some patients with UT infections involving the kidney; this suggests that humoral proteins, including Abs, are being excreted. On the other hand, cystitis patients who lack increased humoral Abs may nevertheless have low titers of urinary Abs, indicating that such Abs are being produced locally in inflamed areas of the bladder mucosa. Immunoglobulins of the class IgA have been demonstrated in urine, but their significance in protection against cystitis is not known. *It is probable that both Abs and nonantibody antimicrobial factors of unknown nature function on the bladder mucosa and thus oppose infection.* There is evidence from animal studies that bacteria adhere to kidney cells by means of pili, thereby permitting colonization which may be a necessary prerequisite for establishing infection. The presence of Abs in the UT could protect against infection by preventing bacterial adherence.

K. Laboratory Diagnosis

The laboratory diagnosis of infections with coliform bacteria is relatively simple. Urine, pus, or other specimens are cultured on blood agar, EMB, MacConkey, or any of a variety of selective and differential media. Colonies become visible within a day or less. A fecal odor is characteristic of *E. coli* and on EMB the flat colonies have a distinctive metallic sheen. Lactose fermentation helps to differentiate *E. coli* from some of the highly pathogenic gram-negative rods along with other biochemical tests.

Fluorescent Ab techniques are useful as presumptive tests for screening for enteropathic *E. coli,* but agglutination tests with pure cultures are essential for final identification.

The diagnosis of UT infections usually depends on quantitative culture of clean-voided or catheterized urine. It has been established that the presence of more than 10^5 organisms per ml in a clean-voided urine specimen indicates true infection. Fewer than 10^3 bacteria per ml usually denotes contamination during urine collection. However, when clinical symptoms are present, bacterial counts between 10^3 and 10^5 require that the culture be repeated. In addition, gram-stained smears of one drop of uncentrifuged urine will reveal the presence of bacteria only if more than 10^5 organisms per ml are present; therefore, the direct gram-stained smear is useful for gaining presumptive evidence of UT infection.

L. Therapy

Most of the enteric bacteria are susceptible to one or more of a number of antibiotics, including the tetracyclines, sulfonamides, chloramphenicol, ampicillin and cephalexin. Nitrofurantoin is frequently employed for treating UT infection due to coliforms.

It is sometimes necessary to correct a predisposing condition in order to permit successful treatment of infections due to gram-negative rods. For example, a congenital anatomic defect in the urinary tract that results in continual exposure of the tract to heavy contamination or that predisposes to infection by causing retention of urine should be corrected surgically; otherwise antibiotic therapy is merely a temporizing measure.

The treatment of patients with UT infections varies with the category of infection. The *E. coli* strains that cause uncomplicated acute infections are almost always sensitive to all of the antibacterial agents generally used for gram-negative infections. Consequently, the less toxic agents should be employed, and sensitivity testing is not required. Recurring infections or chronic bacteriuria are usually caused by organisms that are resistant to antimicrobial agents, hence sensitivity testing should be carried out in these instances.

M. Reservoirs of Infection

The principal reservoirs of *E. coli* are the intestinal tracts of man and animals. Members of the genus *Enterobacter* and some of the other coliforms can exist as free living saprophytes as well as parasites.

N. Control of Disease Transmission

Since the coliforms are widespread in nature the usual measures for preventing bacterial infection are not generally applicable. However, iatrogenic infection due to these organisms can be controlled by careful attention to aseptic techniques. In addition, nursery epidemics due to enteropathic *E. coli* and cross-infections in hospitals can be effectively controlled by careful epidemiologic studies and follow-up.

Klebsiella

The most common species of this genus, *K. pneumoniae,* is found in the alimentary and respiratory tracts of about 5% of normal persons. Although the organism occasionally causes UT infections and chronic infections in various organs, it is better known as a cause of severe hemorrhagic pneumonia, accounting for about 2 to 3% of all cases of acute bacterial pneumonia. The mortality rate in untreated *Klebsiella* pneumonia is high (50%); therefore, *prompt recognition of the infecting organism and early treatment are essential.* It is especially important to distinguish between pneumonia due to *K. pneumoniae* and pneumonia due to other organisms such as *Diplococcus pneumoniae* because the antibiotics appropriate for treatment vary depending on the infecting agent.

The incidence of gram-negative bacillary infections of the respiratory tract (RT) is increasing as a result of various clinical procedures. A recent study of 213 patients admitted to a medical intensive care unit revealed that the RT of 45% of these patients became colonized with gram-negative bacilli, 22% on the first hospital day! About 12% of the 213 patients subsequently developed nosocomial infections. *Klebsiella pneumoniae* was isolated most frequently; other isolates commonly included species of enterobacteria and *Pseudomonas aeruginosa.*

Klebsiella pneumoniae is nonmotile; it produces a large polysaccharide capsule resulting in the formation of mucoid viscous colonies. The capsule is highly antiphagocytic. According to O and K Ag determinations, a large number of serotypes exist. The organism can be identified directly in sputum by means of the capsular swelling test conducted with specific antiserum. It is sometimes impossible to diagnose pneumonias produced by opportunistic gram-negative bacilli early enough to permit effective therapy. Consequently, methods for rapid diagnosis are being sought, such as those to detect bacterial Ag in serum or other body fluids. For example, soluble capsular Ag of *Klebsiella* sp. can be detected in serum by counter immunoelectrophoresis, permitting the diagnosis of *Klebsiella* pneumonia within 1 to 2 hours rather than the 1 to 2 days which is required for isolation and identification of the organism.

Klebsiella infections are difficult to treat because of the marked tissue necrosis and suppuration produced by the organism. The most effective antibiotic for treatment is often cephalothin; however, this varies with the strain. *Penicillin is not effective.*

On rare occasions, other species of *Klebsiella* cause disease of the upper RT; they are *K. ozaenae,* which can cause atrophy of the nasal mucous membranes, and *K. rhinoscleromatis,* which causes granulomatous lesions in the nose and throat.

A related organism, *Donovania (Calymmatobacterium) granulomatis,* is the cause of granuloma inguinale. This disease, which is usually transmitted venereally, is characterized by the development of a slow-spreading ulcer(s) on the genitalia, rectum, or abdominal wall. The ulcer presents both growing and healing areas, and resembles the lesion of a similar disease, *lymphogranuloma venereum* (caused by a *Chlamydia*); however, the buboes characteristic of the latter disease are not found in patients with granuloma inguinale.

Proteus

Organisms of the genus *Proteus* are characterized by the capacity to rapidly degrade urea to ammonia and their failure to ferment lactose. The 4 species are *Pr. vulgaris, Pr. mirabilis, Pr. morganii* and *Pr. rettgeri.* Members of two species, *Pr. vulgaris* and *Pr. mirabilis,* exhibit "swarming motility" on solid agar. For unknown reasons the organisms "swarm" (migrate en masse) in successive directional waves. Swarming overgrowth can be inhibited by adding phenylethyl alcohol or sodium azide to the medium. The characteristic odor of *Proteus* aids in its identification.

Members of the genus *Proteus* are normal intestinal inhabitants, but are also found free-living in soil and water. They are a frequent cause of UT infections, especially *Pr. mirabilis.* The latter is usually susceptible to penicillin and ampicillin, whereas other species of *Proteus* tend to resist these and a number of other antimicrobial agents.

Some strains of *Proteus* share antigenic determinants with some of the rickettsiae. Thus, strains OX2, OX19, and OXK are agglutinated by Abs formed during certain rickettsial infections. Present evidence indicates that there is no genetic relationship between proteus and rickettsiae, but that the sharing of antigenic determinants is merely fortuitous.

Alcaligenes

Another gram-negative rod that is similar in some respects to the coliforms is *Alcaligenes faecalis;* however, this organism belongs to a different family (*Achromobacteriaceae*). Nevertheless, its growth characteristics, source and low pathogenicity justify its consideration along with coliforms. It is a non-lactose-fermenting member of the normal intestinal flora. The organism is a cause of UT infections and occasionally of infections in other parts of the body. The name *Alcaligenes* is derived from the fact that these organisms fail to ferment any of the usual carbohydrates and produce an alkaline reaction in media.

References

Carpenter, C. C. J.: Cholera and other enterotoxin-related diarrheal diseases. J. Infect. Dis. *126*:551, 1972.

DuPont, H. L., Formal, S. B., Hornick, R. B., Snyder, M. J., Libonati, J. P., Sheahan, D. G., LaBrec, E. H., and Kalas, J. P.: Pathogenesis by *Escherichia coli* diarrhea. New Engl. J. Med. *285*:1, 1971.

Edwards, P. R., and Ewing, W. H.: *Identification of Enterobacteriaceae.* Minneapolis: Burgess Publishing Co., 1972.

Jacks, T. M., Wu, B. J., Braemer, A. C., and Bidlack, D. E.: Properties of the enterotoxic component in *Escherichia coli* enteropathogenic for swine. Infect. Immun. *7*:178, 1973.

Johanson, W. G., Pierce, A. K., Sanford, J. P., and Thomas, G. D.: Nosocomial respiratory infections with gram-negative bacilli. The significance of colonization of the respiratory tract. Ann. Intern. Med. *77*:701, 1972.

Kunin, C. M.: *Detection, Prevention, and Management of Urinary Tract Infections.* Philadelphia: Lea & Febiger, 1972.

Sack, R. B., Gorbach, S. L., Banwell, J. G., Jacobs, B., Chatterjee, B. D., and Mitra, R. C.: Enterotoxigenic *Escherichia coli* isolated from patients with severe cholera-like disease. J. Infect. Dis. *123*:378, 1971.

Stirm, S., Orskov, F., Orskov, I., and Mansa, B.: Episome-carried surface antigen K88 of *Escherichia coli* II. Isolation and chemical analysis. J. Bacteriol. *93*:731, 1967.

Taylor, A. L., and Trotter, C. D.: Linkage map of *Escherichia coli* strain K-12. Bact. Rev. *36*:504, 1972.

Chapter 18

Salmonella

Salmonella typhi, 247

Salmonella choleraesuis and Salmonella enteritidis, 253

Members of the genus *Salmonella* of the family *Enterobacteriaceae* comprise several species and hundreds of different serotypes, all of which are pathogens. The taxonomy of the salmonellae is exceedingly complex and the present trend is to attempt to bring order out of chaos by grouping them in 3 species, *Sal. typhi, Sal. choleraesuis* and *Sal. enteritidis,* and to further divide them into serologic types on the basis of their antigenic makeup.

In physical and chemical structure the salmonellae are similar to *E. coli.* Their heat-stable somatic (O) and heat-labile flagellar (H) Ags resemble those of other members of the family *Enterobacteriaceae.* Some strains of salmonellae have a heat-labile K-like envelope Ag called "virulence Ag" (Vi Ag) because the strains possessing it are virulent for mice. The tremendous variety and the myriad of combinations of both O and H Ags account for the large numbers of salmonella serotypes. The complexity of serotypes is further exaggerated by the occurrence of "phase variation" of H Ags that occur in most strains either as phase 1 Ag(s), which are relatively strain specific, or as phase 2 Ag(s), which are group specific. Genetically controlled changes from one phase to another can occur. Strains may be multiphasic, diphasic or monophasic. The Kauffmann-White schema of serotyping introduced in 1934 recognized 44 serotypes. Subsequently the number grew to 211 in 1941 and now exceeds 1400. Fortunately, most strains isolated in clinical practice belong to a small number of serologic types. Serotypes have usually been named for the site where they were first isolated, followed by Arabic numbers to designate O Ags, lower-case Roman letters to designate phase 1 H Ags and Arabic numerals to designate phase 2 H Ags. For example, a serotype of *Sal. enteritidis,* first isolated in Chicago, that has O Ag 28, a phase 1 Ag called r and phase 2 Ags 1 and 5 is designated "ser Chicago 28:r:1,5." The list of serotypes testifies to the widespread distribution of salmonellae, including such names as ser Albuquerque, ser Argentina and so on through the alphabet to ser Yeerongpilly and ser Zanzibar. The salmonellae cause disease in a wide range of animal hosts both natural and unnatural. Although man serves as a natural host only for *Sal. typhi,* the prototype species, and organisms of the paratyphoid group, he can serve as an accidental host for many strains of the other species.

Few bacteria are genetically more diverse than the salmonellae. Variants include those that range from rough to smooth colony-producing strains, from motile to nonmotile species and strains, from Vi Ag-producers to those lacking Vi Ag, and from piliated (fimbriate) to nonpiliated (nonfimbriate) organisms.

Some genetic changes in salmonellae are induced by phages. For example, certain O Ags are the result of lysogenic conversion, and transduction has been shown to transfer the capacity to synthesize both O and H Ags.

Conjugation may occur among different salmonellae or between *E. coli* and salmonellae, resulting in the transfer of genes.

Bacteriocins and multiple drug-resistance factors are frequently transferred among the salmonellae by episomes or plasmids.

The diseases caused by various salmonellae are similar and fall into 3 general patterns: (1) the *enteric fevers,* which are characterized by septicemia and enteritis and are most commonly caused by *Sal. typhi* and certain strains of *Sal. enteritidis (paratyphoid group);* (2) *septicemia* alone, which is most often caused by *Sal. choleraesuis;* and (3) *gastroenteritis,* which can result from any one of more than 1400 serotypes of *Sal. enteritidis.*

Salmonella typhi, the cause of typhoid fever, will be given the most attention and will be discussed first; many of its properties also apply to the other salmonellae, especially the paratyphoid organisms that produce enteric fevers, which are usually milder than typhoid fever.

Salmonella typhi

A. Medical Perspectives

Typhoid fever is the most serious of the various infections caused by salmonellae and in past centuries was one of the most frequent of the water-borne diseases. Typhoid fever and typhus, which have similar symptoms, were first clearly recognized as distinct diseases by Schoenlein (1839). William Budd (1856-1873) recognized the contagiousness of typhoid fever and noted that the mode of spread was principally by ingestion of food, milk and water contaminated with the feces of typhoid patients. Eberth (1880) discovered the organism in tissues and Gaffky first isolated it in pure culture in 1884. Before the era of modern sanitation, typhoid epidemics were a constant threat and a bane of armies during military campaigns. Typhoid fever is still a disease of major importance in the world at large, especially in underdeveloped countries.

Outbreaks occur even in areas where sanitation is generally good. For example, in 1963 an epidemic affecting 280 persons started in the ski-resort town of Zermatt, Switzerland; the next year an outbreak of some 400 cases was reported in Aberdeen, Scotland; in 1967, 30 of 72 members of a fraternity at Stanford University contracted the disease. The epidemiology of typhoid fever is often bizarre; for example, a 1959 outbreak involved a water supply contaminated by the feces of seagulls that had fed on sewage effluents discharged at sea.

In the USA, many thousands died of typhoid fever in the year 1900, whereas the annual number of cases today does not exceed a few hundred and very few deaths result from the infection. Nevertheless, because a few long-term carriers persist in the population, small sporadic outbreaks continue to occur, as, for example, the outbreak at Homestead, Florida, in the early spring of 1973 in which over 100 of its victims were hospitalized.

B. Physical and Chemical Structure

Salmonella typhi possesses a number of Ags in common with other salmonellae, particularly organisms of the paratyphoid group.

Aside from the general structural properties of the salmonellae described in the introduction to this chapter, the only structural feature of *Sal. typhi* deserving comment is the Vi Ag which, when abundant, can render the organism inagglutinable by anti-O serum and resistant to phagocytosis. The Vi Ag is a polymer of N-acetyl D-galactosamine uronic acid. Its precise role in virulence of *Sal. typhi* remains to be elucidated.

C. Genetics

More than 80 phage types have been described; these provide a valuable method for epidemiologic studies. (See the introduction to this chapter for discussion of the genetics of the salmonellae.)

D. Extracellular Products

No medically important extracellular products are known, with the exception of bacteriocins which may help the organisms to compete in the highly mixed flora of the GI tract and thus permit invasion and passage of the organism from host to host.

E. Culture

Salmonella typhi is a non-lactose-fermenting facultative anaerobe with simple nutritional requirements. It grows well on ordinary media under aerobic conditions over a temperature range of 10 to 41°C (optimal 37°) and a pH range of 6 to 8. The organism can grow in bile.

The isolation of *Sal. typhi* and other salmonellae from feces, which contains enormous numbers of other bacteria, requires special methods. Therefore, selective or selective-differential media or enrichment cultures followed by other media are commonly used for the isolation of these organisms. A sample of the feces, or other material, to be tested can be cultured in selenite broth or other enrichment media prior to plating, or it can be streaked directly onto a selective and differential medium such as salmonella-shigella (S-S) medium. MacConkey's medium, eosin-methylene-blue medium or other differential media permit distinction between the non-lactose-fermenting salmonellae and the lactose-fermenting nonpathogens, with the exception of species of the genera *Proteus* and *Pseudomonas*.

F. Resistance to Physical and Chemical Agents

Among nonsporulating bacteria, *Salmonella typhi* and other salmonellae are average in their susceptibility to most physical and chemical agents. They are readily killed by chlorination and most of the commonly used disinfectants. Heating at 55°C is lethal to these organisms; however, they resist freezing and survive well in chilled and frozen foods. They withstand fairly high concentrations of salts and survive in sea water as well as fresh water for weeks. They are notably resistant to drying and can remain alive in dried sewage for weeks.

G. Experimental Models

The mouse has been used for experimental infection with *S. typhi* but is unsatisfactory because the organism is not invasive for this animal and the immunologic responses and disease do not simulate human typhoid fever. Higher subhuman primates such as the chimpanzee provide the closest models for the human disease. The mouse model using *Sal. enteritidis* ser typhimurium does not closely simulate typhoid fever in man.

H. *Infections in Man*

Typhoid fever is the most serious of the enteric fevers due to the salmonellae and is the classical prototype of these infections. It may be mild enough to subside within a week or two after the onset of symptoms, or severe enough to kill the patient within 10 days; however, the usual case lasts for 4 or 5 weeks. The disease begins as a generalized septicemia characterized by a fluctuating bacteremia that is almost constant during the first 1 to 2 weeks.

Infection commonly results from the ingestion of food or fluids contaminated either directly or indirectly (by vectors such as flies) with the excreta of chronic carriers or of typhoid patients. The incubation period varies inversely with the number of organisms ingested and is usually 1 to 2 weeks (range 3 to 30 days). Unusually large infecting doses may provoke early acute gastritis prior to the onset of typhoid fever. Histologic study and work with animal models indicate that the organisms invade through the mucosa of the small intestine. They evidently adhere to and colonize on the epithelial surface and are probably engulfed by mucosal cells and passaged directly to the submucosa. Apparently they do not grow extensively within or destroy the epithelial cells. They multiply in the submucosa and reach the local lymph nodes via lymphatics where they grow, probably in large part within macrophages, which initially are not "immune." Organisms soon reach the blood, presumably following liberation from dying macrophages in the lymph nodes. The first bacteria that reach the blood are rapidly cleared by macrophages of the RES which accumulate and proliferate in large numbers at bacillary foci. This macrophage hyperplasia causes enlargement of lymph nodes and crowds hematopoietic elements in the bone marrow. Later, when the macrophages of the RES are overwhelmed, a persisting bacteremia sets in and an acute febrile illness of 3 to 5 weeks' duration, attended with many symptoms, gradually develops. The temperature rises in a stepwise fashion to a plateau that may sometimes represent extreme pyrexia. Other symptoms include dull frontal headache, prostration, abdominal discomfort and tenderness, skin rash, nonproductive cough, splenomegaly and leukopenia. Usually the symptoms intensify during the 2nd and 3rd weeks and then gradually decline. At the height of illness, mental dullness and delirium may set in and "rose spots," consisting of areas of petechial hemorrhage due to emboli of bacteria clumped by agglutinins, may appear in the skin. By about the 2nd to 3rd week, substantial metastatic lesions rich in macrophages are also present at various sites including the bone marrow, lung, lymphoid elements of the lamina propria of the small intestine and colon, and especially in the biliary tract where the organisms thrive and escape with the periodic discharge of bile to seed the feces with enormous numbers of organisms. Heavy involvement of the solitary lymphoid follicles of the gut and especially the Peyer's patches of the terminal ileum often leads to extensive ulceration. Serious complications include hemorrhage due to erosion of blood vessels in intestinal lesions and the rare (1% of cases) but most dangerous of all complications, intestinal perforation, due to deep ulceration. These 2 complications account for 75% of all deaths. Other complications include femoral thrombophlebitis, cerebral thrombosis, cholecystitis, pneumonia (often a mixed infection), osteomyelitis, meningitis, endocarditis, toxic myocarditis, alopecia and abortion. Hyaline degeneration of certain voluntary muscles and vascular hyperreactivity to epinephrine and norepinephrine develop.

Strong, albeit not solid, lifetime immunity to typhoid fever commonly follows recovery. However, in some 10% of the subjects, relapse occurs about 1 to 2 weeks after defervescence. It is most frequent following cure with antibiotics and can recur 2 or 3 times. Relapses are mild and, since Ab titers to H, O and Vi Ags can be high, presumably result from an inadequate cellular immune response. Mortality in untreated subjects varies markedly with different outbreaks but averages about 10%; it is reduced to about 1 to 2% by chemotherapy.

Chronic carriage, often for a lifetime, develops in 3 to 5% of those who have the disease (particularly adult females), intestinal carriage due to gallbladder infection being more common than urinary carriage. The gallbladder wall of the carrier is heavily infiltrated with lymphocytes and contains hyperplastic lymphoid follicles. Urinary carriage occurs most often in regions where schistosomiasis is endemic.

I. Mechanisms of Pathogenicity

The apparent ability of *Sal. typhi* to grow unrestricted within normal (immunologically immature) macrophages is undoubtedly important in pathogenesis. There is evidence that virulent species of *Salmonella* multiply intracellularly, whereas avirulent species do not. It has been suggested that some unique properties of the cell wall, perhaps the unusual sugars found there, may help the virulent organisms to resist degradation within host macrophages.

The mechanisms by which *Sal. typhi* produces tissue injury and disease are not known. The organism produces no known toxin except endotoxin. Since many of the symptoms of typhoid fever can be produced with endotoxin, it has been generally assumed that endotoxin contributes importantly to pathogenesis. During the course of typhoid fever, the bacteremia is cleared long before symptoms subside. Some investigators have attributed the continued symptoms to the slow release of endotoxin from disrupted parasitized macrophages, even in the absence of extracellular infection. The alternative suggestion has been made that the synthesis and release of endogenous pyrogen from activated macrophages may contribute to symptoms of the disease. The endotoxin theory has not been proved conclusively and is challenged by a number of observations. For example, volunteers made highly resistant to endotoxin before experimental challenge infection have been noted to develop typhoid fever equivalent to the disease in nontolerant control volunteers.

J. Mechanisms of Immunity

Much remains to be learned about the mechanisms of immunity to *Sal. typhi* and other salmonellae, even after decades of study. However, it is the consensus that cell-mediated immunity is of primary importance. There is no correlation between immunity to typhoid fever and the titer of any known humoral Ab; moreover, passive transfer of a substantial degree of immunity with serum has not been demonstrated conclusively. Humoral Abs are formed early during typhoid fever, usually by the second week. They agglutinate *S. typhi* and, together with C, can lyse the organisms. Nevertheless, they do not terminate the disease, which persists for weeks after Abs become demonstrable. Circulating Abs may well destroy extracellular organisms and inhibit the growth and systemic spread of salmonellae. However, the overall ineffectiveness of humoral immunity evidently results from the fact that the bacteria can multiply within nonimmune macrophages where they are sequestered from humoral Abs and C. In such situations, cellular immunity becomes the dominant immune force.

Cellular immune mechanisms have been intensively studied in the mouse-typhimurium model, and to some extent in man. Evidently effective immunity depends on properties of activated immune macrophages which, in contrast to nonimmune macrophages, can kill or inhibit intracellular salmonellae. Although the development of immune macrophages is specific, resulting from stimuli provided by immune lymphocytes incited to activity by specific Ag, their ability to inhibit and kill salmonellae is nonspecific. Evidence that cellular immunity is of paramount importance in mouse salmonellosis is provided by passive transfer experiments which show that protection against infection can be transferred to a nonimmune recipient with lymphocytes from an immunized donor, but not with immune sera. Also, immunization is much more effective when living attenuated bacteria or killed bacteria in Freund's complete adjuvant are used (which favor the development of cellular immunity) than when killed saline-suspended organisms are administered. These data, of course, do not deny the possibility that humoral Abs contribute to overall immunity. Indeed, humoral Abs cytophilic for macrophages, which may be most abundant in the local lesion, may contribute to macrophage activation, thereby aiding in protection. Another possibility is that secretory IgA Abs might contribute to protection against invasion of the organisms.

Vaccines currently used in man against enteric fevers consist of killed saline suspensions of typhoid and paratyphoid bacteria. The usual combined vaccine, called TAB (comprised of a pool of *Sal. typhi,* paratyphoid A, and paratyphoid B), offers limited protection. This is in sharp contrast to the marked and long-lasting immunity engendered by the disease itself. If Freund's complete adjuvant could be added, more effective protection could probably be achieved; however, this adjuvant produces severe granulomatous reactions and cannot be used in man. Suitable adjuvants have not been discovered to date, but new ones are being developed that may be both safe and effective.

K. Laboratory Diagnosis

Because typhoid fever is easily confused with a number of other diseases, laboratory diagnosis is important. It is based on culture of blood, feces and, occasionally, urine or exudates and tests for serum agglutinins. Colonies are readily recognized on selective-differential media and can be picked and identified by biochemical tests and serotyping with known agglutinating antisera. The percentages of positive cultures of blood, stool and urine and of positive agglutination tests are shown in Figure 18-1. A fourfold increase in serum Abs, especially anti-O agglutinins, with known *Sal. typhi* (Widal test), is indicative of typhoid fever, provided the patient has not recently received typhoid vaccine.

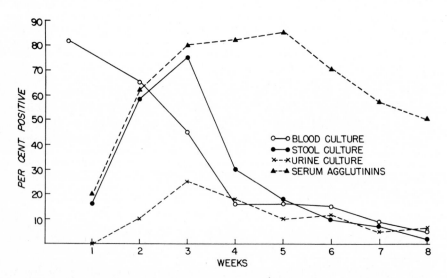

Figure 18-1. Serum agglutination tests and the incidence of positive blood, stool and urine cultures of patients during the course of typhoid fever. (Adapted from: Dubos, R. J., and Hirsch, J. G.: *Bacterial and Mycotic Infections of Man,* 4th ed. Philadelphia: J. B. Lippincott Co., 1965.)

L. Therapy

Chloramphenicol is the chemotherapeutic agent of choice. Since a few strains have developed antibiotic resistance, sensitivity testing is necessary. A number of other antibiotics, including ampicillin, are useful but less effective. Response to therapy occurs slowly over a period of 1 to 5 days, and hemorrhage and perforation may develop despite ongoing therapy. Chloramphenicol suppresses the development of agglutinins, promotes relapses and does not alter the acquisition of carriage. Supportive measures include administration of steroids to combat severe toxemia.

M. Reservoirs of Infection

The only reservoirs of infection are human patients, convalescent carriers and chronic carriers. Since the organisms can survive for weeks in water and food, organisms in excreta reaching food and streams may persist for long periods and be carried for long distances without losing their infectivity.

N. Control of Disease Transmission

Obviously the principal keys to control of typhoid fever are sanitary regulation of food and water supplies, the elimination of carriage and regulation of carriers. Except for disasters such as floods, which disrupt water and food supplies, the major problem relates to typhoid carriers as food handlers. Obviously no carrier should be allowed to handle or prepare food eaten by others. Unfortunately, existing laws make it difficult to treat and regulate carriers. Bacteriophage typing is useful for epidemiologic studies.

Cholecystectomy eliminates carriage in about 85% of the carriers and combined ampicillin-probenecid treatment commonly eliminates carriage in those individuals who are not biliary-tract carriers.

Immunization, especially of adults, which affords a minor degree of protection, may often prevent infection, especially if the exposure dose of organisms is low, and decreases the severity of disease. Organisms killed by mild heat treatment are generally used. The vaccine when given intramuscularly tends to produce fever, severe local inflammation and lymphadenopathy; this can be minimized by the use of small repeated intracutaneous doses. An annual booster is required to maintain the partial immunity afforded by the vaccine. Needless to say, a better vaccine is in the realm of possibility and is sorely needed.

Salmonella choleraesuis and Salmonella enteritidis

Except for being relatively less virulent for man than *Sal. typhi,* salmonellae of the above species are very similar to *Sal. typhi* in most respects.

Consequently, discussion of these organisms will be largely limited to the diseases that they produce.

These salmonellae may be carried by any domestic animal, wild warm-blooded animals and some cold-blooded vertebrates. It has been estimated that there are nearly 4 billion domestic animals in the USA at present, and that about 3% of them are infected with salmonellae. Animal salmonelloses are of tremendous economic importance, amounting to an annual loss of about 10 million dollars in the poultry industry alone. Recent outbreaks of salmonellosis in man have been traced to such reservoirs as pet turtles, chicks, ducklings, dogs, chickens and a variety of other domestic animals.

Septicemia occurs most often in very old, very young or debilitated individuals. *Salmonella choleraesuis* infects man as an accidental host and can cause all 3 types of infection. It can cause local or systemic infection and is the most frequent cause of salmonella infections characterized by septicemia alone. As in typhoid fever, ingested organisms transgress the intestinal epithelium and pass to the lymph nodes and blood stream from whence they establish foci of infection at various sites. However, unlike *Sal. typhi,* they do not infect the bladder nor do they produce lesions in the intestinal epithelium. Mortality ranges from 5 to 20%.

Gastroenteritis is commonly due to *Sal. enteritidis.* Since the organisms are of low virulence for man and large numbers are required to produce disease, the usual source of infection is food in which the organisms have multiplied extensively. Although the disease is the most common of the salmonelloses it is relatively mild and self-limiting. Of the 15,000 to 20,000 cases reported annually to the USPHS, the relatively few that are fatal occur in immunologically compromised individuals. As a rule, the symptoms of "salmonella food-poisoning" usually begin 12 to 48 hours after eating the contaminated food. Nausea, vomiting and diarrhea may be accompanied by slight fever and headache. Mild cases may last less than a day, but even the more severe ones usually terminate within 3 to 5 days. Antimicrobial therapy is seldom required. Fluids and electrolytes should be replaced if extensive diarrhea and vomiting have occurred.

The *pathogenesis* of gastroenteritis probably rests, at least in part, on the activities of endotoxin. The facts that large numbers of bacteria are required to produce disease and that the onset of illness usually follows within hours to a day or two after ingestion of contaminated materials support this concept.

There are reports that salmonella gastroenteritis does not lead to immunity and that repeated infections can occur with the same serotype. However, these suppositions have not been firmly established as facts.

Control of gastroenteritis presents major problems. No effective vaccine is available. Special attention must be paid to methods of food preparation and preservation and every attempt must be made to ensure adequate sanitation in slaughter houses, food-processing plants and restaurants. For example, some salmonellae can remain alive at room temperature for 6 to 8 weeks in salami sausages containing strong brine. Also they may survive in dried materials for months, and for several weeks on apparently clean eggshells. Highly acid or alkaline environments (pH < 4.5 or > 9.0) lead to death of salmonellae, but pH effects vary considerably depending on the nature of the suspending medium, temperature and other factors.

The *incidence* of gastroenteritis is impossible to determine accurately because most cases are mild and many are not reported. In the USA, probably only 1 of every 10 to 20 cases is reported; however, the number reported has increased dramatically over the past decade. This is thought to largely reflect an increase in incidence, as well as improved detection and reporting. The increase may result, in part, from the increasing use of certain processed convenience foods which can harbor salmonellae. The salmonelloses are far from being controlled, and will probably remain a major public health problem for the foreseeable future. When outbreaks occur, extensive epidemiologic studies with phage typing may be required to identify the source of the infection. Serologic typing is of limited epidemiologic value because very few serotypes cause the majority of outbreaks. For example, *Salmonella enteritidis* ser *Typhimurium* is responsible for about a fourth of the reported cases of salmonella gastroenteritis.

The Riverside, California, epidemic of 1969, involving nearly 20,000 cases, reflects some of the problems presented in the control of salmonella gastroenteritis. The source was traced to the municipal water supply, and ultimately to human carriers. The water had been monitored by standard procedures to detect fecal contamination, but was only chlorinated when the tests indicated a certain level of *E. coli* contamination. As a rule, this procedure is adequate because *E. coli* occurs in much greater numbers than salmonellae in fecally contaminated water; however, in this instance the salmonellae were present in large numbers in the water. In fact they were 10 times as numerous as *E. coli*. Nevertheless, routine chlorination would have prevented this epidemic.

Salmonellae are commonly present on foods such as poultry and eggs because they are present in the gastrointestinal tract of the animals. The organisms are able to survive procedures often used to preserve foods, such as freezing (section F). Thus, frozen chickens and turkeys, as well as many other kinds of foods, often contain salmonellae that can multiply during food preparation. Unless care is taken, such foods serve as a source of salmonellosis. A common example is the frozen turkey, which takes a long time to thaw. Many cooks have used the dangerous short-cut of allowing the turkey to thaw at room temperature. This permits the multiplication of salmonellae on the surface of the bird and in the body cavity. Particularly if a partially frozen turkey is roasted, the temperature inside the cavity may not rise enough to kill the organisms.

References

Collaborative Report: A waterborne epidemic of salmonellosis in Riverside, California, 1969. Amer. J. Epidemiol. 93:33, 1971.

Edwards, P. R., and Ewing, W. H.: *Identification of Enterobacteriaceae.* Minneapolis: Burgess Publishing Co., 1972.

Kauffmann, F.: *Serological Diagnosis of Salmonella-Species Kauffmann-White-Schema.* Copenhagen, Munksgaard, 1972.

Prost, E., and Riemann, H.: Food-borne salmonellosis. Ann. Rev. Microbiol. 21:495, 1967.

Roantree, R. J.: Salmonella O antigens and virulence. Ann. Rev. Microbiol. 21: 443, 1967.

Sanderson, K. E.: Linkage map of *Salmonella typhimurium,* Edition IV. Bact. Rev. 36:558, 1972.

Shigella

Members of the genus *Shigella* belong to the family *Enterobacteriaceae*. They are all parasites in the intestinal tracts of their natural hosts, the primates, although dogs occasionally serve as unnatural hosts. The virulent shigellae produce bacillary dysentery in man and the higher apes. *The organisms are shed in the feces and the disease is transmitted by the fecal-oral route and by mechanical vectors, such as flies.*

A. Medical Perspectives

Bacillary dysentery in man is likely to occur in epidemic form whenever sanitation and personal hygiene are lax, for example during military campaigns. It has often played a decisive role in the outcome of battles throughout the centuries. Herodotus reported that the defeat of the Persian Army in 380 B.C. was due largely to dysentery that swept through the Persian troops. The fabulous military success of Alexander the Great has been attributed in part to his insistence that his armies boil their drinking water, thereby guarding against dysentery and certain other enteric infections. Although bacillary dysentery has been recognized for centuries, its

TABLE 19-1

The Genus *Shigella*

Species	Relative Incidence in USA
Sh. dysenteriae	Not found except for rare imported cases
Sh. flexneri	Frequent cause of shigellosis; common in the Southern States
Sh. sonnei	Most common cause of shigellosis; more frequent in the Northern States
Sh. boydii	Rare

causative agent was not discovered until 1898, when Shiga identified the "dysentery bacillus," later named *Shigella dysenteriae*.

During previous centuries, shigellosis took a huge toll of lives among infants in the USA and throughout the world. It was at its maximum in the USA during the era of the outdoor toilet, and pioneer graveyards abound with its victims.

At present, infection with the highly virulent species *Sh. dysenteriae* is rare in the USA, but shigellosis due to other *Shigella* sp. is relatively common (Table 19-1). Outbreaks occur among migrant farm workers and others who live in inadequate housing. Often fecally contaminated water supplies are the source of outbreaks. Nonseasonal endemic disease is important and transmission due to poor personal hygiene is frequent. Outbreaks in orphanages and mental institutions often result from person-to-person transmission. Experimental studies using human volunteers have shown that as few as 200 ingested *Sh. flexneri* organisms can initiate infections in healthy adult males.

Between 11,000 and 16,000 cases of shigellosis were reported to the USPHS annually during the decade from 1962 to 1972 and, like salmonellosis, many more cases were not reported. During this period the yearly death toll due to the disease varied from 60 to 153.

American Indians living on reservations have an unusually high incidence of shigellosis. For example, in 1968 the reported incidence was 212.2 cases per 100,000 among Indians, compared with 4.6 per 100,000 of the entire population of the USA.

In the world at large, shigellosis remains an infectious disease of major importance and in certain underdeveloped countries it still takes its high toll of lives among infants and young children.

B. Physical and Chemical Structure

The shigellae are nonmotile, nonsporing, nonencapsulated gram-negative rods possessing characteristic O Ags. In gram-stained smears, they resemble the coliforms, the rods being about 1 to 3 μm in length and 0.5 μm in diameter. Although flagella are lacking, the organisms possess pili.

C. Genetics

Like other members of the family *Enterobacteriaceae*, the shigellae show marked genetic variability. The variation of greatest importance to the practicing physician is the readiness with which these organisms acquire multiple drug resistance. In fact, resistance transfer factors (RTF) were discovered in shigellae during an epidemic of shigellosis in Japan in 1959, and were subsequently shown to occur in other genera of bacteria. The RTF were first demonstrated in the USA during an outbreak of shigellosis in Georgia in 1968. The causative organism was a strain of *Shigella flexneri* with demonstrated resistance to sulfadiazine, streptomycin, tetracycline, chloramphenicol and ampicillin. In the laboratory, it was shown that this multiple resistance could be transferred to a strain of *E. coli,* previously sensitive to all of these drugs! Shigellae are susceptible to certain bacteriophages and may be altered by lysogenic conversion. Bacteriophage typing has not proven to be of epidemiologic value.

D. Extracellular Products

The marked severity of *Sh. dysenteriae* infections, which have a fatality rate of about 20% in untreated subjects, results in large part from the production of a potent exotoxin (shigella enterotoxin). The toxin is a fairly heat-stable (90°C) protein (mol wt 82,000). It is thought to be identical with the exotoxin described in the early literature as a "neurotoxin." Other species of *Shigella* do not produce this exotoxin.

Studies of the effects of shigella enterotoxin on rabbits indicate that it kills intestinal epithelial cells. Although the toxin produces a watery diarrhea, its mode of action is clearly different from that of the enterotoxins produced by *Vibrio cholerae* (Chapter 20) and *E. coli* (Chapter 17), and remains to be elucidated.

E. Culture

The shigellae are facultative anaerobes that either do not ferment lactose or ferment it very slowly. Their cultural requirements are the same as those of the salmonellae (Chapter 18).

F. Resistance to Physical and Chemical Agents

The salmonellae and shigellae are similar with respect to resistance to environmental factors and to antibiotics. Hence, these properties of the salmonellae, described in Chapter 18, are also applicable to the shigellae. For unknown reasons the organisms do not survive long in fecal specimens.

G. Experimental Models

The infected subhuman primate serves as the best experimental model of human shigellosis. The rabbit is commonly used to study the effects of shigella enterotoxin, which causes paralysis and death when injected intravenously into either rabbits, guinea pigs or mice. The effects of the toxin are neutralized by specific antitoxin. Fatal shigellosis can be induced in weanling guinea pigs deficient in folic acid. Other treatments, such as starvation or antibiotic treatment, that reduce the natural resistance of the guinea pig permit limited infections.

H. Infections in Man

Unlike the nontyphoid salmonelloses, which are commonly transmitted from animals to man, human shigellosis is essentially always transferred from man to man, either directly via the fecal-oral route, or through the agency of mechanical vectors such as the housefly, which gains access to human feces. It is noted for being transmitted via food, fingers, feces, and flies. Also unlike the salmonellae, the *shigellae do not invade beyond the surface integument of the intestine; they gain entrance and grow within epithelial cells of the intestine.*

Shigellosis presents a severe form caused by Sh. dysenteriae *and a less severe form resulting from infections with other shigellae.* In both instances, the onset is abrupt, and usually follows an incubation period of 2 days (range 1 to 6 days) after the ingestion of contaminated food or water. The first symptoms are fever and abdominal cramps, followed by the onset of diarrhea within a few hours. Characteristically, the *stools are watery and contain mucus, pus and blood.* Nausea is common, but vomiting is usually not a prominent symptom. Within a few hours the diarrhea subsides and tenesmus becomes marked.

In Sh. dysenteriae *infections, the diarrhea is severe and may lead to a cholera-like dehydration.* In addition, headache may be severe and *sometimes neurologic symptoms develop.* The disease is either fatal or runs its course within about 10 days. Complications, which are rare, include arthritis, neuritis, conjunctivitis, iritis, vulvovaginitis and chronic colitis.

Dysentery due to other species of Shigella *is usually milder and of shorter duration.* The highest incidence occurs in children 1 to 4 years of age. Recovery may be complete within a few days in some subjects, but usually takes place within a week.

Bacillary dysentery is notable for the high mortality it causes in infants, the aged, and debilitated persons if these subjects are not treated. This is true regardless of the species causing the infection. Antibodies appear in serum during convalescence and can also be demonstrated in the feces.

I. Mechanisms of Pathogenicity

The enterotoxin is important in the pathogenesis of bacillary dysentery caused by *Sh. dysenteriae*. It contributes to ulceration of the intestinal mucosa and to acute inflammation in the lamina propria; a pseudomembrane often forms. Also, endotoxin released from dead organisms probably contributes to pathogenesis.

All of the shigellae possess the unique capacity to gain entrance into intestinal epithelial cells and to multiply within them. It is thought that pili may facilitate localization and possibly entrance of organisms into host cells by attaching to their surfaces (Chapter 9). Apparently the organisms in some manner induce their own engulfment by host cells. Their position within epithelial cells helps to protect them against host defenses. However, they multiply to eventually kill host cells and in so doing attract neutrophils, which engulf and destroy at least some of the extracellular organisms. The dying neutrophils probably contribute to necrosis and ulceration of the mucosa.

Infection is limited to the superficial layers of the intestinal tract and is largely confined to the terminal ileum and colon where small ulcerating abscesses develop. Multiplication of the organisms occurs in the submucosa or lamina propria, but the greatest numbers of organisms are found near the surface of the gut lumen. *The organisms do not invade systemically.*

J. Mechanisms of Immunity

The nature of immunity to shigellosis is not understood. Humoral Abs are formed against the cell wall Ags of shigellae and against the enterotoxin, but the roles they play in protection against natural infection have not been clearly established. Passive transfer of antitoxin affords some protection against the enterotoxin; however, there is no evidence to suggest that circulating agglutinins contribute to immunity. It is possible that coproantibodies, especially sIgA, may contribute to recovery by blocking the adherence of the organisms to gut epithelium and subsequent engulfment.

Administration of killed bacterial vaccines affords no protection against shigellosis. Consequently, efforts are being made to develop effective living vaccines that can be given orally.

K. Laboratory Diagnosis

Bacteriologic diagnosis is made by isolating the organisms from the feces. Blood and urine cultures are of no diagnostic value. Bits of bloody mucus in the feces are most likely to yield positive cultures. Since the organisms die rapidly in feces, *fecal specimens should be cultured promptly follow-*

ing collection. Their microscopic examination often aids in differentiating shigellosis, in which the fecal specimens are usually rich in neutrophils, from salmonellosis or enterotoxin-caused diarrheas, which generate few leukocytes in feces. The general procedures for isolating and identifying shigellae are similar to those used for salmonellae (Chapter 18). The fact that shigellae are always nonmotile is helpful in laboratory diagnosis. Identification is based on biochemical tests and serologic analysis. Serum agglutinins appear late after infection and agglutination tests are of value for retrospective diagnosis.

L.　Therapy

Fluid replacement is the most important aspect of therapy, especially in children; antibiotics are also highly effective. Ampicillin is the antibiotic of choice; chloramphenicol and the tetracyclines may be also used if the infecting strains are sensitive to them.

M.　Reservoirs of Infection

Man is the principal reservoir of human shigellosis. On rare occasions man may contract the disease from subhuman primates. The organisms are usually carried for only a short time (up to 1 month) after recovery from disease; however, an occasional patient develops the state of chronic carriage with intermittent shedding of organisms, which serves to perpetuate the organisms in nature.

N.　Control of Disease Transmission

Isolation of patients and the usual sanitary measures applicable to enteric diseases are the keys for controlling shigellosis. Adequate and prolonged antibiotic therapy during the disease helps to prevent the establishment of the short-term and chronic carrier states. Mass chemotherapy is a useful measure for controlling severe epidemics. Although, in theory, proper hygiene and sanitation could eradicate shigellosis, this goal is difficult to achieve, principally because of the chronic carrier.

References

Calabi, O.: *In vitro* interactions of *Shigella flexneri* with leukocytes and HeLa cells. J. Infect. Dis. *122*:1, 1970.

DuPont, H. L., Hornick, R. B., Dawkins, A. T., Snyder, M. J., and Formal, S. B.: The response of man to virulent *Shigella flexneri* 2a. J. Infect. Dis. *119*:296, 1969.

Edwards, P. R., and Ewing, W. H.: *Identification of Enterobacteriaceae.* 3rd ed. Minneapolis: Burgess Publishing Co., 1972.

Haltalin, K. C., Nelson, J. D., Woodman, E. B., and Allen, A. A.: Fatal shigella infection induced by folic acid deficiency in young guinea pigs. J. Infect. Dis. *121*:275, 1970.

Keusch, G. T., Grady, G. F., Takeuchi, A., and Sprinz, H.: The pathogenesis of shigella diarrhea. II. Enterotoxin-induced acute enteritis in the rabbit ileum. J. Infect. Dis. *126*:92, 1972.

Nelson, J. D., Kusmiesz, H. T., and Haltalin, K. C.: Endemic shigellosis: a study of fifty households. Am. J. Epidemiol. *86*:683, 1967.

Reller, L. B., and Spector, M. I.: Shigellosis among Indians. J. Infect. Dis. *121*:355, 1970.

Chapter 20

Vibrio

Members of the genus *Vibrio,* of the family *Spirillaceae,* are short, curved, gram-negative rods. The nonsporing, rigid cells occur singly or are attached to form spiral aggregates. They usually possess a single polar flagellum. Most species are aerobic or facultatively anaerobic, although a few are strictly anaerobic. Whereas many species are aquatic saprophytes, others are parasitic and some are pathogenic for a wide range of animal hosts, including man. Some species of *Vibrio* are found among the normal flora of the mouth.

Vibrio cholerae

Vibrio cholerae, *the cause of human cholera, is a strict parasite of man,* its only natural host. It can survive for a period of days or weeks in water or other moist environments while en route from one human host to another. Epidemic spread of cholera occurs via water, or less often food, contaminated by human excreta; the infection is endemic in some parts of the world, notably in the Philippines, Pakistan, Bangladesh, India, Africa and Southeast Asia.

A. Medical Perspectives

Few diseases cause more panic than cholera, with its swift spread and high fatality rate. Unless prompt treatment is available, more than half of its victims may die within a few hours to several days after onset of debilitating diarrhea.

Cholera has been known and feared for thousands of years. As early as the 5th century B.C., Thucydides described what was probably a cholera outbreak in Athens, and the disease was reported to be epidemic in the army of Alexander the Great about 320 B.C. Six well-documented great pandemics swept the world during the 19th and early 20th centuries, several of them spreading across the USA. It was during this period that much was learned about the disease and its control.

Some of the most significant advances in understanding the nature of cholera were made by a British physician, John Snow, who is also famous for being the world's first anesthesiologist. This highly perceptive observer studied the cholera epidemics of 1849 and 1854 in London. His paper, "On the Mode of Communication of Cholera," is one of the classics of medical literature. In it, he clearly showed that the 1849 outbreak stemmed from water supplied by the Broad Street pump, a public water source in London. Although the causative agent was not known, he deduced that fecal contamination of the water was responsible for the disease, and furthermore that the causative agent must be self-replicating because it was not lost by dilution in large volumes of water. He even observed that the area of the Thames which supplied the water responsible for the 1854 outbreak was saltier than other areas of the river, a fact that assumed significance in the light of later investigations.

After Koch's discovery of the cholera vibrio in 1883, many pioneering studies based on this organism were conducted. Pfeiffer discovered the phenomenon of antibody-plus-complement lysis of gram-negative organisms (Pfeiffer phenomenon) when he described vibriocidal Abs in 1894. About the same time, Ag-Ab precipitation reactions were first observed, using Abs and soluble Ags of *V. cholerae*.

Prevention of cholera is difficult and the disease has continued to offer a major challenge to the investigator. Even though improvements in sanitation have greatly decreased the incidence and spread of the disease, the World Health Organization (WHO) reported some 42,000 cases and 4,000 deaths during 1966. Furthermore, it is estimated that about 100 individuals are infected for each case reported, suggesting that, on a worldwide basis (excluding mainland China), more than 4 million cases of cholera occurred in 1966! Little wonder that intensive, cooperative research on cholera has received massive support in recent years from many governments and from the WHO. The exciting recent progress made in isolating and characterizing cholera enterotoxin has led to improved prospects for controlling the disease, and promise of advances in understanding the normal physiology of the gastrointestinal tract.

The future of the disease is difficult to predict. However, the mode of spread, the explosive nature of epidemics and the low level of herd immunity, even in endemic areas, *suggest that the disease will continue to be a threat until a method for producing high and durable immunity by artificial immunization is developed.*

B. Physical and Chemical Structure

Like most gram-negative, motile rods, *V. cholerae* possesses distinguishing flagellar (H) and somatic (O) Ags. Its single polar flagellum is composed of a protein that is antigenically the same in all strains. However, this H antigen is also shared by some nonpathogenic vibrios; thus it is of no value in diagnostic tests.

The O Ag is a typical lipopolysaccharide, gram-negative cell wall component. The lipid portions of the complex molecules have endotoxic activities, and the polysaccharide constituents are responsible for antigenic specificity. Cholera vibrios may be grouped into several strains within the species on the basis of their O antigenic makeup.

Receptor sites for phages occur on the surface of cholera vibrios and phage typing is used to identify substrains of vibrios for epidemiologic studies.

C. Genetics

There are several distinct genetic variants of cholera vibrios. Inaba and Ogawa *serotypes* of both classical and El Tor *biotypes* exist. All 4 combinations cause disease; the El Tor generally produces the mildest form. El Tor strains were first described near the turn of the century, and for many years were considered to be nonpathogenic variants of *V. cholerae;* however, their virulence is now well established.

D. Extracellular Products

Vibrio cholerae produces a variety of extracellular enzymes and toxins including *enterotoxin* and the enzymes mucinase and neuraminidase. It has been postulated that such enzymes may contribute to the ability of the vibrios to exist adjacent to the intestinal mucosa; however, this has not been proven.

E. Culture

Cholera vibrios grow readily on a variety of laboratory media and are unique among gram-negative enterics in their preference for an alkaline environment. They grow best at pH values near 8.0 and are rapidly killed by an acid medium. The optimum temperature for growth is 37°C; however, they grow over a wide range of temperatures (14 to 42°C). These vibrios can tolerate concentrations of tellurite salts that kill most other enteric organisms.

F. Resistance to Physical and Chemical Agents

As noted by John Snow more than a century ago, cholera vibrios survive and multiply in fecally contaminated water, especially if the salt concentration is fairly high. In addition to thriving at a high pH and in the presence of tellurite and high concentrations of NaCl, these organisms can also survive in the presence of bile salts. They are, however, readily killed by most disinfectants, drying and heat (56°C, 15 min), as well as by acid. Cholera vibrios have been shown to survive in water for about a month, and on the surfaces of moist fruits or vegetables for as long as 2 weeks. The organisms are susceptible to certain antibiotics including the tetracyclines.

G. Experimental Models

Although man is the only natural host for *V. cholerae,* a variety of animals can be infected experimentally. Infant rabbits and about 35% of mongrel dogs respond to oral administration of the organisms with a disease that resembles cholera in man. Adult guinea pigs and some other animals can also be infected if gastric acidity is neutralized before the organisms are administered.

The canine model has been very instructive. Some of the dogs that develop severe cholera after oral infection recover without treatment. The experimental disease closely mimics cholera in man; intensive, watery diarrhea occurs for 36 to 48 hours. Carriers can be detected among dogs that have recovered from experimental cholera and carriage may last at least 26 months.

The pathogenesis of cholera has been extensively studied in both the rabbit intestinal loop model and the canine Thiry-Vella intestinal loop. In the ligated rabbit loop, for example, sutures are placed around the intestine at varying intervals to form loops, leaving the blood supply undisturbed. Characteristically, large amounts of fluid accumulate within the loop following introduction of living vibrios or certain of their products.

H. Infections in Man

Infections in man, which follow ingestion of the vibrios, are limited to the intestinal tract; *the organisms do not invade systemically.* After an incubation period of a few hours to a few days, the illness begins with a feeling of abdominal fullness and loss of appetite, which are soon followed by onset of diarrhea and vomiting. *The hallmark of cholera is copious, watery diarrhea.* There may be as many as 20 to 30 fluid bowel movements in one day. Flakes of epithelial cells sometimes slough into the watery bowel contents, giving the stools a characteristic appearance; they are referred to as "rice-water" stools because they resemble the water in which rice has been cooked.

The diarrheal fluid is composed principally of water and salt ions, and is low in protein. More than a liter of fluid may be lost each hour, *resulting in rapid and devastating dehydration,* often with a loss of 5 to 10% of body weight within hours. The skin becomes loose, the eyes sunken, and other effects of fluid loss rapidly become apparent. The blood becomes so viscous that circulation is impaired; hypovolemic shock may occur and anuria is common.

Loss of bicarbonate ions in cholera stools and in vomitus is of particular significance, because it can rapidly lead to acidosis. *Consequently, the symptoms and complications of acidosis are often superimposed on the picture of severe dehydration.*

I. Mechanisms of Pathogenicity

The principal factor directly responsible for cell injury and disease is the enterotoxin of V. cholerae. However, other factors produced by the vibrios may contribute to their ability to survive and proliferate within the small intestine where the toxin is produced and exerts its effects. Pili of toxin-producing strains have been described, but whether they aid in attachment of vibrios to the mucosa, which is the target tissue for enterotoxin, is uncertain. The role of endotoxin in pathogenesis is not well established. At present, *there is no compelling evidence that any factor other than enterotoxin is essential in the pathogenesis of cholera.* However, there is some evidence that the capacity to adsorb to the intestinal mucosa may be an attribute of pathogenicity.

Koch (1883) proposed that a bacterial toxin was responsible for the clinical manifestations of cholera, but only during the past decade has the toxin been isolated, characterized, and shown to produce the watery diarrhea typical of cholera.

The enterotoxin has been studied by several groups of investigators. Toxin-containing preparations have been given various names, including choleragen, skin-permeability factor (because of its effects when injected into skin), vascular permeability factor, type-2 cholera toxin, and cholera exotoxin. It now appears that the cholera-producing factor is the same in all these preparations, and that the designation *cholera enterotoxin* will be accepted.

In vitro, the toxin affects cells of various types, all of which possess membrane-bound adenyl cyclase. Hence, in cholera *the intestinal epithelium is the target of the toxin because of localization of the organisms on the mucosa* and not because of any unique susceptibility of mucosal cells to the toxin.

The principal pathogenetic characteristic of the enterotoxin in cholera is its unique diarrheagenic activity. The toxin is a heat-labile ($56°C$, 15 min), acid-labile protein that is degraded by the proteolytic enzyme pronase but not by trypsin. It is antigenic, and under appropriate circumstances stimulates the production of neutralizing Ab (antitoxin). Prevailing evidence indicates that *toxins from various strains of vibrios are antigenically the same.* The toxin is synthesized and secreted well before vibrio lysis, indicating that *it is a typical exotoxin.* Its extreme toxicity and amenability to toxoiding with formalin are properties consistent with those of other bacterial exotoxins. The toxoid has been used experimentally to immunize dogs against cholera.

Enterotoxin attaches to epithelial cells within one minute after application to intestinal mucosa; however, the onset of its action is slow, beginning several hours later. *The toxin presumably affects water and electrolyte transport by mucosal cells, by activating adenyl cyclase.* Adenyl cyclase, a membrane-bound enzyme that is normally stimulated by certain hormones, catalyzes the formation of cyclic adenosine monophosphate (CAMP) from adenosine triphosphate. When intracellular concentrations of CAMP are high, the cell is activated to perform its normal functions; when CAMP concentrations are low, cellular functions are curtailed. Cholera enterotoxin acts like certain hormones in that it stimulates the formation of intracellular CAMP. However, enterotoxin continues to act on the cell, whereas hormone activity is intermittent and controlled. Although the mechanism of action of cholera enterotoxin is not known, it has been postulated that the toxin may be stereochemically similar to a normal hormone that stimulates intestinal cells, and that once attached to the cells it stimulates adenyl cyclase activity continuously until the cell dies.

Elucidation of the mechanism by which cholera enterotoxin produces diarrhea led to the unexpected finding that intestinal epithelial cells normally participate in the flux of water and electrolytes between plasma and the gut lumen. The adenyl cyclase regulation of this function apparently depends on hormone action, and it is postulated that certain prostaglandins may have this hormone function. Thus, very practical researches into the cause and control of a dangerous infectious disease have contributed substantially to understanding the basic physiology of man. Moreover, a very real possibility is that further studies on the mechanism by which enterotoxin interacts with cell components to stimulate adenyl cyclase activity could lead to the development of some simple therapeutic measure for blocking the primary effects of the toxin.

J.   Mechanisms of Immunity

In spite of recent outstanding advances toward understanding the pathogenesis and treatment of cholera, *much remains to be learned about mechanisms of immunity to this disease.* Initially it was thought that immunization with toxoid might give strong and long-lasting immunity, as with diphtheria and tetanus toxoids. *However, the situation is not analogous,* because, in cholera, the infection and the enterotoxin are limited to the lumen of the intestine. Very little toxin is absorbed into the circulation, and its target (the intestinal mucosa) is not exposed to appreciable quantities of humoral Abs. Moreover, extensive field trials with vaccines of killed organisms have shown that the resulting immunity, which is of short duration (about 6 months), is strictly type specific. This is in contrast to antitoxic Abs which are not type specific.

Further evidence that antitoxic Abs are not fully protective, at least under natural conditions, has been gained from studies showing that humoral vibriocidal Abs, which are present in a large proportion of the population in endemic areas, increase in titer with the subject's age and increasing immunity, whereas antitoxic Abs do not. Apparently, repeated antigenic stimulation, which both maintains and increases the vibriocidal humoral Ab response, occurs from time to time. In addition, during one epidemic period studied, there was a correlation between the presence of vibriocidal Abs and protection against infection. This does not necessarily mean that vibriocidal humoral Abs are protective; alternatively it is possible that a certain level of antigenic stimulation by vibrios resulted in both vibriocidal and protective Abs of unknown nature. In contrast to vibriocidal Abs, which increased in titer with increasing age, the level of demonstrable toxin-neutralizing Abs decreased with age. This finding suggests that antibacterial immunity can afford complete protection against reinfection with *V. cholerae,* and that the reexposed individual is not stimulated to produce antitoxic Abs, even if there is repeated contact with the organism. Also, in subjects in whom antitoxic but not vibriocidal Abs were detectable, infection resulted even though it led to less severe disease. Serum antitoxin levels following cholera are variable and are often low, probably because little toxin is absorbed systemically; the antitoxin may remain detectable in the serum for about 12 to 18 months following the disease.

It is probable that local coproantibodies in the intestine are of primary importance in protection against cholera. It has been known for some time that coproantibodies play a role in recovery and that a majority of the immunoglobulins on the mucosa are sIgA. Studies are under way to determine the amounts, immunoglobulin classes and specificities of local coproantibodies against *V. cholerae* and their modes of action. These studies have provided strong support for the hypothesis that coproantibodies prevent the adsorption and colonization of vibrios on the mucosal surface.

K. Laboratory Diagnosis

During epidemics, the clinical picture of cholera virtually provides the diagnosis, and quick confirmation can be made if examination of the stool by darkfield microscopy is possible. *The vibrios exhibit a characteristic, darting motility which is abrogated by adding a drop of specific antiserum.* On gram-stained smears they appear as comma-shaped, gram-negative rods. (The old name for this organism, *V. comma,* described the shape of the vibrios.)

Cholera vibrios, which are present in enormous numbers in the stool during infection, are isolated by using selective media that allow growth of the vibrios and discourage other intestinal flora. Monsur's medium is one example of such a medium. It contains salts and other nutrients; its high pH and the presence of tellurite are inhibitory for many organisms other than *V. cholerae.*

Alkaline peptone water has long been used to enrich growth of the vibrios before streaking them on solid media. Fluorescent Ab techniques can also be employed to identify the vibrios after 4 to 10 hours' growth in peptone broth cultures.

Positive identification of cultured organisms depends on serologic tests using anti-O sera. Bacteriophage typing, which is useful for epidemiologic studies, is of no aid in diagnosis.

L. Therapy

Since the pathologic effect of *V. cholerae* is simple and readily reversible, namely, severe dehydration without appreciable tissue injury, *the benefits of therapy are prompt, dramatic and essentially completely successful. With adequate therapy the death rate from cholera can be reduced from as high as 75% to less than 1%.* Treatment consists of replacing the volume of fluid lost with a sterile solution containing appropriate electrolytes. A "5-4-1 solution" (i.e., 5 gm NaCl, 4 gm $NaHCO_3$, and 1 gm KCl per liter of water) is commonly given intravenously.

The especially designed "cholera cot" is a help in determining the amount of fluid lost. This bed provides a hole under the buttocks so that the copious diarrheal fluid can be collected directly in a bucket placed under the bed and then measured (Fig. 20-1).

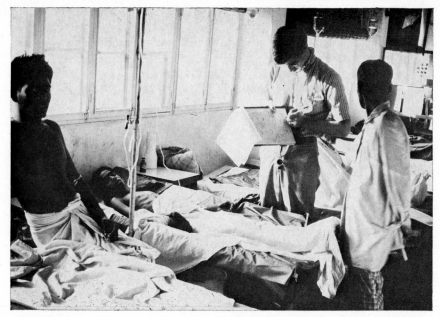

Figure 20-1. Cholera cot used in treating patients with acute cholera. Note the bucket beneath the cot which serves as a collecting vessel for the massive diarrhea. Fluid is replaced in volumes equal to that of the diarrheal fluid. (Courtesy Dr. S. H. Richardson.)

The recent success in developing oral therapy to substitute for intravenous therapy represents a tremendous achievement. It was based on the finding that addition of glucose or glycine to the electrolyte solution enhances the absorption of ingested water and ions. Following initial rehydration by intravenous infusion if necessary, the glucose and salts solution is fed by mouth or introduced through a stomach tube. In Bangladesh, where cholera is a major problem, this simplified method cut the cost of treatment from $42 to 63 cents per patient.

Tetracyclines and certain other antibiotics are effective; they shorten the course of the illness and also the period during which vibrios are excreted. Nevertheless, *survival depends on immediate replacement of fluid and ion losses.*

M. Reservoirs of Infection

Man is the only reservoir for V. cholerae. Usually, the vibrios are transmitted, via water, from patients or from convalescent carriers up to 20 days after onset of the disease. Long-term carriage, which is common in typhoid fever and many other diseases, is infrequent in cholera. However, there is evidence that the *vibrios may be carried in the gallbladder for long periods of time and shed under certain conditions.*

N. Control of Disease Transmission

Prevention of cholera depends on adequate sanitation; the disease is virtually unknown in countries where sanitation is good. Unfortunately, there are large areas of the world where it will not be possible in the immediate future to provide adequate sanitation. Consequently, efforts are being made to develop better vaccines. It is hoped that immunization with toxoid, when it becomes available, will help control the disease. At present, killed cholera vaccines afford limited protection for some 6 months to about 85% of those immunized.

The WHO is waging a constant battle against cholera, which is one of the 6 quarantinable diseases governed by WHO rules on international travel. Any traveler who has been in an area where cholera is endemic or epidemic is subject to quarantine unless he can show proof of immunization within the past 6 months.

The WHO is also constantly working to improve sanitation and to help provide noncontaminated water supplies in underdeveloped areas. This organization faces many sociologic, financial and political problems. The following account illustrates their complexity: A team of workers from WHO visited one village in India where endemic cholera was present. They found that each villager dipped water from the well with his own bucket, which was usually allowed to rest in fecally contaminated mud around the well before dipping. This practice kept the water supply continually contaminated. It was a simple matter to prevent contamination of the well by installing a belt-driven pump and covering the well. However, a year later the team returned, only to find that, once more, buckets were being dipped into the well. The pump was not being used because the villagers, who were Hindus, had found that the belt was made of cowhide.

Although from a medical and scientific standpoint, cholera should be easy to control on a worldwide basis, it will probably be a long time, if ever, before this goal is achieved.

Other Vibrios of Medical Importance

Two other species of the genus *Vibrio* are of minor medical importance; they are *V. fetus* and *V. parahaemolyticus. Vibrio fetus,* which is similar to *V. cholerae,* is a common cause of abortion in cattle and sheep and can produce sepsis and abortion in human beings. *Vibrio parahaemolyticus* causes outbreaks of food poisoning. This halophilic vibrio of fish is transmitted to man by ingestion of raw fish. Food poisoning caused by *V. parahaemolyticus* has been reported most often in Japan where raw fish dishes are popular; however, it also occurs occasionally in the USA.

References

Carpenter, C. C. J.: Cholera and other enterotoxin-related diarrheal diseases. J. Infect. Dis. 126:551, 1972.

Feeley, J. C., and Oseasohn, R. O., eds.: Workshop on the immunology of cholera. J. Infect. Dis. 121 (Suppl.):S1-S150, 1970.

Freter, R.: Parameters affecting the association of vibrios with the intestinal surface in experimental cholera. Infect. Immun. 6:134, 1972.

Peterson, J. W., LoSpalluto, J. J., and Finkelstein, R. A.: Localization of cholera toxin in vivo. J. Infect. Dis. 126:617, 1972.

Pierce, N. F., Banwell, J. G., Gorbach, S. L., Mitra, R. C., and Mondal, A.: Convalescent carriers of Vibrio cholerae. Ann. Intern. Med., 72:357, 1970.

Pierce, N. F., Kaniecki, E. A., and Northrup, R. S.: Protection against experimental cholera by antitoxin. J. Infect. Dis. 126:606, 1972.

Richardson, S. H., Evans, D. G., and Feeley, J. C.: Biochemistry of Vibrio cholerae virulence I. Purification and biochemical properties of P/F cholera enterotoxin. Infect. Immun. 1:546, 1970.

Verwey, W. F., ed.: Current problems in cholera. Tex. Rep. Biol. Med. 27 (Suppl. 1):177-316, 1969.

Waldman, R. H., Bencic, Z., Sinha, R., Deb, B. C., Sakazaki, R., Tamura, K., Mukerjee, S., and Ganguly, R.: Cholera immunology. II. Serum and intestinal secretion antibody response after naturally occurring cholera. J. Infect. Dis. 126:401, 1972.

Pseudomonas

Members of the genus *Pseudomonas* of the family *Pseudomonadaceae* are abundant in soil and water. These organisms, commonly called pseudomonads, have extensive oxidative capabilities and play important roles in degradative cycles in nature. Most of them are free-living; certain species, especially *Ps. aeruginosa,* are frequent among the normal flora of the human intestinal tract and are found occasionally on the skin and in saliva. Although a few species are obligate parasites and pathogens for plants and animals, most species that parasitize animals represent facultative parasites, and none is an obligate parasite of man. *Pseudomonas aeruginosa* is the species that most commonly assumes the role of a facultative human parasite, and this chapter is centered primarily on a discussion of this organism.

Like many other nonpathogenic gram-negative rods, *Ps. aeruginosa* acts as an opportunistic pathogen, most often in the hospital environment. *It is among the most common causes of nosocomial infections and also is one of the most feared of the opportunists because the infections that it causes are difficult to treat and are often fatal.*

A. Medical Perspectives

Pseudomonas aeruginosa was recognized many years ago as the cause of "blue-pus infections" (Gessard 1882); recently these infections have increased greatly in incidence because of increasing numbers of highly susceptible patients, including both the elderly and those with underlying diseases, especially malignancies, chronic uremia, cystic fibrosis and liver disease. Individuals treated with immunosuppressive drugs, such as patients with connective tissue diseases and recipients of organ grafts, patients on anticancer drugs and patients with serious burns contribute importantly to the numbers at risk of opportunistic infections. In addition, the use of certain devices has provided new avenues of entrance for the pseudomonads; for example, intravenous catheters allow direct entry, and intermittent positive-pressure machines for respiratory support sometimes become contaminated with large numbers of pseudomonads which are consequently introduced into the patient's lungs. The high resistance of many pseudomonads to some of the widely used disinfectants, as well as to many antibiotics, compounds the problem. There is every indication that pseudomonas infections will remain a serious problem, at least until more effective immunoprophylactic, immunotherapeutic or chemotherapeutic agents are developed to combat them.

B. Physical and Chemical Structure

Organisms of the genus *Pseudomonas* are gram-negative, nonsporing, occasionally encapsulated rods of varying length (average 1.5 to 3.0 μm $\times$ 0.5 μm). In stained smears they cannot be distinguished from the coliforms. Most strains are motile by means of a single polar flagellum. The organism has a typical gram-negative endotoxin-containing cell wall, and an outer toxic slime layer. Serologic typing of *Pseudomonas* strains has been attempted, and work is in progress toward developing an international standard typing schema. Type specific cell-wall lipopolysaccharides (LPS) exist, but typing is difficult because many wild-type strains contain multiple LPS antigens.

C. Genetics

Mutations that create difficulties in identifying *Ps. aeruginosa* include the loss of flagella and loss of the ability to produce the characteristic pigment, pyocyanin. Among the important genetic attributes of this species are the possession of episomal or plasmid resistance transfer factors (Chapter 4) and the production of pyocins (bacteriocins). The latter are rod-shaped protein particles that resemble phage tails. Pyocins attach to specific receptors on the cell walls of sensitive strains of host bacteria and kill them. The specificity of attachment permitting pyocin typing of strains has been of great aid in epidemiologic studies.

D. Extracellular Products

Pseudomonads are notorious for their ability to synthesize and secrete a large number of extracellular enzymes. In nature, these secreted enzymes serve to degrade many substances; some of the degradation products are probably used as nutrients by the organisms. Many species and strains are proteolytic. Among the enzymes secreted by *Ps. aeruginosa* are collagenase, elastase, lecithinase, lipase, protease and hemolysin. At least 2 exotoxins, designated A and B, are also produced.

Both water-soluble and chloroform-soluble pigments are produced by *Ps. aeruginosa,* the most important being the deep-blue, chloroform-soluble pigment, pyocyanin, and the yellowish-green, water-soluble pigment, fluorescein. Certain of the pigments have strong antibacterial activities against a wide range of gram-positive and gram-negative organisms, and against some fungi. The early name given the organism, *Bacillus pyocyaneus* or *Ps. pyocyaneus,* was coined to designate the blue color lent to pus by pigments produced by the organisms.

E. Culture

Pseudomonads are aerobes, utilizing *only* oxidative metabolism. They are readily cultured because they are not nutritionally fastidious and grow over a wide range of temperature (5 to 43°C). Their ability to use a wide variety of nutrients allows them to grow in materials that support few or no other bacteria. They can survive or even grow in unlikely media such as disinfectant solutions, and often can be isolated from water faucets, sinks, thermometers and similar locales, where they multiply using the meager nutrients present.

Some species of the genus *Pseudomonas* are psychrophilic and can grow at refrigerator temperatures. Hence, they can multiply in refrigerated blood, saline solutions and foods. Transfusion of stored blood or intravenous fluids contaminated with *Pseudomonas sp.* has caused lethal shock resulting from toxins of the bacteria.

F. Resistance to Physical and Chemical Agents

Pseudomonads are relatively resistant to quaternary ammonium compounds, benzalkonium chloride, hexachlorophene and many other disinfectants. However, they are susceptible to ethylene oxide or heat (55°C for 1 hr). Although most of the pseudomonads are susceptible to certain antibiotics, resistance tends to develop readily.

G. Experimental Models

Experimental pseudomonas infections have been studied in mice and various other laboratory animals. The pathogenicity of different strains of *Ps. aeruginosa* for guinea pigs and mice varies greatly; some strains kill in 24 to 48 hours, whereas others may not kill for weeks or are not lethal. The toxicities of extracellular products of *Ps. aeruginosa* have also been examined; exotoxins secreted by the organisms have the greatest lethal toxicity for mice. It has been reported that antitoxin protects mice against otherwise lethal doses of exotoxin(s). Laboratory animals have been used to study the effects of active and passive immunization on pseudomonas infections in burn wounds; variable results have been obtained.

H. Infections in Man

The most common diseases caused by *Ps. aeruginosa* involve infections of the urinary tract and of wounds. Other diseases produced by the organism include otitis media, meningitis, endocarditis, necrotizing pneumonia and necrotizing lesions of the skin and eye.

The major cause of death of burn patients is infection with *Ps. aeruginosa*. Areas of injured skin, moist with inflammatory exudate or dressings, offer ideal conditions for multiplication of the ubiquitous *Ps. aeruginosa*. The source of infection may be from the patient's normal flora (endogenous) or exogenous from the hospital environment. Often, the infection begins during the 1st week after the burn, and extends via lymphatics to local subcutaneous tissues during the 2nd to the 4th week. Characteristically, there is *hemorrhagic necrosis* of the subcutaneous tissues, sometimes without appreciable suppuration. Late during infection, the organisms may enter the blood stream, resulting in septicemia and bacteremic shock that are usually fatal.

Other routes by which pseudomonads invade are the urinary and respiratory tracts. The organisms are often introduced via urinary catheters, tracheostomy apparatus, nebulizers, or respiratory support equipment. Alternatively, they may be introduced into the blood directly by means of intravenous catheters and injected materials. Meningitis caused by *Ps. aeruginosa* usually is the result of introducing this organism during lumbar puncture.

I. Mechanisms of Pathogenicity

Little is known about the pathogenesis of infections due to pseudomonads. The lesions are hemorrhagic, necrotizing and ulcerative, with large numbers of organisms present in surrounding tissue. Secreted proteolytic enzymes are thought to be responsible for the characteristic hemorrhagic skin lesions produced by *Ps. aeruginosa.* As the infection progresses, neutrophils are conspicuously absent, evidently because the organisms produce strong antiphagocytic components including the slime layer and LPS cell wall Ags. *Pseudomonas aeruginosa* presents a great array of potentially harmful substances, and no single factor has been shown to be the key to virulence. However, to be virulent a strain must possess both the ability to grow in fresh serum and the capacity to produce necrosis on intradermal injection. An extracellular toxin causes increased permeability of small blood vessels. Several extracellular enzymes may contribute importantly to tissue damage; for example, the hemolysin damages cell membranes, the elastases injure vessel walls, the collagenase degrades collagen, and the lecithinase is toxic for many cells, including granulocytes which it lyses. The proteolytic enzymes produced not only appear to make the major contribution to the development of necrotic lesions, but also may increase the invasiveness of the organisms. It is likely that endotoxins also contribute to pathogenesis.

J. Mechanisms of Immunity

Even though *Ps. aeruginosa* possesses a large armamentarium of potential virulence factors, it is important to note that it does not invade and cause disease unless some abrogation of normal defenses takes place. Except in special circumstances it is probable that a simple breach in the integuments is insufficient to allow infection and must be accompanied by a depression or block of certain other factor(s) of host resistance. In burn patients, for example, systemic as well as local depression of antimicrobial defense probably occurs. The necrotic tissue in burned skin hampers local defense mechanisms and provides a favorable environment for bacterial growth; however, the mechanisms involved in nonspecific depression of systemic defense following burns have not been defined. Other circumstances predisposing to pseudomonas infection include suppression of other bacteria of the normal flora with broad-spectrum antibiotics, debilitating malignant disease, or nonspecific depression of immune responses caused by steroid or antimetabolite therapy.

Humoral Abs appear to be important in defense against *Ps. aeruginosa,* as evidenced by passive transfer of immunity with human gamma globulin containing specific Abs. However, the important immunogens have not been clearly defined and the approaches to immunoprophylaxis and immunotherapy in man by use of vaccines and antisera have been largely empirical. Recent evidence indicates that the majority of isolates from human disease are resistant to the bactericidal action of convalescent serum, but that anti-LPS Ab in the presence of the first 4 components of C exerts strong opsonic effects in promoting phagocytosis and killing by neutrophils.

10

K. Laboratory Diagnosis

Although *Ps. aeruginosa* grows on most ordinary media, blood agar is commonly used for bacteriologic diagnosis. The colonies are usually apparent because of diffusion of the blue-green pigments into the surrounding medium. Pure cultures have a characteristic peculiar sweetish odor caused by the metabolic product trimethylamine. The fluorescent pigments produced occasionally also aid in identification of the organisms in the laboratory and in direct diagnosis of pseudomonas infection in the patient. For example, examination of a burn with ultraviolet light may reveal fluorescence produced by infecting *Ps. aeruginosa* before the infection becomes clinically overt; a concentration of 10^3 pseudomonas organisms per cm^2 can be visually detected under a Wood's light, whereas invasive sepsis of burn wounds is not likely to occur until the concentration reaches $10^5/cm^2$ or higher.

Difficulties in identification arise with strains that lack pigments or flagella. In these instances, biochemical tests are particularly important. Whereas the *Enterobacteriaceae* ferment many sugars, obligately oxidative pseudomonads cannot ferment carbohydrates.

Serotyping, phage typing and pyocin typing are of some use as tools for epidemiologic studies, but not for diagnosis.

L. Therapy

Antibiotic therapy is difficult but can be effective against pseudomonas infections; sensitivity testing is absolutely essential. Carbenicillin, colistin and gentamicin are currently the antibiotics of choice. The benefits of passive immunotherapy with specific antisera and of combined active and passive immunotherapy are under investigation.

M. Reservoirs of Infection

Reservoirs of *Pseudomonas sp.* are ubiquitous; the patient himself or any other human being may serve as a source of infection. In addition, *Ps. aeruginosa* thrives in or on medical and surgical equipment, solutions, food, water and a variety of other materials.

N. Control of Disease Transmission

Prevention is the best method for coping with pseudomonas infections. *Patients at risk should be managed with great attention to aseptic techniques, and with minimal use of broad-spectrum antibiotics.* Sterilization, rather than "disinfection," of equipment is essential.

A promising method for preventing pseudomonas infection is being developed in studies of burn patients. Multiple doses of a polyvalent killed vaccine are given sequentially, beginning as soon as the patient is admitted to the hospital. This results in the rapid acquisition of specific Abs before infection can become established. This procedure of active immunization appears to be effective for decreasing the incidence and severity of pseudomonas burn infections, although its evaluation has not been completed.

O. Infections Caused by Species of the Genus Pseudomonas Other than Ps. aeruginosa

Diseases similar to those caused by *Ps. aeruginosa* can result from infection with less common pseudomonads, including *Ps. maltophilia, Ps. stutzeri, Ps. multivorans* and several others.

Pseudomonas mallei (old name *Actinobacillus mallei*) causes a disease called *glanders* in its natural hosts—horses and related animals. Man can be infected accidentally by contact with diseased animals, but this seldom occurs at present because glanders is rare among the horse population. Without antibiotic treatment, human infections are often fatal.

Melioidosis, a disease similar to glanders, is caused by *Ps. pseudomallei. Pseudomonas pseudomallei* resembles *Ps. aeruginosa* in many respects; however, some strains produce a yellow pigment. Human melioidosis occurs most often in Southeast Asia, where the organism is found in wild rats and other animals and in soil and water. It is usually transmitted from rats to man by the bites of fleas or mosquitoes, but can also be contracted from contaminated food and water. In recent years, cases of melioidosis have appeared in the USA in a number of military service personnel returning from endemic areas. In contrast to the opportunistic pathogen *Ps. aeruginosa, Ps. pseudomallei* is a primary pathogen and melioidosis often occurs in healthy young people. The disease frequently involves the lungs and takes various forms, ranging from an acute septicemia, that may be rapidly fatal, to chronic infections with widespread granulomatous lesions in lymph nodes and other tissues. Treatment with broad-spectrum antibiotics and sulfonamides is usually effective; however, it may be necessary to continue therapy for many weeks.

References

Alexander, J. W., Fisher, M. W., and MacMillan, B. G.: Immunologic control of pseudomonas infection in burn patients. Arch. Surg. *102*:31, 1971.

Burdon, D. W., and Whitby, J. L.: Contamination of hospital disinfectants with *Pseudomonas* species. Brit. Med. J. *2*:153, 1967.

Franklin, M., and Franklin, M. A.: *A Profile of Pseudomonas.* Clifton, N. J.: Beecham Pharmaceuticals, 1971.

Gilardi, G. L.: Infrequently encountered *Pseudomonas* species causing infections in humans. Ann. Intern. Med. *77*:211, 1972.

Heckly, R. J.: *Microbial Toxins,* Vol. III. Bacterial protein toxins. T. C. Montie, S. Kadis, and S. J. Ajl, eds. New York: Academic Press, 1970.

Howe, C.: Melioidosis. *Infectious Diseases,* P. D. Hoeprich, ed. Hagerstown, Md.: Harper & Row, 1972.

Liu, P. V.: The role of various fractions of *Pseudomonas aeruginosa* in its pathogenesis. III. Identity of the lethal toxins produced *in vitro* and *in vivo*. J. Infect. Dis. *116*:481, 1966.

Stanier, R. Y., Palleroni, N. J., and Doudoroff, M.: The aerobic pseudomonads: a taxonomic study. J. Gen. Microbiol. *43*:159, 1966.

Young, L. S., and Armstrong, D.: Human immunity to *Pseudomonas aeruginosa*. I. *In vitro* interaction of bacteria, polymorphonuclear leukocytes and serum factors. J. Infect. Dis. *126*:257, 1972.

Chapter 22

Bacteroides and Fusobacterium

The normal human adult excretes approximately 10^{11} bacteria per gram of feces, a majority of which are strictly anaerobic, gram-negative, nonsporing, pleomorphic rods, predominately of the genus *Bacteroides,* family *Bacteroidaceae.* These organisms are also normal inhibitants of the mouth and vagina. They have little pathogenic potential in normal hosts, but as opportunists cause infections, particularly in persons who are immunologically compromised. Predisposing conditions include malignant neoplasms, diabetes mellitus and corticosteroid therapy. *A characteristic of bacteroides is that they frequently cause mixed infections in conjunction with other microbes.* Some 30 species of *Bacteroides* exist, most of which may cause human infections; however, *Bacteroides fragilis* is most frequently encountered.

The taxonomic designations of the gram-negative nonsporeforming anaerobic rods are changing. Morphologic criteria have been used in the past, but many strains have atypical morphologic characteristics. Consequently, the genera listed in Table 22-1 have recently been reclassified on the basis of their biochemical activities. Although this may change the genus name, the specific epithet (e.g., *fragilis*) remains the same. In addi-

TABLE 22-1

Some Medically Important Species of the Genera *Bacteroides* and *Fusobacterium**

Genus and Species	Characteristics†
Bacteroides fragilis	Resistant to penicillin (1 μg/ml), also to kanamycin, neomycin, and polymyxin
Bacteroides oralis	Sensitive to the above antibiotics
Bacteroides melaninogenicus (Bacteroides nigrescens)	Produces black pigment on blood agar
Fusobacterium fusiforme	Ferments glucose to butyric acid; long, thin cells with tapered ends; may grow as filaments in culture
Fusobacterium necrophorus (also known as Sphaerophorus funduliformis)	Ferments glucose to butyric acid; pleomorphic; often beta-hemolytic and produces lipase

* This group of organisms is referred to as the *Bacteroides-Fusobacterium* (*B-F*) group.

† Most strains.

tion to the organisms listed in Table 22-1 and discussed in this chapter, the following anaerobic organisms may also cause infection: *Bacteroides corrodens, Leptotrichia buccalis, Dialister* sp., *Vibrio sputorum, Butyrivibrio fibrisolvens,* and others.

For convenience, the abbreviation "B-F" or "B-F group" will be used in the following discussion to designate species of Bacteroides *and* Fusobacterium, *the closely related gram-negative anaerobes most often implicated in human disease.*

A. Medical Perspectives

Infections with *Bacteroides* sp. and other anaerobic bacteria of low pathogenicity often go undiagnosed. This probably has resulted from a general lack of appreciation of the opportunistic potential of these organisms, as well as the failure to properly conduct anaerobic culture of specimens from such infections. The increasing use of forms of therapy that predispose to infections with *Bacteroides* sp. and other anaerobes makes it imperative that they be recognized and identified, because the diseases that they cause may be fatal. A recent study of patients with bacteroides bacteremia revealed that 15 of 39 patients (38%) died of their infections! *With proper diagnosis and treatment, bacteroides infections need not be fatal.*

B. Physical and Chemical Structure

Members of the B-F group contain endotoxin in their gram-negative cell walls. Most of them lack flagella and are nonmotile. At present, antigenic analysis of these organisms is not used in laboratory diagnosis.

C. Genetics

Little is known about the genetics of B-F organisms.

D. Extracellular Products

No extracellular products of medical importance are known.

E. Culture

Care must be taken to avoid exposing media to air before anaerobic cultures are made, in order to guard against oxygen absorption and the formation of toxic organic peroxides. Plates of blood agar, brain-heart infusion agar, hemolyzed blood-agar with menadione, or other media are inoculated and incubated under anaerobic conditions. Liquid media should be freshly prepared or heated at 100°C for 20 min prior to use, to drive off dissolved oxygen. Tubes of liquid media serve best if they are incubated anaerobically or covered with a layer of melted petroleum jelly and paraffin to exclude contact with air. Thioglycollate broth or media containing chopped meat provide anaerobic conditions in the lower portions of the tube.

Bacteroides species yield visible growth within 2 to 10 days. They often produce a foul odor as the result of their anaerobic metabolism, and gas may be demonstrable in the cultures.

F. Resistance to Physical and Chemical Agents

Extreme susceptibility to oxygen is a notable characteristic of most of these nonsporing anaerobes. Resistance of some species to certain antibiotics is the basis of selective media used to isolate the organisms.

G. Experimental Models

Organisms of the B-F group are not markedly pathogenic for laboratory animals except for an occasional strain of *Fusobacterium necrophorum*.

H. Infections in Man

The B-F group of organisms can infect virtually any tissue in which anaerobic conditions exist. Thus, they are usually isolated from patients suffering from mixed infections such as those complicating colectomy, colostomy, appendicitis, cholecystectomy, gunshot wounds, rectal abscess, puerperal or postabortal sepsis, necrotizing pneumonia, lung abscess and brain abscess. These organisms produce the typical symptoms of gram-negative sepsis, including shock in about 25% of cases. Infection with these anaerobes should be suspected whenever there is foul-smelling pus, a black discharge, necrotic tissue, or infection in a bite wound inflicted by either a human being or an animal. Thrombophlebitis occasionally develops near the site of infection, and emboli may be shed into the circulation.

Lung infections with anaerobes usually follow invasion of normal flora from the mouth and upper respiratory tract, and occur in the immuno-logically compromised patient. The onset is often insidious, and symptoms such as malaise, cough and low-grade fever may occur over a period of weeks or months before the physician is consulted. In such cases, an un-derlying malignant disease is often found to be the predisposing factor.

Fusospirochetal disease occurs when B-F organisms and spirochetes of the normal flora infect together. This may occur following injury to mu-cous membranes, as a result of other infections, or in compromised hosts. The most common example is ulcerative gingivostomatitis (trench mouth) and the associated condition, Vincent's angina, in which ulcerative lesions develop in the tonsillar areas. Trench mouth and Vincent's angina usually are associated with dietary deficiencies, particularly deficiencies of vitamins B and A. Fusospirochetal infections also produce ulcerative lesions else-where, including lung abscesses.

I. Mechanisms of Pathogenicity

Little is known about the mechanisms of pathogenicity of B-F infections. It can be postulated that endotoxins of the gram-negative cell walls play a role, especially in those patients who develop shock. The necrotizing nature of the lesions may reflect the activities of proteolytic enzymes and other extracellular products of the anaerobes. This concept is supported by the occurrence of foul-smelling, putrid discharges that ostensibly re-sult from proteolysis of tissues.

J. Mechanisms of Immunity

The normal human being has a high level of innate immunity against B-F species and never becomes infected in spite of being host to billions of normal flora organisms. It is only when normal defenses are abrogated that B-F organisms invade their hosts. Nevertheless, little is known about the nature of immunity to organisms of the B-F group.

K. Laboratory Diagnosis

Special care must be taken in collecting and transporting specimens to the laboratory, as well as in culture techniques. Normal flora of body orifices always include many gram-negative anaerobes; therefore, it is necessary to avoid contamination of specimens with normal flora. Also, the B-F organisms are strict anaerobes, and are readily killed by excessive exposure to oxygen during transport and culture.

Direct microscopic examination is often a valuable aid in diagnosis; both wet mounts and gram-stained smears should be prepared. Specimens are inoculated heavily into chopped meat or some other anaerobic broth medium, and onto solid agar plates, and incubated anaerobically (Section D). Since mixed infections are the rule, pure cultures must be obtained from the primary cultures for biochemical identification of the organisms. Identification of species is usually based on colony characteristics, biochemical reactions, and patterns of susceptibility to antibacterial agents.

Of course, aerobic cultures of clinical specimens should also be prepared, since both aerobic and anaerobic microbes may occur in these mixed infections.

L. Therapy

Drainage of lesions and surgical debridement to eliminate anaerobic foci are essential, and may be sufficient to limit the disease without other therapy. However, antibiotic treatment is important and necessary for more serious infections, especially those with associated bacteremia.

The antibiotic sensitivity of B-F organisms varies with the species, as well as with strains. *Bacteroides fragilis* is noted for its resistance to penicillin, which is in contrast to other members of this group. Tetracyclines may be effective; however, many strains are now resistant to tetracycline. Currently, most strains are sensitive to Clindamycin and to chloramphenicol, which are the antibiotics of choice for acute infections. Because the mortality is high in B-F sepsis, chloramphenicol therapy should be initiated while culture and sensitivity testing are being done.

M. Reservoirs of Infection

The reservoir of infection is man, particularly the alimentary tract of the infected host.

N. Control of Disease Transmission

Control of B-F infections rests on their prevention. This is best achieved by avoiding or correcting predisposing conditions; for example, by using great care in treating patients with immunosuppressive agents, particularly with respect to the suppression of antibacterial immunity. Prophylactic treatment of patients with wounds that permit the entrance of normal flora into injured tissues is especially important.

References

Bodner, S. J., Koenig, M. G., and Goodman, J. S.: Bacteremic bacteroides infections. Ann. Intern. Med. *73*:537, 1970.

Finegold, S. M.: Isolation of anaerobic bacteria. In *Manual of Clinical Microbiology*. J. E. Blair, E. H. Lennette, and J. P. Truant, eds. Bethesda, Md.: American Society for Microbiology, 1970, pp. 265-279.

Hermans, P. E., and Washington, J. A., II: Polymicrobial bacteremia. Ann. Intern. Med. *73*:387, 1970.

Holdeman, L. V., and Moore, W. E. C.: Gram-negative nonspore-forming anaerobic bacilli. In *Manual of Clinical Microbiology*. J. E. Blair, E. H. Lennette, and J. P. Truant, eds. Bethesda, Md.: American Society for Microbiology, 1970, pp. 286-289.

Prevot, A. R.: *Manual for the Classification and Determination of the Anaerobic Bacteria* (Trans. by V. Fredette). Philadelphia: Lea & Febiger, 1966.

Smith, L. D., and Holdeman, L. V.: *The Pathogenic Anaerobic Bacteria*. Springfield, Ill.: Charles C Thomas, 1968.

Chapter 23

Brucella

The genus *Brucella* of the family *Brucellaceae* contains 3 major species, *Br. abortus, Br. melitensis* and *Br. suis,* which cause natural disease, primarily in cattle, goats and swine, respectively. Since these organisms are obligate parasites the animal hosts serve as the major reservoirs of infection for man. Human beings become infected by contact with diseased animals or by the ingestion of contaminated milk and dairy products.

A. Medical Perspectives

Human brucellosis (undulant fever) was first described in 1863 by Marston, who recorded attacks of the disease experienced by others and by himself during his tour of duty as a British Army surgeon on the Island of Malta. The disease was subsequently referred to as Malta fever. In 1887, Bruce isolated *Br. melitensis* at necropsy from British soldiers who had died of Malta fever. The species *Br. abortus* was first isolated by Bang in 1897 in Denmark from cows suffering from infectious abortion (Bang's disease); Traum, an American investigator, isolated *Br. suis* from a premature swine fetus in about 1914. Recently a new species, *Br. ovis,* has been isolated from infected sheep following abortion; another species *Br. canis* has been described as a cause of abortion in dogs.

Brucellosis is a worldwide endemic disease in goats, cattle and swine as well as in many wild cloven-hoofed animals including deer, elk and Alaskan caribou. In addition, mules, horses, sheep, camels, buffaloes, reindeer, dogs, hares and chickens sometimes acquire the disease naturally. In the USA alone, annual livestock losses due to brucellosis are appraised at about 100 million dollars. It has been estimated that, in the USA, 5% of all female cattle, 15% of all cattle herds and about 1 to 3% of swine are infected.

In domestic mammals it is probable that infection commonly results from ingestion of contaminated food or, less frequently, water. The infection spreads to the mammary glands. Spread to the genital organs, and particularly the placenta, is common and is the cause of abortion. The organisms are shed in milk, urine, feces and vaginal secretions. Virgin heifers, which are relatively resistant to brucellosis, become susceptible following pregnancy. In cows the organisms have a marked viscerotropism for the fetal portion of the placenta, the placental fluids and the chorion. This remarkable localization of the organism is apparently due to high local concentrations of erythritol which stimulate the growth of the organisms, even within phagocytic cells. Erythritol appears to be the main biochemical determinant of infectious abortion due to brucellae (Section I). As a rule, females with clinical brucellosis have high titers of agglutinins in their sera as well as in their milk; these Abs can be detected by agglutinin tests.

Human brucellosis occurs most often among individuals who are engaged in occupations concerned with livestock and dairy products such as farming, veterinary medicine, and the processing of meats and dairy products. Cattle and swine represent the principal natural reservoirs of human brucellosis in the USA, whereas the goat is the chief source of the disease in countries where goat's milk is a common human food. Human brucellosis is still a substantial medical problem in some areas of the world. It is estimated that only about 1 case in 5 is diagnosed and reported. During the period 1962 to 1971 the number of human cases of brucellosis reported annually to the USPHS ranged from 183 to 411. This low incidence of the disease in the USA represents a remarkable public achievement. It is unlikely that brucellosis will again become a significant problem if constant vigilance for controlling the disease among farm animals is maintained and pasteurization of milk is enforced. The problem is further mitigated by the fact that the mortality rate in untreated persons with brucellosis of 2 to 3% can be reduced essentially to zero when appropriate diagnostic and therapeutic procedures are practiced.

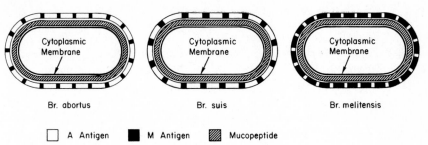

Br. abortus   Br. suis   Br. melitensis

☐ A Antigen   ■ M Antigen   ▨ Mucopeptide

Figure 23-1. Diagrammatic representation of the ratio of A and M antigens in brucellae.

B. Physical and Chemical Structure

Organisms of the genus *Brucella* are small, pleomorphic, nonmotile, sometimes encapsulated, nonsporing aerobic, gram-negative rods that tend to assume a "coccobacillary form" (0.3 to 2.3 μm in length). *Brucella* species share a common Ag with *Vibrio cholerae* which explains why individuals vaccinated against cholera form agglutinins that react with the brucellae. Cross-agglutination reactions with *Francisella tularensis* have also been reported. The 3 major species of *Brucella* contain 2 dominant Ags designated A and M. *Brucella abortus* contains approximately 20 times as much A Ag as M Ag; in contrast, *Br. melitensis* possesses about 20 times as much M Ag as A Ag. *Brucella suis* exhibits an intermediate antigenic pattern although it resembles *Br. abortus* in having a predominance of A Ag. The distribution of these Ags in the various species is depicted in Figure 23-1. Monospecific anti-A and anti-M sera can be prepared by absorption with appropriate brucellae. It has been proposed that the A and M Ags are composed of glucose, glucosamine, galactose, and hexuronic acids. Brucellae also contain cell wall endotoxins that are similar to those of other gram-negative bacteria. Capsules can be demonstrated on smooth and mucoid variants.

C. Genetics

Isolates of various species of *Brucella* exhibit the classical smooth-to-rough dissociation pattern. The S→R mutation is associated with a loss of virulence, a tendency toward spontaneous agglutination and a decrease in the Ags which stimulate agglutinins specific for smooth strains. The attenuated vaccine strain, *Br. abortus* 19, an intermediate mutant, is immunogenic despite its avirulence for cattle and low virulence for man.

D. Extracellular Products

The brucellae do not produce any extracellular products of known medical importance. The only apparent toxin produced is an endotoxin.

E. Culture

The brucellae are aerobic and will not grow under strict anaerobic conditions. They grow slowly at 37°C in trypticase soy broth or on standard blood agar media pH 6.6 to 6.8. In contrast to the other brucellae that infect man, *Br. abortus* requires 5 to 10% CO_2 for primary isolation from clinical specimens. The 3 major species of the brucellae are differentiated on the basis of their growth patterns in the presence of thionine and basic fuchsin, CO_2 requirement, H_2S production and A and M Ag patterns.

F. Resistance to Physical and Chemical Agents

Brucellae are readily killed by heat and the usual antiseptics and disinfectants, but are relatively resistant to drying. They can remain viable in contaminated raw milk for as long as 10 days at 4°C and persist in unpasteurized cheese and butter for periods up to 4 months. Brucellae can survive for weeks to months in dust, tissues of dead animals, feces, soil, water and urine.

G. Experimental Models

Experimentally infected monkeys develop a nonprogressive disease with undulating temperature patterns; mice and rats are highly resistant. The guinea pig is susceptible to many strains of brucellae, especially *Br. melitensis,* which is often fatal for this animal.

H. Infections in Man

Although man is highly susceptible to infection with virulent brucellae, immunity is readily acquired and most infections remain inapparent. Virulence for man varies widely among strains. Evidently man has little or no natural immunity to virulent brucellae and essentially all of the immunity he acquires, albeit sometimes weak, is developed as a response to primary infection.

In naturally acquired brucellosis the organisms can infect via broken skin, the oropharynx, the alimentary tract or the conjunctivae. Thus ingestion, contact and inhalation are the major means of disease transmission. The organisms are seen within macrophages and to a lesser extent within endothelial cells and fibroblasts. After multiplication at the local site of penetration the organisms spread to the lymphatics, lymph nodes and blood stream. Ultimately small granulomatous lesions become established in many organs including the spleen, liver, kidneys and bone marrow. Brucellosis may express itself as an acute, subacute or chronic disease, but seldom takes a fulminating fatal course.

Acute brucellosis usually has an incubation period of 10 to 14 days (range 4 to 45 days). An undulating daily fever pattern is common, although it is not consistently found in patients in the USA. An initial septicemia occurs. Positive blood cultures can usually be obtained during the first 14 to 21 days of the disease; they tend to become negative as the patient develops agglutinins, C-F Abs and opsonins. *Relapses are hallmarks of this disease; when they occur the body temperature is elevated and blood cultures usually become positive again.* Positive, delayed-type skin reactions can usually be elicited with brucellergen, a protein-containing bacillary extract, after the 3rd to the 6th week of the disease. Patients with clinical brucellosis usually exhibit a low-grade fever, which often peaks in the afternoon and early morning (undulant fever), and complain of headache, fatigue, night sweats, weakness, insomnia, anorexia, constipation and generalized aches and pains. Pain on motion of the spine may occur due to a localized spondylitis of one or more of the vertebral bodies. Some 5% of patients exhibit enlarged cervical nodes and about 30% have splenomegaly. Hepatitis is common and jaundice is sometimes seen. Orchitis, if it occurs, is ushered in by a chill followed by high fever. In most patients the primary disease undergoes remission in 3 to 5 months. In a few individuals, brucellosis exhibits a more chronic and extended course.

Chronic brucellosis usually produces weakness, fatigue and vague aches and pains, as well as mental depression, in spite of lack of characteristic abnormal physical findings. Irritability, anxiety and mental depression may become profound and sometimes present major problems in management. The chronic form of brucellosis can last for 1 to 20 years with relapses of varying degrees of intensity; complications involving many tissues and organs may occur. Fortunately the most serious complications, endocarditis and meningoencephalitis, are rare. Abortion due to brucellosis is extremely rare in human beings.

I. Mechanisms of Pathogenicity

The manner by which the brucellae cause tissue injury is not known but presumably depends, in part at least, on delayed hypersensitivity and possibly endotoxin. The brucellae are primarily intracellular parasites within macrophages and in accord with expectation the chronic lesions are granulomas composed of epithelioid cells, giant cells and lymphocytes. *Brucella suis,* in particular, can produce granulomas exhibiting central necrosis and caseation. Virulence varies greatly among strains of brucellae, but little is known about the factors determining virulence. Since smooth strains are virulent and rough strains are not, cell wall composition is presumed to be related to virulence. The capacity of virulent organisms to metabolize erythritol, a growth-promoting substance, appears to be a virulence factor enabling certain strains (but not others) to infect the ungulate placenta, which is rich in erythritol. For unknown reasons, virulent strains can survive and grow within macrophages better than avirulent strains. In certain strains this property of virulence is enhanced by growing the organisms in media supplemented with placental fluid.

J. Mechanisms of Immunity

Immunity acquired as a result of natural infection is only partial and, as a consequence, either superinfection, reactivation or reinfection can occur. The low level of acquired immunity is also in accord with the usual relapsing nature and chronicity of the disease. Apparently, bactericidal serum Abs and neutrophils can effectively destroy organisms that are not engulfed and sheltered (at least for a time) by other cells, principally macrophages. In accord with the prediction supported by these circumstances, there is no correlation between serum Abs and acquired immunity in brucellosis, but, instead, *strong evidence that the main mechanism of acquired immunity is cellular.* Although it has been observed that immune macrophages can inhibit the intracellular growth of brucellae *in vitro* more effectively than normal macrophages, there is also evidence that virulent brucellae possess a toxicity for macrophages which can be neutralized by immune serum. *Consequently it may be that the maximum expression of acquired immunity rests on an interplay between cellular and humoral immune forces.* The Ags responsible for acquired immunity are not known. Antiendotoxin Abs are not protective.

K. Laboratory Diagnosis

The clinical diagnosis of brucellosis is often difficult to establish. The disease is commonly categorized among the "fevers of unknown origin." In order to make a definitive diagnosis it is necessary to cultivate the brucellae from samples of blood or aspirates of bone marrow or lymph nodes. It is especially difficult to culture brucellae from patients with subacute or chronic infections. Evidently the intracellular position of the organisms within macrophages is responsible for the frequent failure of blood culture, especially in chronic brucellosis. Clinical specimens are inoculated into trypticase soy broth incubated in the presence of 10% CO_2, and examined for growth of typical brucellae at 4-day to 5-day intervals. *The primary culture should be incubated for 4 to 6 weeks before being discarded as negative!* When growth occurs subcultures are made on a trypticase soy-blood-agar medium and incubated under 10% CO_2. Species identification can be made by employing the tests listed in Table 23-1 as well as with monospecific antiserum (anti-A or anti-M). *Cultures of brucellae should be handled with care because of the high risk of laboratory infection.*

TABLE 23-1
Characteristics of Brucella Species

	Br. abortus	Br. melitensis	Br. suis
CO_2 requirement	+	−	−
Glucose	+	+	+
Urea	−	−	+
Carbamate	−	+	−
Thionine 1:800	+*	−	−
Basic fuchsin 1:200	−†	−	+
Crystal violet 1:400	−	−	+
Azure A 1:1,000	+	−	+
Nitrite sensitivity	−	+	−

* = zone of inhibition greater than 4 mm.
† = zone of inhibition less than 4 mm.
Adapted from Pickett, M. J., Nelson, E. L., and Liberman, J. D.: J. Bacteriol. 66:210, 1953; Pickett, M. J., and Nelson, E. L.: J. Bacteriol. 69:333, 1955.

Agglutination tests are performed on patients' sera with phenolized suspensions of heat-killed smooth organisms. Agglutinin titers above 1:80 to 1:160 are generally interpreted to indicate past or present infection; rising titers in early disease are particularly significant. *It should be emphasized that patients who have received a brucellergen skin test or cholera vaccine will usually have serum agglutinins for brucellae.* Because of the value of agglutination tests the brucellergen skin test should not be used routinely as a diagnostic aid. In some patients, brucellae Abs of the "blocking" type which fail to produce agglutination occur. A positive test for blocking Abs even though agglutinins are lacking is presumptive evidence of brucellosis. These Abs that appear in chronic disease may be detected by substituting 5% serum albumin for 0.85% NaCl diluent. Antibodies that precipitate with brucella extracts appear late in acute disease; they persist as long as the disease remains active and are the best indicator of an active clinical infection.

L. Therapy

The course of acute brucellosis can be shortened and the complications minimized by the use of a 3-week therapeutic regimen of tetracycline. This schedule must be repeated if a relapse occurs; however, more than 2 courses

of tetracycline are seldom administered. If patients suffer from severe toxemia, depression, anorexia and a generalized debilitated condition, adreno-
corticoid therapy is recommended as an adjunct to antibiotic therapy. Tetracycline therapy is effective in chronic forms of the disease. Herxheimer-
like reactions are sometimes encountered during chemotherapy.

Many attempts have been made to desensitize patients with repeated injections of increasing doses of brucellae Ags based on the premise that a
significant component of the symptom complex is due to a systemic delayed
sensitivity reaction. While there may be some merit to this procedure, it is
very difficult to evaluate and is time consuming. Moreover, it is fraught
with the possibility of violent local and systemic reactions and is not generally recommended.

M. Reservoirs of Infection

The major reservoirs of human brucellosis in the USA are infected
cattle and hogs. Goats are a major reservoir in countries where goat milk
is used extensively. The organism is highly infectious and laboratory infections are easily acquired.

N. Control of Disease Transmission

Brucellosis in cattle can be controlled moderately well by vaccinating
calves with an attenuated live vaccine such as strain 19 or BA-19. Another
promising vaccine strain is called Rev 1. In addition, the segregation and
slaughter of serologically positive animals provide a highly effective control
measure. The role that wild animals might play in obstructing efforts to
eradicate infection in herds of domestic animals has not been assessed.

Human brucellosis among urban populations in the USA has been essentially eradicated by pasteurization of milk. However, this does not help to
minimize the occupational risk of those individuals who are exposed to
infected animals and dairy products made from raw milk.

Appropriate human vaccines could be of value in protecting individuals
at high occupational risk; nevertheless, public health authorities in the
USA have not recommended immunization with the vaccines currently
available. However, human brucellosis has allegedly been reduced 10-fold
as a result of widespread vaccination in Russia. As one would expect, a
search for safer and better vaccines is in progress.

References

Bhongbhibhat, N., Elberg, S. S., and Chen, T. H.: Characterization of *Brucella* skin-
test antigens. J. Infect. Dis. *122*:70, 1970.
Chen, T. H., and Elberg, S. S.: Immunization against brucella infections: serological and immunological studies on a soluble antigen from *Brucella melitensis*.
J. Infect. Dis. *120*:143, 1969.

Feeley, J. C.: Somatic O antigen relationship of brucella and *Vibrio cholerae*. J. Bacteriol. *99*:645, 1969.

Golden, B., Layman, T. E., Koontz, F. P., and Mergner, W. J.: *Brucella suis* endocarditis. South. Med. J. *63*:392, 1970.

Human Brucellosis—United States 1968. Morbidity and Mortality Reports. *18*:114 (April 5), 1969.

Jones, L. M., and Berman, D. T.: Antibody response, delayed hypersensitivity, and immunity in guinea pigs induced by smooth and rough strains of *Brucella abortus*. J. Infect. Dis. *124*:47, 1971.

Pearsall, N. N., and Weiser, R. S.: *The Macrophage*. Philadelphia: Lea & Febiger, 1970.

Smith, H., and Pearce, J. H., eds.: *Microbial Pathogenicity in Man and Animals*. Cambridge, England: Cambridge University Press, 1972.

Zinneman, H. H., Seal, U. S., and Hall, W. H.: Some molecular characteristics of blocking antibodies in human brucellosis. Arch. Intern. Med. (Chicago) *93*:993, 1964.

Chapter 24

Yersinia and Pasteurella

Yersinia pestis, 298

Yersinia pseudotuberculosis, 308
Pasteurella, 308

The genus *Yersinia* of the family *Brucellaceae* comprises 2 species, *Yersinia pestis* (formerly *Pasteurella pestis*) and *Y. pseudotuberculosis* (formerly *Pasteurella pseudotuberculosis*). Closely related organisms of the genus *Pasteurella* are *Past. multocida* and *Past. hemolytica*. All are parasitic and most are pathogenic for their natural hosts; all tend to produce hemorrhagic lesions and septicemia, some more so than others (hemorrhagic septicemia group). *Yersinia pestis,* the cause of plague, is the only human pathogen of great importance among species of these 2 genera.

Yersinia pestis

Man and the domestic rat, the principal source of human plague, are highly susceptible accidental hosts of *Y. pestis;* the *natural hosts,* which constitute the permanent reservoir, are relatively resistant wild rodents.

A. Medical Perspectives

Although plague is a minor health problem in the world today, the ever-present threat of future outbreaks stands as a grim reminder that, *during centuries past, periodic epidemics of this fearsome pestilence extracted the greatest toll of human lives of any epidemic disease.* In fact, plague was one of the major reasons that population control was not needed in past centuries. During the period 600 B.C. to A.D. 1800, more than 196 major epidemics and pandemics occurred causing well over 200 million deaths. In some epidemics, as many as 50% of entire populations were killed. The 50-year Justinian pandemic of the 6th century took 100 million lives and the "black plague" epidemic of the 14th century claimed the lives of one-fourth of the population of Europe (25 million). For some unknown reason the disease was relatively quiescent during most of the 18th and 19th centuries only to reappear with its usual fury near the beginning of the 20th century; mortality during the Hong Kong epidemic of 1894 was 95%. In India alone, 10 million died of plague between 1898 and 1918. Good descriptions of plague epidemics are given in Boccaccio's *Decameron* and Defoe's *Journal of the Plague Year in London.*

The swiftness and destructiveness of the great plague epidemics of the past (most had a major pneumonic component) are difficult to imagine. Petrarch (1348), who wrote about one such epidemic in France, emphasized that future generations would be unable to comprehend ". . . the empty houses, the abandoned towns, the squalid countryside, the field littered with dead, and the dreadful silent solitude which seems to hang over the whole world." *The enormity of the impact of this one disease on the course of human history can never be accurately evaluated.* It has caused wars to begin and wars to cease, has brought about major social upheavals and has contributed to the rise and fall of nations. For example, it played a major role in the fall of the Roman Empire and dealt the final blow to the feudal system.

The causative organism was discovered by Yersin (1894) during the Hong Kong epidemic. Although it had been noted repeatedly during thousands of years that both rats and human beings sicken and die during plague epidemics, the reasons for the association were not clear until Ogata (1897) suggested and Simond (1900) and the English Plague Commission (1906) proved that the rat flea transmits the causative organism from rat to rat and from rat to man. Plague antiserum was used therapeutically in Yersin's time and a vaccine was introduced by Haffkine in 1896.

During the last 100 years, *Y. pestis* spread widely from Asia, Africa and Europe to other parts of the world, including the USA (San Francisco in 1900). It has spread throughout sylvatic regions in the West, particularly New Mexico, and other limited areas in the USA to establish permanent reservoirs in relatively resistant wild rodent hosts, including rabbits (sylvatic plague). Although plague in man commonly results from the bites of insects (usually rat fleas) and involves local lymph nodes (*bubonic plague*), the organisms may enter the blood stream following the bite and produce a primary septicemia; a massive lung infection may develop and the disease is passed rapidly from man to man via sputum droplets (*pneumonic plague*). In contrast, animal plague almost always results from insect bites and is never pneumonic in type.

The epidemiology of plague is fascinating and stands as a classic model of an insect-transmitted disease in an accidental host; it is a "darling" of the epidemiologist. Its complexity is not surprising in view of the large number and variety of rodent hosts (some 200 species and subspecies) and insect vectors involved and the numerous ecologic factors, including meteorologic conditions, that influence their relative numbers and activities. *Yersinia pestis* can survive arctic winters in hibernating rodents with latent disease which reactivates when these animals awaken. The incidence of sylvatic plague among rodents fluctuates with changes in population balances between rodents having varying degrees of susceptibility to the organism. A high percentage of surviving rodents in areas of sylvatic plague develop immunity to *Y. pestis*. This allows for waves of epidemics among sylvatic hosts as new generations of young susceptible animals arise. *Evidently permanent reservoir areas are only maintained providing relatively resistant hosts are among the fauna of the area; in areas where all hosts, such as domestic rats, are highly susceptible the reservoir tends to diminish and disappear.* As expected, permanent sylvatic reservoirs can exist in areas untouched by man or the domestic rat.

The ecologic balances that determine rat epizootics and associated human epidemics are exceedingly delicate and triggering conditions are stringent. Human plague is contracted principally from populations of rodents that have close liaison with man (liaison hosts, commensal hosts). Domestic rats (house rats, barn rats, sewer rats) and semiwild mice, including the multimammate mouse (*Mastomys coucha*) and the spiny mouse *Acomys cahirinus,* which become house guests during inclement weather, constitute the principal sources of human infections. *In general the domestic rat reservoir does not become established unless the population of rats surpasses a certain level and the population of fleas on the rats reaches a certain density (rat-flea index).* Consequently, climates and seasons favoring the propagation of rats and fleas promote epizootics and, in turn, human epidemics which follow in their wake. Since dense populations of domestic rats are found principally in urban environments, epidemics of plague are largely confined to towns and cities.

Human plague is most common in unsanitary surroundings. Epidemics present a *pre-epidemic phase* during which a few cases gradually appear, an *epidemic phase* when cases appear in large numbers and a *declining phase* during which the incidence of new cases declines sharply. Transmission from rat to rat and from rat to man is due to 2 species of rat fleas which parasitize 3 species of domestic rats, *Rattus norvegicus* (gray or brown rat), *Rattus rattus* (black rat) and *Rattus alexandrinus* (Egyptian rat). Fleas made hungry by death of their hosts or blockage of their proventriculus by bacilli growing there and in the midgut avidly seek new hosts, including humans, to feed upon. They are especially effective in transmitting the disease because, during their vigorous but futile efforts to feed, they repeatedly regurgitate ingested blood loaded with bacilli into the wound that they inflict. The organisms may grow and persist in the flea for several months, especially at low temperatures. Obviously the flea is both a biologic vector and a reservoir.

Because *Rattus rattus* is more susceptible to *Y. pestis* than *Rattus norvegicus* and lives in closer association with man than its fierce Norwegian cousin, it is the more effective reservoir for inciting epidemics. On the other hand, *Rattus norvegicus* is probably more important than *Rattus rattus* in maintaining a semipermanent reservoir among rats because the latter is too susceptible to the disease. During long interepidemic periods, sylvatic rodents constitute permanent reservoirs for maintaining the organism in nature and serve as sources of reinfection of rat populations.

Under ordinary circumstances, prevention of human plague epidemics is not difficult and can usually be effected by preventing the establishment of plague reservoirs in domestic rat populations. It is accomplished by suppressing local populations of permanent reservoir hosts and rats, together with constant surveillance to prevent the transmission of disease *per saltum* from distant reservoirs to local rat populations. Control has been excellent in recent decades and annual plague deaths in the world at large have been limited to hundreds. Permanent sylvatic reservoirs are difficult to control and probably can never be eliminated, even by extreme measures. This, together with the fact that modern transportation permits rapid transmission of infection for thousands of miles through the agency of rats, fleas and contaminated materials, means that plague epidemics will always remain as a public health threat. However, with today's epidemiologic knowledge and tools for controlling rats and insect populations together with vaccines and effective chemoprophylactic agents, all of which our forefathers lacked, *it is difficult to envision why future epidemics of any magnitude should occur in developed countries*. The greatest risks of future epidemics lie in underdeveloped countries where there is danger of overpopulation with attending social and economic chaos and their sequelae, poverty and poor sanitation. Of course, an unforeseen "Wellesian event" could take place even in a developed country and it is well to remain mindful of the fact that, for unknown reasons, *plague epidemics have had a relentless way of disappearing and reappearing over the centuries. The rise and fall of past epidemics and pandemics may have been related to the composition of rat populations and virulence of organisms.* The decline of plague in Europe during the 18th and 19th centuries may have been due to the fact that the fierce Norwegian rat largely replaced its cousin, the black rat; the black rat is the reservoir par excellence for human plague because of its companionability with man and the intense epizootics that it supports. Rapid passage of the organism in this highly susceptible host permits it to reach the acme of virulence which, in turn, may favor the establishment of the pneumonic form of plague in man. Most of the severe epidemics and pandemics of the past have had a large component of pneumonic plague characterized by "vomiting of blood" and unusually high mortality.

Sporadic cases of plague will probably increase in regions of the USA where sylvatic reservoirs exist; sylvatic infection is transmitted in many ways including bites of insects and rodents, skinning of animals, and consumption of rodent meat. There is special danger when epizootics occur among highly susceptible wild animals such as prairie dogs. Physicians in areas of sporadic plague should be alert to its presence. Moreover, in this day of air travel, plague and many other exotic diseases of distant regions may be encountered by a physician practicing anywhere in the world.

B. Physical and Chemical Structure

Yersinia pestis is a pleomorphic, nonsporing, nonmotile, gram-negative, enveloped, ovoid rod measuring some 0.5 to 0.8 μm. $\times$ 1.5 to 2 μm. It occurs singly, in pairs and in chains and exhibits bipolar staining with polychrome stains. Pleomorphism is enhanced by growth in unfavorable environments such as on an agar medium containing 3% NaCl.

At least 18 Ags have been detected in *Y. pestis* including endotoxin and several other toxins. However, no serotypes have been described and the precise roles that various bacterial components play in pathogenesis and immunity are not known. The envelope of *Y. pestis* consists largely, if not entirely, of a heat-labile antiphagocytic protein, and is commonly, but not invariably, present in virulent organisms. Its antiphagocytic activity may be due in part to its ability to interfere with the opsonic activity of C by directly activating and consuming C2 and C4. The envelope protein is synthesized *in vivo* and is abundant in young cultures incubated aerobically at 37°C, but not at 28°C. It is not formed during the organism's growth in the flea. Two associated antiphagocytic Ags, V and W, occur, probably as a complex. The V-W complex Ags are present in virulent and avirulent strains, and are produced only at 37°C. They are destroyed at 80°C for 30 min; V Ag is a protein (mol wt 90,000) and W Ag is a lipoprotein (mol wt 145,000). Antigen V, but not W, has been shown to be a protective immunogen in mice.

Among the several toxins produced by *Y. pestis,* one called "murine toxin" is toxic for mice and rats, but not for all animal species. It consists of 2 extractable protein toxins, a 240,000-mol wt cell membrane protein (toxin A) and a 120,000-mol wt cytoplasmic protein (toxin B). It is possible that in their natural state the 2 components exist as a complex molecule or alternatively that they represent the monomeric and dimeric forms of a single molecule. Murine toxin acts selectively on the mitochondria of certain organs of susceptible animals, but not others. It is not toxic for the mitochondria of resistant animals. It binds to mitochondrial protein, causes mitochondrial swelling and inhibits mitochondrial respiration. Toxicity for mitochondria correlates well with toxicity for the animal species from which the mitochondria are derived. For a discussion of animal toxicity see Section I.

C. Genetics

A number of colonial types of *Y. pestis,* including smooth and rough, have been described. However, colonial morphology is not meaningful in terms of virulence. For example, virulent isolates from the same patient form both R and S colonies; moreover, these virulent organisms can be rendered avirulent by subculture without change in colony morphology. Mutants resistant to streptomycin have been demonstrated.

D. Extracellular Products

The only known extracellular products of possible medical importance are bacteriocin (pesticin I), coagulase, and a fibrolytic factor, all of which may be related to virulence.

E. Culture

Yersinia pestis is a slow-growing organism (generation time 4 hours) with simple nutritional requirements. It grows on common laboratory media over an extremely wide range of temperature (5 to 45°C) with an optimum range of 25 to 30°C; the range of pH values for growth is about 6.0 to 8.0. Following growth, the pH may rise to 8.8 to 9.0. Surface growth on solid media may require hematin or reducing agents. The organism ferments certain sugars without producing gas; it is aerobic and facultatively anaerobic. Colonies on 0.1% blood agar are small, round, viscous and granular and have irregular margins; they are pigmented due to accumulation of red cell pigments. The organism will grow in pure bile.

F. Resistance to Physical and Chemical Agents

Yersinia pestis exhibits the usual resistance to physical and chemical agents possessed by most vegetative bacteria. It is killed within minutes by sunlight, drying, moist heat above 50°C and the common disinfectants. When present in certain animal materials such as flea feces and dried sputum, *Y. pestis* may survive under natural conditions for weeks to months, especially at low temperatures. The organism remains viable for months in frozen human and animal cadavers. Cultured organisms store well at refrigerator temperatures, and can be preserved for many years by lyophilization.

G. Experimental Models

Many species of animals are susceptible to plague, but adult birds are totally resistant. Since bubonic plague in man and that in animals are similar, various species of animals have been used as models of human disease including mice, guinea pigs, rats, rabbits and monkeys. The favored animal for diagnostic work, the guinea pig, is extremely susceptible; one organism can cause fatal infection. Disease in animals induced with infected fleas usually takes one of two forms depending on host resistance, namely, lymph node (bubonic) infection with septicemia or without septicemia. In septicemia the blood bacillary load may reach 100 million/ml; in contrast the load is much lower in man, which reduces the chances of insect transmission of plague from plague patients to healthy human beings or animals. A third form of plague is septicemia without ostensible lymph node involvement.

H. Infections in Man

Although *Y. pestis* infects man by many routes, including the conjunctivae and mucous membranes of the respiratory and digestive tracts, infection usually results from organisms introduced into the skin by infected rat fleas. Under unusual circumstances, bubonic plague may be transmitted from man to man by the human flea *Pulvex irritans*.

Bubonic plague is characterized by sudden onset usually marked by low fever, restlessness, prostration, slurred speech, mental confusion, abdominal pain, vomiting and other symptoms. The incubation period is 2 to 5 days. Since fleas commonly bite the legs, the draining lymph nodes involved are usually in the popliteal and/or inguinal regions. Sometimes a discernible primary lesion develops at the site of infection in the form of a small vesicle. If the exposed individual possesses some degree of immunity, a local lesion will not form or will be transitory. In nonimmune individuals the infecting organisms multiply rapidly and soon reach the draining lymph nodes, where they produce extensive hemorrhagic and necrotizing lesions. The resulting exquisitely tender and painful swollen lymph nodes ("buboes") are firm and movable; they present gray areas of coagulation necrosis in the medulla which often suppurate.* Necrosis evidently results from plague toxins. Perilymphatic tissues are intensely edematous.

It is probable that bacilli always reach the blood early, in small numbers at least, and can be cultured from blood in 60 to 80% of persons infected. The extent of bacteremia fluctuates markedly during the course of the disease and frequently develops into a fulminating septicemia involving the spleen, meninges, skin and lung. Lung complications occur in about 5% of patients with bubonic plague and hemorrhages often develop in the skin and mucous membranes. Clotting in small vessels and consumption coagulopathy are presumed to be responsible for hemorrhage. Septicemia leads to hemoconcentration, circulatory failure and death. The mortality rate in persons with untreated bubonic plague without septicemia is 25 to 50% and in those with septicemia is near 100%; the overall mortality is 60 to 90%. In the event of natural recovery from bubonic plague, healing of lymph node and splenic lesions is slow and organisms may persist for weeks.

Primary *septicemic plague* sometimes develops before lymph nodes become involved. It is presumed to result from the direct introduction of bacilli into the blood stream by feeding fleas and is almost always fatal.

Pneumonic plague, which is characterized by swift spread and near 100% mortality, is sometimes contracted by persons caring for bubonic plague patients with pneumonic complications. *Under suitable conditions one case can start an epidemic of pneumonic plague even in a nonendemic area.* Passage of pneumonic plague from one person to another by droplet infection appears to be favored by high virulence, high humidity and low atmospheric temperatures. Such conditions contributed to the massive Manchurian epidemic of pneumonic plague in 1910-1911 that took a toll of 60,000 lives. The onset is abrupt and the symptoms include generalized pain and headache, rigor, nausea, respiratory difficulty, fever, and a cough yielding blood-tinged frothy sputum filled with bacilli. At terminus the patient develops extreme cyanosis and death results from suffocation.

I. Mechanisms of Pathogenicity

Little is known about the virulence of *Y. pestis* for animals, let alone man. *The factors of virulence are so complex that the identification of even the key determinants of virulence is difficult.* For example, whereas full animal virulence demands both envelope protein and murine toxin, either or both of these components may be lacking in strains of lesser virulence. *An observation of singular interest is that virulence tends to fall rapidly during the decline phase of rat epizootics and human epidemics and remains low during interepidemic periods.* Presumably this is due to the selective pressure of rising herd immunity against virulent organisms during

---

* The term "bubo" is derived from the Greek word "bubon" meaning groin. It is currently used to designate swollen lymph nodes irrespective of their location.

an epizootic and is in keeping with the observation that rapid passage of avirulent strains through fully susceptible animals restores virulence. Animal studies have led to the thesis that the determinants of full virulence are linked with or constitute the attributes of toxinogenicity, encapsulation, production of V-W Ags, and calcium dependence in culture, and the ability to synthesize purines, to form pigmented colonies on hemin-containing media, to resist phagocytosis by neutrophils and free macrophages, and especially to grow within macrophages.

Ability to survive and multiply within macrophages seems to be the major attribute of virulence and is probably related to the V-W complex, other surface Ags, and possibly toxins. For unknown reasons, only virulent organisms grow freely in the chick embryo and kill it. The roles that the bacteriocin, pesticin I, coagulase and fibrinolysin may play in virulence are unknown.

Plague toxins, including murine toxin, endotoxin, and other toxins, undoubtedly contribute to tissue injury and death from plague. The hemorrhagic and degenerative lesions seen in the organs of bacteria-free fetuses carried by plague patients and the "toxic death" which occurs in plague patients subsequent to "bacterial sterilization" effected by chemotherapy are evidently due to toxins. However, the particular toxins involved and their modes of action are not known. Since species vary in their susceptibility to the toxins, animal studies can only suggest what the modes of action of murine toxins may be in man.

The histopathology seen in human plague is similar in many respects to that seen in animals injected with murine toxin and includes edema, hemorrhage, hemoconcentration, serosanguineous effusions in body cavities, and foci of coagulation necrosis in lymph nodes and other organs. Many of these lesions may represent secondary changes and the cells that are the primary targets of toxin remain to be defined.

J. Mechanisms of Immunity

The mechanisms involved in immunity to plague differ among different hosts making it difficult to interpret animal results in terms of human immunity. There is no evidence of racial differences in human immunity to plague and all individuals are equally and fully susceptible to primary infection. However, *most plague survivors acquire strong and durable immunity,* and many kinds of Abs are produced. Although antisera convey partial protection against infection, the classes, specificities and activities of the Abs concerned are not known. Antitoxic Abs do not contribute significantly to immunity and serum Abs and C do not lyse plague organisms. Apparently enveloped organisms resist both phagocytosis and killing by free phagocytes including neutrophils and macrophages. They are more readily engulfed by fixed than by free macrophages. Nonenveloped organisms are engulfed by normal monocytes and grow intracellularly where they synthesize envelope Ag and become more virulent. It is not known whether the macrophages of immune animals engulf and destroy or inhibit organisms more readily than do the macrophages of nonimmune animals. Although acquired immunity has been presumed to be due largely to the opsonic activity of Abs against the envelope protein and V and, possibly, W Ags, this is uncertain. *Instead, the ability to grow within normal monocytes suggests that antimicrobial cellular immunity may be an important component in immunity, a possibility that does not appear to have been explored.*

Vaccines in current use consist of live attenuated organisms or formalin-killed virulent bacilli. They afford only partial protection and booster doses every 3 to 6 months are necessary to maintain effective immunity. It will be difficult to devise more effective vaccines until a better understanding of the mechanisms of acquired immunity are at hand.

K. Laboratory Diagnosis

The organisms are commonly present in abundance in lymph node biopsy material or aspirates, abscesses and blood. In pneumonic plague they are present in the sputum. Direct smears stained with polychrome stain can be highly suggestive of plague. Blood agar, glycerol agar, or, if the specimen is contaminated with other organisms, azide-antibotic-dye selective medium is useful for primary culture. Small delicate colonies develop after 24 to 48 hours at 30°C. Identification is based on cultural and fluorescent Ab tests together with inoculation of guinea pigs, either subcutaneously or if the specimen is highly contaminated with other organisms, by rubbing the material on an area of freshly shaved skin. Other organisms can be easily mistaken for plague bacilli; hence, the guinea pig test is valuable. In guinea pigs, death occurs in from 2 to 5 days and typical postmortem changes include congested viscera, enlarged spleen, granular liver, and pleural effusion. Specific phage is also useful for identifying *Y. pestis*.

L. Therapy

Early diagnosis and treatment are the keys to therapeutic success; unfortunately diagnosis is often missed or is delayed in sporadic cases because plague is not suspected. *Therapy initiated later than 12 to 15 hours after the appearance of fever is often of little or no value, especially in pneumonic plague.* The drugs of choice are the tetracyclines and chloramphenicol. Sulfonamides should be avoided if possible and should not be used alone. Streptomycin is highly bactericidal but should be used cautiously. If given it should be combined with tetracycline to obviate the development of streptomycin resistance. Also, in some patients, the administration of large doses of streptomycin has precipitated fatal shock resembling a generalized Shwartzman reaction, presumably because of large amounts of endotoxin and other toxins liberated from the dying bacteria. Drugs are often given by both the intravenous and oral routes and combinations of drugs are sometimes used. Early drug therapy reduces mortality in bubonic disease by about 80%, but is much less effective in pneumonic plague. Serum therapy, which reduces mortality in bubonic disease by about 50%, is no longer used. Supportive treatments to counteract failure of peripheral circulation and pulmonary function are important elements of therapy. Abscesses should not be drained because of danger of massive spread of organisms.

M. Reservoirs of Infection

As outlined in previous sections, the principal *reservoirs of human bubonic plague in man are domestic rats and rat fleas, and sylvatic rodents and the insect vectors that they harbor (principally fleas).* In special situations, plague patients and the human fleas that infest them, and dogs and cats and their fleas can serve as sources of human bubonic plague. *The reservoir of pneumonic plague is the plague patient.*

Chronic carriage in man is not known to exist, but temporary carriage in the throat has been demonstrated during convalescence and in immune contacts; the role of carriers as reservoirs is unknown.

N. Control of Disease Transmission

As stated in Section A, control of disease transmission in man hinges largely on control of domestic rat and sylvatic reservoirs. Fortunately, this can be accomplished now without resort to the extreme practices of the past, such as the burning of homes. The use of insecticides should precede the destruction of rodents for otherwise the dispossessed fleas seek human hosts and temporarily pose a greater threat to man than if the rats are left unmolested. Mass vaccination and chemoprophylaxis are also useful for preventing or halting epidemics, and vaccination of high-risk individuals in endemic areas is valuable for preventing sporadic plague. Except for the limited instances in which the flea infesting man serves as a vector, measures for preventing man-to-man transmission are largely routine and include quarantine of patients, the use of masks and gloves by attendants of plague patients, and chemoprophylaxis.

Yersinia pseudotuberculosis

Yersinia pseudotuberculosis seldom causes disease in the USA; however, in Europe it causes a nonfatal mesenteric lymphadenitis that mimics acute or subacute appendicitis. Rarely, it produces a septicemic disease that may be fatal. In either case, the infection responds to antibiotic therapy.

Pasteurella

The pasteurellae, particularly *Past. multocida,* are parasites and pathogens for an unusually wide range of animal species. *They cause tremendous losses of livestock but only occasionally infect man as an accidental host.* The organisms are commonly carried in the URT of animals as strains of low virulence. *In animals they are opportunists par excellence and tend to promptly invade mucosae and increase in virulence with resulting septicemia whenever host defenses are lowered.* An example is "shipping fever" or "stockyard fever" due to *Past. multocida* and *Past. hemolytica.* Virulent strains of *Past. multocida* cause epizootics of *hemorrhagic septicemia,* particularly in the tropics and subtropics. The organisms can act as secondary invaders to cause subacute and chronic infections in animals.

Man infrequently carries pasteurellae in his URT, and human *infection, although rare, occurs often enough that physicians should remain alert to its pathogenic potential. Most infections result from the bites of dogs, cats, rats, other animals or, sometimes, man.* The infected bite wounds are painful and tend to suppurate and undergo necrosis. The organisms can spread by contiguity or via lymphatics and the blood stream to produce distant diseases including meningitis, osteomyelitis and pneumonia. In recent years, more cases of human infection have occurred in Oregon than elsewhere in the USA. The susceptible mouse is used in diagnosis. Penicillin is the therapeutic drug of choice.

References

Cartwright, F. F.: *Disease and History.* New York: Thomas Y. Crowell Co., 1972.

Gibbon, E.: *The History of the Decline and Fall of the Roman Empire.* New ed. London: W. Allason, 1816.

Hecker, J. F. C.: *The Epidemics of the Middle Ages.* London: Sydenham Society, 1844.

Holmes, M. A., and Brandon, G.: *Pasteurella multocida* infections in 16 persons in Oregon. Public Health Rep. *80*:1107, 1965.

Janssen, W. A., and Surgalla, M. J.: Plague bacillus: survival within host phagocytes. Science *163*:950, 1969.

Kadis, S., and Ajl, S. J.: Site and mode of action of murine toxin of *Pasteurella pestis.* In *Microbial Toxins.* Vol. III, *Bacterial Protein Toxins.* T. C. Montie, and S. Kadis, eds. New York: Academic Press, 1970, p. 39.

Marshall, J. D., Quy, D. V., and Gibson, F. L.: Asymptomatic pharyngeal plague infection in Vietnam. Am. J. Trop. Med. *16*:175, 1967.

Reed, W. P., Palmer, D. L., Williams, R. C., Jr., and Kish, A. L.: Bubonic plague in the Southwestern United States. Medicine *49*:465, 1970.

Williams, R. C., Jr., Gerwurz, H., and Quie, P. G.: The effects of fraction I from *Yersinia pestis* on phagocytosis *in vitro.* J. Infect. Dis. *126*:235, 1972.

Wilson, G. S., and Miles, A. A.: *Topley and Wilson's Principles of Bacteriology and Immunity.* 5th ed. Baltimore: Williams & Wilkins Co., 1964.

Chapter 25

Francisella

A single species of the genus *Francisella, Francisella tularensis,* (family: *Brucellaceae*) produces disease in animals and man. This organism (formerly known as *Pasteurella tularensis*) was named after Tulare County, California, where the organism was first isolated by McCoy and Chapin in 1912 from ground squirrels exhibiting a plague-like disease. However, the association of the animal disease with clinical disease in man was not established until Francis started a series of investigations in 1919. The term *tularemia* was coined by Francis to indicate that in man the organism can invade the blood and become generalized.

A. Medical Perspectives

Tularemia, also known as rabbit fever, deer-fly fever and Ohara's disease, is an endemic disease of wild animals that is transmitted to man by direct contact or by insect vectors; man serves as an unnatural or accidental host. The most characteristic manifestations of disease in man include a necrotizing cutaneous or mucous membrane lesion at the site of inoculation, coupled with regional lymph node enlargement, septicemia, and a relatively high fever.

Francisella tularensis is highly virulent for man but fortunately man-to-man transmission has never been documented. Wild cottontail rabbits are the principal reservoir of *Fr. tularensis* in the USA and accordingly the disease is most prevalent in hunters, linemen, butchers and housewives, who are most likely to come in contact with infected rabbits or their ecto-parasites. Human tularemia is naturally restricted because of conditions necessary to transmit the disease to man. Accordingly, human cases occur sporadically and usually in small numbers. Nevertheless, since the mortality rate of untreated persons with tularemia is between 6 and 7% early diagnosis and treatment are of utmost importance.

B. Physical and Chemical Structure

Francisella tularensis is a pleomorphic gram-negative, nonmotile, non-sporing rod ranging in size from 0.3 to 0.9 μm; coccoid and short bacillary forms usually predominate. There is only one antigenic type based on the specificity of agglutinins and acquired immunity, although several distinct Ags are present in the cell wall. It appears that these bacteria have one protein Ag in common with members of the genus *Brucella*. Like other gram-negative bacteria, *Fr. tularensis* cell walls contain lipopolysaccharide.

C. Genetics

Smooth strains are virulent and as a rule rough strains are avirulent. Virulent cultures usually contain a few mutant cells of low virulence. The live vaccine strain (LVS) of *Fr. tularensis* is an attenuated strain that can induce substantial immunity in man.

D. Extracellular Products

No exotoxins have been identified, although living cells of virulent *Fr. tularensis* produce acute toxicity and death in rabbits when injected intravenously in large numbers ($> 10^8$); heat-killed organisms are devoid of this toxicity.

E. Culture

Francisella tularensis is a strict aerobe that grows between 24 and 39°C; the optimum temperature is 37°C and the optimum pH is 6.9. It is a relatively fastidious microbe and requires a rich medium plus blood, glucose and cystine; any organism that grows on plain nutrient agar cannot be *Fr. tularensis*.

11

F. Resistance to Physical and Chemical Agents

Francisella tularensis is highly susceptible to heat and the routine anti-bacterial agents, including the common disinfectants. The organism is particularly sensitive to drying and does not survive well in old cultures.

G. Experimental Models

Domestic rabbits, as well as common laboratory animals, are extremely susceptible to infection. As few as 1 to 5 organisms of a virulent strain may be lethal.

H. Infections in Man

The most prevalent form of tularemia, accounting for $> 80\%$ of human cases, is *ulceroglandular* disease. The primary lesion usually occurs on the fingers or hands as a consequence of contact with the tissues of infected animals. The organism is highly virulent and can even invade skin that appears to be unbroken. After 3 or 4 days a papule appears at the site of exposure and subsequently transforms into an ulcer by the seventh or eighth day. By this time the infection has extended to the regional lymph nodes.

The *oculoglandular* type of tularemia is the consequence of infecting the eyes with contaminated blood or by rubbing the eyes with contaminated fingers. Local ulceration of the conjunctivae occurs with spread to regional lymph nodes. The prognosis is generally favorable if the infection is diagnosed and treatment is instituted promptly. Localized lymph node involvement without a primary skin lesion is termed *glandular* tularemia. Systemic infection that develops without a primary ulcer or localized lymphadenitis is referred to as the *typhoidal* form. The *pulmonary* form can result from inhalation of aerosols generated in the laboratory in the course of handling virulent cultures or may be secondary to hematogenous dissemination. This form of tularemia causes mucoid sputum, hemoptysis, dyspnea, pleuritic pain and cyanosis.

On rare occasions the ingestion of contaminated meat or water can cause primary lesions in the *gastrointestinal* tract. Other rare forms of disease include endocarditis, pericarditis, peritonitis, osteomyelitis, meningitis and appendicitis.

Marked fever is characteristic of tularemia; temperatures of 104 to 105°F may persist for as long as 4 weeks in the untreated patient. Splenomegaly is usually evident clinically, and an evanescent macular or papular rash may be present on the trunk and extremities in early disease.

I. Mechanisms of Pathogenicity

The hallmark of tularemia is an infectious granulomatous lesion that undergoes necrosis; often with attending suppuration of draining lymph nodes. The granulomas resemble tubercles when present in liver, spleen, lung or kidney. Although the organism is not known to secrete any toxins, it is highly toxic for macrophages, which probably explains the marked necrosis that occurs in the granulomas produced. Delayed sensitivity may also contribute to tissue damage.

J. Mechanisms of Immunity

Specific acquired immunity to tularemia appears to be primarily cellular in nature, although there may well be an interplay with some form of humoral immunity directed against toxic components of the organism. It is of interest that BCG-vaccinated mice express significant nonspecific resistance against many infectious agents, e.g., *Listeria monocytogenes* and *Salmonella typhimurium,* but not against virulent *Fr. tularensis.* This suggests that acquired immunity in tularemia is complex and depends on more than simply the presence of activated macrophages. Immunity following infection is relatively solid, although second infections have been reported.

K. Laboratory Diagnosis

Francisella tularensis usually can be cultured from the mucocutaneous ulcer or regional lymph nodes; blood cultures are commonly negative. It can also be cultured from the sputum of patients with the pneumonic form of disease. The organism is highly infectious and *clinical laboratories should not attempt to culture it unless they have appropriate laboratory facilities for handling dangerous infectious material.*

Serum agglutinins are usually present after the second week of illness and are particularly useful in diagnosis if a rise in titer is observed.

Infected individuals develop delayed-type sensitivity; therefore, a skin test with an extract of the organisms results in a delayed skin reaction. The test is specific and may be of diagnostic value in some instances.

L. Therapy

Streptomycin is bactericidal for *Fr. tularensis* and is the therapeutic drug of choice; tetracyclines are also effective.

M. Reservoirs of Infection

Man usually contracts tularemia by contact with the tissue of infected animals. Sources of infection include wild rabbits, carnivores, ungulates, birds, squirrels, woodchucks, muskrats, skunks, foxes, opossums, mice, snakes, ticks and fleas. The Rocky Mountain tick (*Dermacentor andersoni*), the western wood tick (*D. variabilis*), the eastern dog tick (*D. occidentalis*) and the Lone Star tick (*Amblyomma americanum*) function as constant reservoirs of infection because the organism can be transmitted transovarially. One species of deer fly (*Chrysops discalis*) and a species of mosquito present in Sweden (*Aedes cinereus*) also can transmit tularemia to man. Contaminated water sometimes causes infection.

N. Control of Disease Transmission

The attenuated live vaccine (LVS vaccine) is highly effective in man and should be employed for immunizing individuals at risk, especially laboratory workers who handle the organism.

Since wild rabbits are the major source of human tularemia in the USA, hunters should be especially wary of lethargic rabbits. Care should be taken in cleaning game, because skinning infected rabbits is the way that tularemia is contracted most often. It is important that laws preventing the sale of wild rabbits by meat markets be instituted and enforced.

Antibiotic prophylaxis with streptomycin may be indicated following known exposure to *Fr. tularensis*.

References

Buchanan, T. M., Brooks, G. F., and Brachman, P. S.: The tularemia skin tests. Ann. Intern. Med. *74*:336, 1971.

Claflin, J. L., and Larson, C. L.: Infection-immunity in tularemia: specificity of cellular immunity. Infect. Immun. *5*:311, 1972.

Day, W. C., and Berendt, R. F.: Experimental tularemia in *Macaca mulatta*: Relationship of aerosol particle size to the infectivity of airborne *Pasteurella tularensis*. Infect. Immun. *5*:77, 1972.

Eigelsbach, H. T., Tulis, J. J., McGavran, M. H., and White, J. D.: Live tularemia vaccine. J. Bact. *84*:1020, 1962.

Miller, R. P., and Bates, J. H.: Pulmonary tularemia. Am. Rev. Resp. Dis. *99*:31, 1969.

Pollitzer, R.: History and incidence of tularemia in the Soviet Union: A review. The Institute of Contemporary Russian Studies, Fordham University, Bronx, New York 10458, 1967.

Saslaw, S., Eigelsbach, H. T., Wilson, H. E., Prior, J. A., and Carhart, S.: Tularemia vaccine study. Ann. Intern. Med. *107*:689, 702, 1961.

Van Metre, T. E., and Kadull, P. J.: Laboratory-acquired tularemia in vaccinated individuals: a report of 62 cases. Ann. Intern. Med. *50*:621, 1959.

Young, L. S., and Sherman, I. L.: Tularemia in the United States: recent trends and a major outbreak. J. Infect. Dis. *119*:109, 1969.

Haemophilus

The organisms belonging to the genus *Haemophilus* (Family: *Brucellaceae*) are small gram-negative, nonmotile, nonsporing aerobic bacilli. Some of the species are highly fastidious and require hemin and nicotinamide nucleoside for growth. The important potential pathogens for man include *H. influenzae, H. aegyptius, H. parainfluenzae, H. aphrophilus* and *H. ducreyi.* Several species are among the normal flora of man; one such species, *H. hemolyticus,* produces beta hemolysis and may be confused with colonies of β-hemolytic streptococci. Several species are parasites of animals. A venereal disease in rabbits is caused by *H. caniculus; H. suis* acts synergistically with swine influenza virus to produce influenza in swine.

Haemophilus influenzae

A. Medical Perspectives

Haemophilus influenzae was first isolated by Pfeiffer in 1892 from several patients suffering from influenza; subsequently it was referred to as "Pfeiffer's bacillus." It is of special interest that *H. influenzae* was considered to be the cause of viral influenza until the 1918 pandemic, which accounts for the species designation. In retrospect, *H. influenzae*, like staphylococci, streptococci and pneumococci, was involved in causing serious secondary infections of the respiratory tract during epidemics of viral influenza. The naming of *H. influenzae* was based on erroneous data and has caused much confusion; accordingly, it is necessary to emphasize to students that *H. influenzae is not the cause of influenza*.

The discovery of Shope (1931) that swine influenza is caused by a virus acting in concert with *H. suis* raised the possibility that synergism might also exist in the human influenza system. However, no data have been obtained to support this possibility.

The role of *H. influenzae* as an important cause of meningitis in children was described by Slawyk in 1899 and its importance in obstructive bronchitis in infants and children was recognized by Lemierre in 1936.

B. Physical and Chemical Structure

Haemophilus influenzae is typically a small, short, plump, gram-negative rod (0.5 to 0.7 × 1.3 μm). It may grow in chains resembling filaments and exhibits extreme pleomorphism. Virulent strains almost invariably possess capsules that are best demonstrated after 6 to 8 hours of incubation in broth cultures. Encapsulated organisms growing for 6 to 12 hours on a transparent agar medium (Levinthal's medium) exhibit iridescent colonies when viewed in obliquely transmitted light. As a rule, cultures 24 hours old undergo autolysis and iridescence is usually absent.

Encapsulated strains of *H. influenzae* possess capsular polysaccharides which comprise 6 serologic types (a, b, c, d, e, f). Isolates can be typed by using specific antisera in the classical capsule swelling test. Serologic specificity of the individual types also can be demonstrated by appropriate agglutination or precipitin tests. It has been observed that *type a H. influenzae* cross reacts with type 6 *D. pneumoniae,* whereas *type b H. influenzae* cross reacts with types 6, 15, 29 and 35 *D. pneumoniae*. In addition, *type c H. influenzae* cross reacts with pneumococcus type 11.

A labile surface protein (M) antigen, a somatic P substance and an endotoxin also have been described.

C. Genetics

Clinical isolates (virulent) are unstable and readily lose their capsules during subculture, indicating that nonencapsulated mutants quickly dominate. Accordingly, the rate of spontaneous S→R mutation is high. Experimentally, capsular types and antibiotic resistance of organisms have been altered by DNA transfer utilizing the principle of transformation.

D. Extracellular Products

Haemophilus influenzae does not produce any known soluble toxins. It does, however, secrete a large amount of capsular polysaccharide which accumulates in detectable quantities in the blood and spinal fluid during the acute phase of the disease; soluble capsular polysaccharide neutralizes the early specific Abs formed thus blocking the opsonic action of the first Ab made and delaying the effector limb of specific acquired immunity.

E. Culture

Haemophilus influenzae is highly fastidious and requires a culture medium with a rich base, such as brain-heart infusion, plus blood. For example, rabbit defibrinated blood (5 to 10%) is added to a hot (80° to 90°C) enriched melted agar medium which disrupts the red blood cells and "chars" the hemoglobin giving the plates a chocolate appearance. The colonies on chocolate agar are small (0.5 to 0.7 mm) and colorless, resembling small droplets of moisture. *Haemophilus influenzae* requires the heat-stable hemin (X factor) and the heat-labile nicotinamide nucleoside (V factor) that are supplied by the blood in "chocolate" agar. The heating of the blood in the preparation of chocolate agar liberates hemin from the red blood cells and also inactivates enzymes in fresh blood that can degrade nicotinamide nucleoside.

Colonies of *H. influenzae* growing in the near vicinity of a staphylococcal colony are larger than those growing at a distance. This is referred to as the *satellite phenomenon* and is due to the V factor supplied by the staphylococci; this property can be an aid in the identification of *H. influenzae*.

The pH optimum for growth is 7.6, and some strains grow better on primary isolation in the presence of 5 to 10% CO_2 than without CO_2.

F. Resistance to Physical and Chemical Agents

Haemophilus influenzae is highly susceptible to desiccation and to the common disinfectants. It is readily killed by exposure at 55°C for 30 minutes.

G. Experimental Models

Virulent *H. influenzae* strains produce a fatal infection in mice if the inoculum is suspended in mucin and injected ip. Experimental bronchopneumonia and meningitis have been produced in monkeys with strains virulent for mice.

H. Infections in Man

The most common diseases produced by *H. influenzae* are pharyngitis, laryngotracheitis, epiglottitis, pneumonia, bronchiolitis, otitis media and meningitis. As a rule, these are mainly diseases of children and occur only rarely in adults.

Pharyngitis, caused by *H. influenzae,* is common in children and may persist for several days unless the patient is treated. The throat is usually inflamed and hyperemic.

Laryngotracheitis is a serious localized infection of the upper airway of children that can result in obstruction; a croupy-type cough is associated with intense localized edema and progressive occlusion of the trachea. *Tracheotomy is often necessary because progression of this disease is rapid and can lead to death within 24 hours.*

Epiglottitis may also result in obstruction that must be relieved by tracheotomy.

Primary pneumonia due to *H. influenzae* is also mainly a disease of children. *Secondary pneumonia* due to the organism may be a serious superimposed complication of pertussis or rubeola in children; in addition, it may occur secondary to viral influenza or measles in adults.

Bronchiolitis due to *H. influenzae* in children can be extremely severe and is characterized by a persistent nonproductive cough, wheezing and dyspnea. *This illness is potentially serious and must be recognized and treated promptly because it can be rapidly fatal.*

Otitis media, caused by *H. influenzae,* is relatively common in children but uncommon in adults. Clinically it is indistinguishable from otitis media due to *Strep. pyogenes, Staph. aureus* or *D. pneumoniae.* It is usually necessary to aspirate fluid from the middle ear and culture it in order to establish the presence of *H. influenzae.*

Haemophilus influenzae is the most common cause of *meningitis* in children between the ages of 6 months and 2 years, but is a progressively less frequent cause of meningitis during the remaining years of childhood. Meningitis due to *H. influenzae* may also follow head injuries or surgical operations in children as well as adults. Approximately 95% of the cases of meningitis are produced by type b; only a few cases are caused by type a. The typical clinical signs of acute bacterial meningitis are produced by *H. influenzae* except in very young infants who may only exhibit swelling of the fontanels. *Meningitis due to H. influenzae is an extremely serious disease and demands prompt diagnosis and treatment; essentially all untreated patients die of the disease. In addition, a disturbing number of infants reveal some residual brain damage even in those instances in which diagnosis is prompt and treatment is apparently optimal.*

I. Mechanisms of Pathogenicity

The main virulence factor of *H. influenzae* appears to be the capsule, which has marked antiphagocytic properties. Infections normally originate in the URT and may be limited to various sites in the respiratory tract. If the disease progresses, a bacteremia usually occurs and, as a consequence, meningitis may result in a small percentage of patients. Organisms may also localize in joints or, in rare instances, on heart valves. Suppuration is the rule; accordingly, lesions are dominated by neutrophils and organisms enmeshed in fibrin. No extracellular toxins or other harmful bacterial products have been identified; consequently the mechanisms by which the organism produces injury are unknown.*

J. Mechanisms of Immunity

The main mechanism of specific acquired immunity involves Abs specific for the capsular polysaccharides, that act as opsonins. In addition, with progressing age, bactericidal complement-dependent Abs can be demonstrated in the sera of an increasing percentage of individuals over 4 years old. It is of interest that the incidence of *H. influenzae* meningitis, as a function of age, is inversely related to the bactericidal activity of blood (Fig. 26-1). Accordingly, after maternal Ab is largely catabolized, a pe-

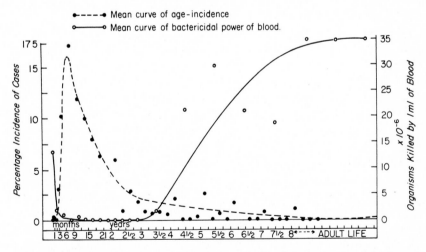

Figure 26-1. The relation of age incidence of influenzal meningitis to the bactericidal power of human blood at different ages against a smooth meningeal strain of *H. influenzae*. Adapted from Fothergill, L. D., and Wright, J. J. of Immunology, 24:281 (1933).

* An unidentified component which is toxic for tracheal organ cultures has recently been described.

TABLE 26-1
Properties of Some Species of Haemophilus

Species	V Factor (Nicotinamide Nucleoside) Requirement	X Factor (Hemin) Requirement	Hemolysis (Blood Agar)	Reservoir
H. influenzae	+	+	−	Man
H. aegyptius	+	+	−	Man
H. haemolyticus	+	+	+	Man
H. parainfluenzae	+	−	−	Man
H. parahaemolyticus	+	−	+	Man
H. aphrophilus	−	+	−	Man
H. ducreyi	−	+	+	Man (genital)
H. haemoglobinophilus	−	+	−	Dogs (genital)
H. caniculus	+	+	+	Rabbit (genital)
H. suis	+	+	−	Swine

riod of marked susceptibility exists (2 months to 3 years) until specific immunity is acquired naturally.

K. Laboratory Diagnosis

It is possible to identify *H. influenzae* in specimens such as spinal fluid, sputum and exudate by the capsular swelling test in which antisera specific for the capsular polysaccharides are used. A ring precipitin test for capsular polysaccharide in spinal fluid may be performed by layering the fluid over specific *H. influenzae* type b (the most common type) rabbit antiserum. It should be emphasized that, in gram-stained smears, an inexperienced observer can confuse *H. influenzae* with *D. pneumoniae* or *N. meningitidis*.

Culture should be carried out on enriched "chocolate" agar or a comparable medium. *Haemophilus influenzae* can be differentiated from related species on the basis of lack of hemolysis on blood agar plates and its X and V factor requirements (Table 26-1). Capsular swelling tests provide serologic confirmation of cultural identification.

L. Therapy

Essentially all strains of *H. influenzae* are highly sensitive to ampicillin and, as a rule, this drug is effective except in those patients with meningitis who have complications, e.g., subdural empyema. Chloramphenicol plus sulfadiazine also has been demonstrated to be a successful therapeutic regimen for meningitis. Tetracyclines are effective for respiratory infections but are less reliable for meningitis.

M. Reservoirs of Infection

Man is the only known reservoir of *H. influenzae.*

N. Control of Disease Transmission

Man is the only known natural host of *H. influenzae.* Spread of infection is by droplet transmission from infected individuals or carriers to susceptible persons. There appears to be an increasing number of adults who lack Abs specific for *H. influenzae,* indicating lack of exposure to the organism; this could be the result of the widespread use of antibiotics. Renewed interest in the problem of *H. influenzae* infections has prompted investigations into the feasibility of developing a vaccine containing type b capsular polysaccharide. Vaccination could have a great potential for protecting infants from meningitis and its irreversible sequelae. In addition it could prove to be of future value for immunizing adults, provided a substantial increase in the incidence of meningitis occurs among individuals lacking Ab to *H. influenzae.*

Haemophilus aegyptius

Haemophilus aegyptius was first observed by Koch in smears from infected eyes of patients in Egypt (1883). In 1887, Weeks of New York isolated the microbe in pure culture; thereafter it has been known as the Koch-Weeks bacillus. *Haemophilus aegyptius* resembles *H. influenzae* in many ways, including the mutual presence of cross-reactive Ags as well as the requirement for X and V factors. However, the definitive work of Pittman and Davis clearly established that it is a separate species.

Haemophilus aegyptius is responsible for a highly communicable form of a purulent conjunctivitis commonly referred to as "pink eye." In contrast to *H. influenzae,* it is not virulent for mice even if suspended in mucin. It has been shown to produce typical conjunctivitis in human volunteers but fails to infect the common laboratory animals.

Laboratory diagnosis depends on culturing and identifying the organism. As a rule, sulfonamides are effective chemotherapeutic agents although ampicillin and chloramphenicol are the logical drugs of choice in severe infections.

Haemophilus parainfluenzae

Haemophilus parainfluenzae requires the V but not the X factor for its growth. It is probably a member of the normal flora, but under special circumstances can be responsble for subacute bacterial endocarditis. The organism may be involved in some respiratory infections, but is more likely a secondary invader and normally plays a minor role in such infections.

Haemophilus aphrophilus

This organism is commonly present in the normal respiratory tract. It is an uncommon cause of pneumonia, but may be involved as a secondary invader. In addition, it may produce bacterial endocarditis on rare occasions.

Haemophilus ducreyi

Chancroid or soft chancre is an acute localized venereal disease caused by *H. ducreyi*. The chancre-like lesion found on the external genitalia is basically an ulcer with a ragged and irregular margin that is commonly tender and swollen. In addition, the inguinal nodes may be enlarged and painful and may undergo suppuration (buboes).

Haemophilus ducreyi is a short, plump, gram-negative rod that may exhibit bipolar staining. In stained smears of exudates from lesions the organisms usually appear singly, in small clusters and in long lateral columns between inflammatory cells or shreds of mucus. Only occasional organisms are found intracellularly. *Haemophilus ducreyi* can be cultured with some difficulty on enriched blood agar incubated at a slightly reduced oxygen tension.

Chancroid is more common in Negroes than in Caucasians, although its true incidence is not known. The organism is usually transmitted by sexual intercourse; it can be acquired from sexual partners who have no clinical evidence of an active infection. About 2 to 5 days after contact with an infected partner, a localized ulcer appears at the site of initial infection. Mild systemic symptoms may occur as a consequence of regional lymph node involvement such as headache, fever, malaise or anorexia.

Laboratory diagnosis involves examining a stained smear of the exudate from under the edge of the lesion and demonstrating a preponderance of typical gram-negative rods resembling *H. ducreyi*. A culture should be taken, although it is difficult to isolate the organism from the lesion. The majority of patients with chancroid will give a positive delayed-type reaction to a skin test with killed *H. ducreyi* injected intradermally. The skin test is of limited value because specific sensitivity persists for years even after the disease has been cured. The nature of the lesions and mode of transmission demand that the possibility of syphilis be ruled out by appropriate serologic tests and darkfield examination.

The drug of choice for treating chancroid is sulfisoxazole (Gantrisin). Chloramphenicol and the tetracyclines are also effective chemotherapeutic agents. If buboes are large they should be aspirated during treatment to prevent spontaneous rupture.

References

Collier, A. M., Connor, J. D., and Nykan, W. L.: Systemic infection with *Hemophilus influenzae* in very young infants. J. Pediat. *70*:539, 1967.

Denny, F. W.: Effect of a toxin produced by *Hemophilus influenzae* on ciliated respiratory epithelium. J. Infec. Dis. *129*:93, 1974.

Feingold, M., and Gellis, S. S.: Cellulitis due to *Haemophilus influenzae* type B. New Engl. J. Med. *272*:788, 1965.

Johnson, W. D., Kaye, D., and Hook, E. W.: *Hemophilus influenzae* pneumonia in the adult. Am. Rev. Resp. Dis. *97*:1112, 1968.

Newman, R. B., Stevens, R. W., and Gaafar, H. A.: Latex agglutination test for the diagnosis of *Haemophilus influenzae* meningitis. J. Lab. Clin. Med. *76*:107, 1970.

Sanderson, E. S., and Greenblatt, R. B.: The cultivation of *Haemophilus ducreyi* and preparation of an antigen for intracutaneous diagnosis. Southern Med. J. *30*:147, 1937.

Sell, S. H. W., and Karzon, D. T. (eds.): *Hemophilus influenzae.* Nashville, Vanderbilt University Press, 1973.

Turk, D. C., and May, J. R.: *Hemophilus influenzae.* Its Clinical Importance. London, English Universities Press, Ltd., 1967.

Wehrle, P. F., Hathies, A. W., Leedom, J. M., and Ivler, D.: Bacterial meningitis. Ann. N. Y. Acad. Sci. *145*:488, 1967.

White, D. C.: Respiratory systems in the hemin-requiring *Hemophilus* species. J. Bact. *85*:84, 1963.

Bordetella

The genus *Bordetella* (Family: *Brucellaceae*) contains 3 species of medical importance, namely, *Bord. pertussis, Bord. parapertussis* and *Bord. bronchiseptica.*

The organisms belonging to the genus *Bordetella* are small, ovoid, nonmotile (except *Bord. bronchiseptica*), nonsporing, gram-negative rods. *Bordetella pertussis,* the causative agent of pertussis (whooping cough), is the most important species; *Bord. parapertussis* produces a comparatively mild disease resembling whooping cough, and *Bord. bronchiseptica* is responsible for producing respiratory infections in several animal species. A mild whooping-cough-like disease in children, caused by *Bord. bronchiseptica,* occurs on rare occasion.

Bordetella pertussis

A. Medical Perspectives

The first, classic description of pertussis was written by de Baillou (1578):

> The lung is so irritated so that every attempt to expel that which is causing trouble, it neither admits the air nor again easily expels it. The patient is seen to swell up, and as if strangled hold his breath tightly in the middle of his throat. . . . For they are without this troublesome coughing for the space of four or five hours at a time, then this paroxysm of coughing returns, now so severe that blood is expelled with force through the nose and through the mouth. Most frequently an upset of the stomach follows.

Bordetella pertussis was first isolated by Bordet and Gengou in 1906. Naturally acquired pertussis is a highly contagious disease; the attack rate among nonimmunized children exposed to the disease is approximately 90%. However, an effective vaccine is available; vaccination, antimicrobial drugs and proper management has reduced the mortality rate in the USA from 12.5 (1920) to 0.3 (1950) per 100,000. Currently about 200,000 cases of pertussis occur in the USA each year.

B. Physical and Chemical Structure

Bordetella pertussis is similar morphologically to *Haemophilus influenzae;* it is a small rod (0.5 × 1.0 μm) that commonly exhibits bipolar staining. Virulent strains form capsules on culture. Several Ags have been isolated from virulent strains; the outermost Ag is an agglutinogen; a second surface Ag (the hemagglutinating Ag) agglutinates human and fowl RBC. Thermolabile K antigens provide the basis for the serotypes. The cell wall contains a heat-stable lipopolysaccharide that is similar to the O Ags of the enteric gram-negative bacteria. In addition, an immunogenic Ag, a heat-labile toxin, a leukocytosis-promoting factor (LPF) and a histamine-sensitizing factor (HSF) have been described. Pilus-like structures are alleged to be present on phase I but not phase IV organisms.

C. Genetics

Fresh isolates from patients in the catarrhal stage of pertussis are in the smooth encapsulated, fully virulent phase (phase I); phase IV is a term used for the rough avirulent form. Intermediate phases, designated II and III, are also recognized. If virulent strains are subcultured repeatedly these phase variations regularly occur, demonstrating that a virulent encapsulated strain readily mutates to nonencapsulated variants that ultimately outgrow the encapsulated parent strain *in vitro*. These *in vitro* phase changes, which represent a typical S→R mutational shift from virulence to avirulence, also occur in the course of human infection (Section H).

D. Extracellular Products

A heat-labile toxin resembling an exotoxin has been obtained from culture filtrates and lysates of both S and R organisms. *It has been reported that virulent phase I organisms contain 10 times more toxin than the avirulent phase IV organisms.* This toxin, which is of low potency compared to the classical exotoxins, produces necrosis in the skin of rabbits and is lethal for mice. There is evidence to suggest that the toxin may play a major role in the pathogenesis of whooping cough.

E. Culture

Bordetella pertussis is a relatively fastidious, facultatively aerobic organism that grows well on the glycerine-potato-blood agar originally devised by Bordet and Gengou. In contrast to *H. influenzae,* it does not require hemin and nicotinamide nucleoside. The colonies are smooth, glistening and dome-shaped; they tend to be opaque or pearl-like and produce a fuzzy type of hemolysis. Phase I colonies are mucoid and tenacious.

F. Resistance to Physical and Chemical Agents

Bordetella species are average in their susceptibility to the common disinfectants as well as to drying. They are readily killed by heating at 55°C for 30 minutes.

G. Experimental Models

Experimental infections have been produced in chimpanzees, monkeys, dogs, rabbits, rats, mice and ferrets. Intranasal instillation of *Bord. pertussis* in mice results in an interstitial pneumonia. Infections of chimpanzees produce a lymphocytosis and a characteristic paroxysmal cough simulating human pertussis.

H. Infections in Man

Pertussis, a common disease of childhood, can be divided into 3 stages, namely, the catarrhal stage, the paroxysmal stage and the convalescent stage.

The *catarrhal stage,* which lasts about 7 to 14 days, begins about 10 to 15 days after contact with an infected person; it is characterized by coryza, sneezing, a mild cough and a low-grade fever. During this stage, phase I organisms predominate; as immunity is acquired the less virulent phase II and III organisms begin to emerge. Toward the end of this stage the leukocyte count commonly rises to about 20,000 to 30,000 with $> 60\%$ lymphocytes.

The *paroxysmal stage* (patients with uncomplicated disease are afebrile) usually lasts between 1 to 6 weeks and is characterized by a violent, repetitive cough; the coughing commonly forces the air out of the lungs; this is followed by an inspiratory "whoop," the expulsion of thick, mucoid sputum and vomiting. Small localized areas of necrosis appear in the bronchial epithelium and patchy interstitial pneumonia usually develops. The viscous, ropy, mucinous bronchial secretions are extremely difficult to expel and cause local obstruction leading to areas of emphysema and atelectasis.

The *convalescent stage* normally lasts for about 2 to 3 weeks with a gradual decline in the severity of coughing.

Bronchopneumonia, due to secondary infection, occurs in 1 to 10% of patients; the organisms most frequently responsible for secondary infections include, *D. pneumoniae, Staph. aureus, H. influenzae* and *Strep. pyogenes.*

Neurologic symptoms, which may appear at the peak of the paroxysmal stage, occur most frequently in infants and young children with bronchopneumonia. In a study of a series of 35 hospitalized patients, Byers and Rizzo reported that 17% of infants developed some permanent CNS damage. Schacter found that 27.5% of a series of 200 children with uncomplicated whooping cough exhibited subsequent retardation; even a higher percentage displayed character disorders. Other serious neurologic complications include convulsions, coma, paralysis, blindness and psychic disorders. About 50% of children who develop coma do not survive. Late sequelae are epilepsy, spastic paralysis and mental retardation.

I. Mechanisms of Pathogenicity

Bordetella pertussis exhibits marked cell tropism in that it grows preferentially on the ciliated epithelial cells in the bronchi. Since the organisms seldom if ever invade the mucosa, it is believed that the heat-labile exotoxin is responsible for the epithelial necrosis that takes place. It is likely that copious production of mucus plus a toxin-induced depression of mucociliary clearance is responsible, at least in part, for the cough. *The profound lymphocytosis is caused by a protein component referred to as lymphocytosis-promoting factor (LPF).* Purified preparations of LPF also contain histamine-sensitizing factor (HSF); they are probably distinct components. The heat-stable endotoxin may also contribute to the disease, but its role is uncertain.

There is convincing circumstantial evidence to indicate that allergic symptoms may be superimposed on whooping cough and aggravate the symptoms during the paroxysmal stage; HSF could be involved in this pathogenetic mechanism.

It has been proposed that some type of neurologic alteration may be responsible for the whoop because the paroxysmal cough persists long after the organisms have been eradicated. The observation that pertussis vaccine produces β-adrenergic blockade in mice, thus making the lung hyperreactive to injury, supports the neurologic hypothesis.

Bordetella pertussis possesses many potent biologically active components that could contribute to pathogenesis. However, the relative contributions of these substances remain to be elucidated.

J. Mechanisms of Immunity

Active acquired immunity following whooping cough is not permanent. However, even a waning immunity can probably attenuate subsequent infections to the point where they do not resemble whooping cough. Indeed, it is the consensus that repeated subclinical or mild infections probably act as boosters to maintain immunity thus making it appear that immunity is life-long after only a single bout of whooping cough. It is noteworthy that, although passive immunity in newborn infants due to maternal Ab is comparatively weak, it apparently attenuates the disease in young infants when present.

A protective Ag has been described in the cells of virulent phase I organisms. The heat-labile exotoxin is also a potential immunogen.

Immunity may wane to a low level with age; as a consequence, the disease may recur in a severe form in the aged. The antiadhesion activity of s IgA Abs probably accounts for prophylactic immunity.

K. Laboratory Diagnosis

Material for culture is obtained by employing a special nasal swab made from a flexible wire with a small cotton swab at one end. The swab is passed through the nose to the pharyngeal wall and held in place until the patient coughs. The swab is withdrawn, passed through a drop of penicillin solution (inhibits contaminants), placed on a Bordet-Gengou agar plate. The drop is then streaked in the conventional manner. Characteristic colonies appear after 2 days' incubation at 37°C. Alternatively, a cough plate can be used in which the patient coughs onto an exposed agar plate. Final identification can be made by employing a specific agglutination test with appropriate antiserum.

A direct identification can be made by staining the organisms in nasopharyngeal smears with specific fluorescein-labeled Ab.

L. Therapy

Chloramphenicol is the antimicrobial drug of choice for the treatment of patients with severe pertussis; tetracyclines are also used. In most instances, the clinical response to antimicrobial treatment is slow and questionable. However, the bacterial phase of the disease can be arrested by antimicrobial therapy. Persons with mild forms of whooping cough do not require specific treatment.

Hyperimmune human globulin injected early in the course of the illness can attenuate the disease and is recommended for infants under 2 years of age.

It is highly important to replace water and salt loss in patients who suffer severe and frequent vomiting. Prompt detection and treatment of complications, such as secondary bacterial infections of the lungs or middle ear, are of utmost urgency.

M. Reservoirs of Infection

Man is the only known reservoir of infection.

N. Control of Disease Transmission

Bordetella pertussis is endemic throughout the world; epidemics tend to occur in cycles ranging from 2 to 5 years when critical numbers of susceptible children accumulate in a population. Long-term chronic carriers of *Bord. pertussis* have not been observed. It is difficult to explain the maintenance of this pathogen based only on clinically recognized infections. Presumably, many mild cases of the disease go unrecognized and serve to maintain the organism in the human population.

Active immunization of all infants and children with the triple vaccine DPT (diphtheria-pertussis-tetanus) affords good protection against pertussis. Killed phase I cells of *Bord. pertussis* are included in this vaccine. Immunization should be started in children at 2 months of age, followed by a booster dose of vaccine at 1 year of age; subsequent booster doses should be given at 3 and 5 years of age. The degree of protection tends to parallel the serum agglutinin titers at the time of exposure. Vaccination presents a minor risk because of the possibility of severe or fatal *vaccine encephalopathy*. Pittman has estimated that the incidence in the USA is about one fatal reaction in 5 to 10 million doses of vaccine administered. *It is of singular interest that* Bord. pertussis *has marked adjuvant activity and enhances the Ab response to the other Ags in DPT.*

Bordetella parapertussis

This gram-negative rod resembles *Bord. pertussis* except that it develops larger colonies. *Bordetella parapertussis* is the cause of a mild whooping-cough-like disease that, as a rule, does not require specific therapy. The organism possesses somatic Ags that cross-react with Ags of *Bord. pertussis* and *Bord. bronchiseptica.* Apparently DPT vaccine does not immunize against either *Bord. parapertussis* or *Bord. bronchiseptica.*

Bordetella bronchiseptica

This organism is a common cause of sporadic and epidemic pulmonary infections in rabbits and guinea pigs. Colonies of *Bord. bronchiseptica* are small, round and glistening. In contrast to the other species of *Bordetella,* this organism is motile.

Based on cross-immunity experiments, *Bord. bronchiseptica* is more closely related to *Bord. pertussis* and to *Bord. parapertussis* than the latter are related to each other. *Bordetella bronchiseptica* produces a whooping-cough-like disease in children on rare occasions.

References

Additional standards: Pertussis vaccine. Federal Register *33*:1818, 1968.

Bordet, J., and Gengou, O.: Le microbe de la coqueluche. Ann. Inst. Pasteur *20*:731, 1906.

Byers, R. K., and Rizzo, N. D.: A follow-up study of pertussis in infancy. New Eng. J. Med. *242*:887, 1950.

Christie, A. B.: Infectious Diseases, Epidemiology and Clinical Practice. Edinburgh and London, E. and S. Livingstone, Ltd., 1969.

de Baillou, G.: Whooping cough. *In* Classic Descriptions of Disease, 2nd ed. Edited by R. H. Major. Springfield, Ill., Charles C Thomas, 1939.

Eldering, G., Hornbeck, C., and Baker, J.: Serologic study of *Bordetella pertussis* and related species. J. Bact. *74*:133, 1957.

Geller, B. D., and Pittman, M.: Immunoglobulin and histamine-sensitivity response of mice to live *Bordetella pertussis.* Infect. Immun. *8*:83, 1973.

Holt, L. B.: The pathology and immunology of *Bordetella pertussis* infection. J. Med. Microbiol. *5*:407, 1972.

Kendrick, P. L., Gottshall, R. Y., Anderson, H. D., Volk, V. K., Bunney, W. E., and Top, F. H.: Pertussis agglutinins in adults. Public Health Rep. *84*:9, 1969.

Linneman, C. C., Jr., Bass, J. W., and Smith, H. D.: The carrier state in pertussis. Amer. J. Epidem. *88*:422, 1968.

Morse, J. H., and Morse, S. I.: Studies on the ultrastructure of *Bordetella pertussis.* J. Exp. Med. *131*:1342, 1970.

Munoz, J., and Bergman, R. K.: Histamine-sensitizing factors from microbial agents, with special reference to *Bordetella pertussis.* Bact. Rev. *32*:103, 1968.

Nagel, J.: Isolation from *Bordetella pertussis* of protective antigen free from toxic activity and histamine sensitizing factor. Nature *214*:96, 1967.

Pittman, M.: *Bordetella pertussis*—bacterial and host factors in the pathogenesis and prevention of whooping cough. *In* Infectious Agents and Host Reactions, p. 239. Edited by S. Mudd. Philadelphia, W. B. Saunders Co., 1970.

Sato, Y., Arai, H., and Suzuki, K.: Leukocytosis-promoting factor of *Bordetella pertussis.* II. Biological properties. Infect. Immun. *7*:992, 1973.

Schachter, M.: Le pronostic neuropsychologique des enfants d'une coqueluche precoce non compliquee. Proxis *42*:464, 1953.

Zellweger, H.: Pertussis encephalopathy. Arch. Pediat. *76*:381, 1959.

Listeria

Listeria monocytogenes, a facultative parasite and pathogen of the genus *Listeria,* family *Corynebacteriaceae,* infects many species of mammals and birds as well as crustaceans and ticks. It is the only member of the genus that is pathogenic for man. The organism is a saprophyte; it is widely distributed in nature and has been isolated from streams, sewage, mud, silage, and vegetation as well as from the animals that it infects.

A. Medical Perspectives

Listeria monocytogenes was first isolated and characterized in 1926 by Murray, Webb and Swann during an epizootic among guinea pigs and rabbits. The propensity of this organism to induce a monocytosis led to its species name. The first case of human infection with *L. monocytogenes* was described and identified by Nyfeldt in 1929. More than 1500 cases have since been reported. Subsequently, this microbe has been shown to cause disease in such diverse animals as goats, lemmings, foxes, horses, cows, domestic fowl and wild birds. In animals, genital tract infection of the pregnant female with subsequent perinatal infection of the offspring is a characteristic syndrome associated with listeriosis; it also occurs in human beings.

In man, listeria acts as an opportunistic pathogen. Meningitis is the most common form of human listeriosis in the USA. Other forms of human disease include febrile pharyngitis with cervical and generalized lymphadenopathy. As in many opportunistic infections in man, listeriosis is being recognized with increasing frequency. In 1971, 104 cases were reported to the Center for Disease Control. Since 1967, when optional reporting of listeriosis began, 472 cases have been reported. The case rate and mortality rate are highest among infants under 4 weeks of age (attack rate 0.9/100,000) and in adults over 40 years of age (attack rate 0.1/100,000 between the ages of 55 to 64 years). Because of the relatively high incidence of animal infections the animal reservoir is extensive and control of human infection rests on methods that prevent transmission of the disease from animals to man. Better means for diagnosing human listeriosis are needed in order to advance our understanding of its epidemiology and to institute more effective measures for its control.

B.   Physical and Chemical Structure

Listeria monocytogenes is a pleomorphic, nonsporing, gram-positive rod, ranging in size from 0.2 to 0.4 μm $\times$ 0.5 to 2 μm. It possesses peritrichous flagella and exhibits a characteristic tumbling motility when grown in broth culture. The organism possesses a heat-labile flagellar (H) Ag and a heat-stable somatic (O) Ag. Four main serologic types plus a few minor subtypes are recognized. Serotypes 1b (31%) and 4b (38%) account for most cases of listeriosis in man.

A chloroform-soluble lipid that can be extracted from *L. monocytogenes* has been termed "monocytosis-producing agent"; when injected into mice this lipid extract induces a marked monocytosis. However, it has not been shown that the substance has a similar effect on human beings. When grown in media containing 10% serum and 5% glucose the organism produces a mucopolysaccharide capsule.

C.   Genetics

Nonmotile mutants readily develop and may mutate back to motile forms. As a rule the organism grows as a short rod in smooth colonies and as a long filamentous form in rough colonies; it exhibits marked pleomorphism in transitional strains. Aside from variation in antigenic types and colonial forms, little is known about genetic variability of the organism. After several subcultures it usually becomes avirulent for mice. Passage through mice can select for virulent mutants; virulence of laboratory strains is usually maintained by this method,

D.   Extracellular Products

There are no known extracellular products of medical importance.

E.   Culture

Listeria monocytogenes is facultatively anaerobic. It grows on blood agar media over a wide range of temperature (4 to 37°C) and often exhibits a narrow zone of β-hemolysis; consequently, colonies of *L. monocytogenes* may be confused with colonies of β-hemolytic streptococci. *Listeria monocytogenes* is difficult to distinguish from related diphtheroids on morphologic grounds; however, a test for motility is helpful because diphtheroids are never motile. It is of interest that the isolation of *L. monocytogenes* from clinical specimens containing small numbers of organisms is facilitated by storing them at 4°C in glucose broth for several days or even weeks before culturing. Presumably, some cellular division or upgrading in the physiologic state of the organisms occurs as a result of storage at 4°C.

F.   Resistance to Physical and Chemical Agents

Although *L. monocytogenes* can be considered to be "average" in terms of susceptibility to routine sterilization and disinfectants, it has remarkable survival properties in soil and organic materials.

G.   Experimental Models

Mice, rabbits and guinea pigs are susceptible to listeriosis. About 10^4 organisms cause a lethal infection in a mouse. The organism has been used extensively in studies on the mechanisms of cellular immunity, employing the mouse model.

H.   Infections in Man

Culturally proven listeriosis is preponderantly a disease of immunologically immature or compromised individuals. The most common infection in adults is a leptomeningitis that may or may not be associated with bacteremia. In a series of 105 patients with listeriosis, 56 had meningitis. Immunologically normal adults may develop the disease upon sufficient exposure; for example, cutaneous listeriosis has been reported in veterinarians after carrying out bovine obstetrical procedures. *A marked monocytosis is characteristic of listeriosis, in man as well as animals.*

Infections of the newborn range from meningitis that becomes apparent within 4 weeks postpartum to disseminated disease in aborted, premature and stillborn infants; some infected neonates die within a few days after birth. Infants born with disseminated listeriosis are usually critically ill with cardiorespiratory distress, vomiting and diarrhea; hepatosplenomegaly may be evident. Disseminated listeriosis, which has been given names such as "granulomatosis infantiseptica," "miliary granulomatosis" and "pseudotuberculosis," was described by Henle in 1893. Necropsy of infants with this form of listeriosis reveals widely disseminated abscesses and granulomas of varying sizes involving the liver, spleen, adrenal glands, lungs, pharynx, CNS, GI tract and skin. Whereas the meconium of a normal newborn infant does not contain bacteria, the meconium of a neonate with listeriosis contains numerous organisms; hence a gram-stained smear and culture of the meconium should be performed whenever there is gross contamination of the amniotic fluid with meconium, or particularly if a mother has an unexplained fever at the onset of labor.

Listeriosis in a pregnant woman may be asymptomatic or symptomatic; symptomatic infections are characterized by malaise, chills, mild diarrhea, back pain, and itching of skin. Infections that are asymptomatic prior to delivery can become symptomatic a week to a month after delivery. However, the disease in the mother is usually benign and self-limiting.

I. Mechanisms of Pathogenicity

The basic disease process characteristically involves the RES, and is marked by septicemia leading to granulomas, necrosis and suppuration. It is probable that delayed sensitivity contributes to the tissue damage observed. The fact that most infections are inapparent offers further evidence that *L. monocytogenes* is primarily an opportunistic pathogen.

J. Mechanisms of Immunity

Extensive experimental data indicate that *cellular immunity is the main mechanism of acquired immunity in listeriosis.* Some nonspecific systems such as lysozyme and β-lysin probably also contribute to resistance; however, there is abundant evidence from animal experiments that functioning thymus-derived lymphocytes and activated macrophages are the *sine qua non* of resistance to *L. monocytogenes* (see Fundamentals of Immunology).

K. Laboratory Diagnosis

A definitive diagnosis depends on isolation and identification of *L. monocytogenes;* no useful serologic tests are available. Listeriosis should always be considered when cultures from patients with meningitis, conjunctivitis, endocarditis, bacteremia or polyserositis lead to clinical laboratory reports, such as "diphtheroids" or "nonpathogens." The best chances of success in isolating *L. monocytogenes* can be achieved by holding specimens in glucose broth at 4°C (Section E) and subculturing at weekly intervals.

L. Therapy

The overall mortality rate in untreated persons with listeriosis is 70%. Useful chemotherapeutic drugs include sulfonamides, penicillin, tetracyclines and erythromycin; however, penicillin G and erythromycin are the drugs of choice. In meningitis, intravenous infusions of penicillin G plus oral erythromycin are commonly given; their use is generally continued for 5 to 7 days after clinical signs have abated. Listeriosis in the pregnant female is usually treated by administration of tetracycline and erythromycin. An equally successful therapeutic regimen for fetal listeriosis has not been devised.

M. Reservoirs of Infection

The organisms are widespread in nature and cause disease in many species of animals. Contact with fluids of infected animals, ingestion of contaminated milk and inhalation of contaminated dust probably represent the major sources of human infections. In 1971, the United States Department of Agriculture reported 231 cases of bovine listeriosis in 154 herds and 125 cases in sheep and goats from 48 herds. It is a puzzling observation that cases of disease in animals occur most frequently in the spring, the period when human listeriosis is infrequent; the numbers of human cases peak between June and September.

N. Control of Disease Transmission

Prevention of human listeriosis requires pasteurization of milk and elimination of diseased animals by slaughter. Effective control is hampered by difficulties in recognizing the infection, both in animals and in man.

References

Gray, M. L., and Killinger, A. H.: *Listeria monocytogenes* and listeric infections. Bact. Rev. *30*:309, 1966.

Moore, R. M., and Zehmer, R. B.: Listeriosis in the United States—1971. J. Infect. Dis. *127*:610, 1973.

Mouton, R. P., and Kampelmacher, E. H.: Listeria infections of the human skin. *In* Proceedings of the Third International Symposium on Listeriosis. Bilthoven, July 13-16, 1966.

Pearson, L. D., and Osebold, J. W.: Effects of antithymocyte and antimacrophage sera on the survival of mice infected with *Listeria monocytogenes*. Infect. Immun. *7*:479, 1973.

Seebiger, H. P. R.: Listeriosis. New York, Hafner, 1961.

Simpson, J. F., Leddy, J. P., and Hare, J. D.: Listeriosis complicating lymphoma: report of four cases and interpretive review of pathogenic factors. Am. J. Med. *43*:39, 1967.

Mycobacterium

The genus *Mycobacterium* of the family *Mycobacteriaceae* contains a large number of species, both saprophytes and parasites. Organisms of this genus are notable for their lipid-rich cell walls and "acid-fast" staining properties. They are widely distributed in nature and most species have extraordinarily simple nutritional requirements. Pathogenic species attack a wide range of natural hosts throughout the animal kingdom.

Man is the sole natural host of *Mycobacterium tuberculosis* and *Mycobacterium leprae,* the two most important species pathogenic for man. The cow is the natural host for the closely related species *Mycobacterium bovis* which, when transmitted to man as an accidental host, is essentially as pathogenic as *M. tuberculosis.* The *Aves* are the natural hosts of *M. avium* which only rarely, if ever, causes disease in man. Disease in man occasionally occurs due to the facultative parasites *M. ulcerans* and *M. marinum.* Certain other species of mycobacteria, designated by the group terms "atypical," "unclassified" or "anonymous" mycobacteria, can occasionally cause tuberculosis-like diseases in man; most of them are probably facultative parasites. As tuberculosis has waned in developed countries, mycobacteriosis due to the "atypicals" has increased in relative importance. Nonpathogenic mycobacteria are of no special medical interest aside from the fact that some of them are members of the normal flora and may be mistaken for pathogens. *Mycobacterium tuberculosis* stands as the prototype of the pathogenic mycobacteria and will be discussed in the greatest detail.

Mycobacterium tuberculosis

A. Medical Perspectives

Tuberculosis is favored by overpopulation, poverty, ignorance and hereditary predisposition. The most common form of infection, pulmonary tuberculosis (phthisis, consumption), is a chronic wasting disease, which in its early stages is often mistaken for chronic bronchitis. The Greek word "phthisis" means "consumption of the flesh." Symptoms commonly include fatigue, weight loss, night sweats, coughing, and spitting of blood.

In the world as a whole, tuberculosis has always ranked as the leading killer among the infectious diseases of man. However, in developed countries the death rate has declined steadily since about the middle of the 19th century, and precipitously since the advent of highly effective drug therapy in 1952. The reasons for this decline in death rate, which began even before the infectious nature of the disease was fully accepted, are not clearly apparent but probably reflect evolutionary changes in innate immunity of host populations and in virulence of the parasite, as well as improved standards of living. Unfortunately, the case rate has not declined as markedly as the death rate and in recent years appears to be rising.

The origin of tuberculosis antedates the recorded history of man; evidence of the disease, such as the distortions of the spine described by Pott, have been found in the statuary and bones of Egyptians dating as far back as 7,000 years. Asia, Africa and the Middle East were evidently early spawning grounds of many infectious diseases, including tuberculosis.

Tuberculosis probably waxed and waned in Europe during the middle ages, but no records exist to indicate that it reached epidemic proportions until the mid-17th century, after which its incidence declined and rose again to reach a major peak in the mid-19th century. The disease was so prevalent in Europe during the 18th and 19th centuries that "paleness" became fashionable and Alexander Dumas wrote that since everyone has consumption, especially the poets, "It is good form to spit blood from sheer emotion." At that time tuberculosis was thought to be hereditary and the notion grew that it was linked with genius, probably because genius seldom comes to light except by sacrifice and overwork. Among those who have died of tuberculosis are Thoreau, Stevenson, Schiller, Keats, Chopin and the dean of tuberculosis physicians himself, Laennec. In 1815 Thomas Young estimated that tuberculosis caused the premature death of one fourth of the inhabitants of Europe and in 1882 Robert Koch, the discoverer of *M. tuberculosis,* wrote that, in Europe, tuberculosis killed one third of all persons of middle age!

The manifestations of tuberculosis are many and varied; consequently, they were not easily recognized to reflect a single causation. Until late in the 19th century the concept, proposed by Laennec in 1819, that lung and miliary lesions were manifestations of one and the same disease continued to be challenged by men of great competence, such as the famous pathologist Virchow. It is of singular interest that Laennec invented the stethoscope for the express purpose of listening to lung sounds of patients with tuberculosis.

Although Galen, in the 2nd century, proposed that pulmonary tuberculosis is transmitted by the "breath," this concept was abandoned by the Romans. That tuberculosis was not a communicable disease remained the consensus of medical men until the mid-19th century! However, in 1865 the French army surgeon Villemin firmly established the infectious nature of both human and bovine tuberculosis by infecting rabbits and guinea pigs. Robert Koch cultivated and identified *M. tuberculosis* as the causative agent of the disease in 1882, and received the Nobel prize in 1905.

The number of cases of active clinical tuberculosis in the world today probably exceeds 50 million, at least 25 million of which are infectious. Each year the number of new cases approximates 5 million and the number of deaths may be as high as 3 million.

In advanced countries, tuberculosis is no longer the sinister and dreaded "white plague" of centuries past and sanatoria that once had long waiting lists are now virtually empty. However, in underdeveloped areas the tuberculosis problem is still immense; in some countries 25% of all deaths among young adults are due to the disease.

Currently in the USA there are at least 25 million infected individuals, as indicated by positive reactions to tuberculin tests; of these, about 250,000 have active disease. At present, only about 3 to 5% of young adults are tuberculin positive. The infection rate is highest in urban populations, but is, in general, markedly lower today than in past decades when infection rates in large cities sometimes exceeded 95%. It is of singular interest that an infection rate of 80% was reported recently in one slum area of a large city! About 6 thousand died of tuberculosis in 1971 in the USA, and 35,000 new cases of clinical disease were discovered. Alcoholism and drug addiction with associated malnutrition strongly predispose to the development of active disease. The highest incidence of active cases and the highest mortality rate in the USA are among males, especially elderly, single males residing in slum areas in large cities.

Economic losses due to tuberculosis can be staggering because of the prolonged course of the disease and the high cost of care and treatment. The tragic social and economic consequences of the disease have been especially profound in past years. Home life was commonly disrupted by the absence of a parent in the household and most families became financially impoverished. This state has been greatly mollified in recent years because ambulatory treatment with drugs is usually possible.

The future short-term outlook for the control of tuberculosis in developed countries is good, despite the problem of emerging drug-resistant strains. However, since many factors serve to determine infection rates, case rates, effectiveness of therapy and mortality rates, the long-term outlook for tuberculosis, even in a single country such as the USA, is difficult to predict. If, as seems reasonably certain, the long-continued control of tuberculosis within a region will eventually lead to the development of a more susceptible population, the difficulty of controlling the disease may increase with passing generations.

B. Physical and Chemical Structure

Mycobacterium tuberculosis is a nonmotile, nonsporing, nonencapsulated, slender, pleomorphic rod measuring about 0.4 μm $\times$ 3 μm. The organisms are sometimes curved and in stained preparations often have a beaded appearance due to volutin bodies and unstained vacuoles. They stain with great difficulty, but, once stained, retain stains even when such drastic destaining methods as treatment with acid-alcohol are employed—hence the term "acid-fast." The acid-fast staining procedure commonly employed is the *Ziehl-Neelsen* method. Although the properties determining acid-fastness are unknown, physical integrity of the cell is essential. *Mycobacterium tuberculosis* tends to stain weakly gram-positive; however, its chemical composition more closely resembles the gram-negative than the gram-positive bacteria.

The cell wall of *M. tuberculosis* contains enormous quantities of lipids and waxes (up to 60% of the dry weight of the cell), which evidently account, in part at least, for many of the organism's unique properties. These include its high resistance to physical and chemical agents and to intracellular killing by phagocytes, its hydrophobic character, its slow growth, its acid-fastness, and its marked adjuvant and granulomagenic activities. The cell's hydrophobic surface promotes phagocytosis by neutrophils and by macrophages, which are attracted chemotactically to the organism.

The roles that lipids and waxes play in tissue responses and sensitivity reactions in tuberculosis remain uncertain despite extensive investigation. However, it is of interest that the so-called "wax D" of the cell walls, which is composed of mycolic acids and a glycopeptide, has adjuvant and directive effects on the immune response similar to those of whole bacilli. When wax D is mixed with tuberculoproteins it directs the immune response to the proteins largely along the path leading to delayed sensitivity. An old but interesting phenomenon observed over 40 years ago is as follows: when a foreign protein, such as egg albumin, is mixed with tubercle bacilli, especially when Freund's incomplete adjuvant mixture is also included, the immune response to the protein is strongly directed toward the development of the delayed type of sensitivity. On the other hand, injection of free uncomplexed proteins alone, including tuberculoproteins, leads to Arthus and immediate-type sensitivities.

The adjuvant activity of wax D appears to be due to a cell wall peptidoglycolipid existing on the cell surface as a network of fine branching filaments (130 Å in diameter); the filaments are unique to organisms of the genus *Mycobacterium* (see cover illustration).

The tubercle bacillus also contains the so-called *cord factor,* which may contribute to virulence (Section I). Although little is known about the Ags of different mycobacteria, many species share common Ags. This is evidenced by cross-reactions displayed in Ouchterlony gel diffusion tests and in skin sensitivity tests conducted with proteins (tuberculins) derived from various mycobacteria. Human and bovine tubercle bacilli are closely related and their respective tuberculins (bacillary proteins) are essentially of equal potency for eliciting cutaneous tuberculin reactions in individuals infected with either of the two organisms. Other mycobacteria, such as the "atypical mycobacteria," are so distantly related to *M. tuberculosis* that individuals infected with most of these organisms commonly give only weak or negative reactions to standard tuberculins derived from *M. tuberculosis*.

C. Genetics

Little is known about the mechanisms responsible for genetic change in *M. tuberculosis,* especially in the important areas of medical interest, virulence and antibiotic resistance. Bacteriophages for *M. tuberculosis* have been described, but their role in genetic change is unknown. Freshly isolated strains of *M. tuberculosis* from untreated patients with pulmonary tuberculosis have not been found to vary significantly in their virulence for experimental animals. However, isolates from persons having skin tuberculosis (lupus vulgaris) and from patients treated with isonicotinic acid hydrazide (INH) are often of low virulence for animals. Organisms of reduced virulence have also been obtained by long subculture under suboptimal growth conditions that evidently provide growth advantage to avirulent mutants, e.g., the bacillus of Calmette and Guerin (BCG) and the human avirulent strain, H37Ra.

D. Extracellular Products

Little is known about extracellular products of *M. tuberculosis* or the possible role that such substances may play in pathogenesis. Being a facultative intracellular parasite, the shed substances, surface components, or metabolic activities of *M. tuberculosis* could exert toxic effects on the macrophage; in particular, large numbers of growing bacilli within macrophages appear to be cytotoxic. However, no soluble external component likely to produce cytotoxicity has been described.

E. Culture

Although *M. tuberculosis* can grow on very simple synthetic media, it is common practice in diagnostic work to use a complex medium, such as Lowenstein-Jensen medium, because small inocula are sensitive to trace amounts of various toxic components present in synthetic media. Since trace amounts of free fatty acid are stimulatory for growth, known amounts of fatty acid and serum albumin are sometimes added to synthetic media; the albumin binds the fatty acid with an affinity that is proper for maintaining a level of dissociated free fatty acid suitable for growth. Synthetic media containing Tween 80 (a wetting agent) plus albumin are useful for quantitative experimental work since they promote dispersed growth of these hydrophobic organisms.

Mycobacterium tuberculosis is a slow-growing strict aerobe. Its shortest generation time is about 12 to 18 hours and visible growth under the best of conditions is commonly not achieved before 1 to 2 weeks or more; usually at least 3 weeks are required before growth from clinical specimens becomes apparent. Increased CO_2 tension enhances growth, which occurs over a pH range of 6.0 to 8.0. The temperature growth range is 30 to 42°C (optimum 37°C). Colonies are characteristically buff-colored, wrinkled and dry.

F. Resistance to Physical and Chemical Agents

Mycobacterium tuberculosis is highly resistant to drying in the presence of organic matter and survives in dried sputum for days to weeks. It is also highly resistant to acids, alkalies and dye-stuffs. Phenols are among the best disinfectants and moist heat treatment equal to that of pasteurization is required to destroy the organism.

G. Experimental Models

Tuberculosis is largely a disease of domesticated animals and man. Its rarity in wild animals probably rests primarily on lack of adequate patterns of transmission and/or lack of close contact between diseased and healthy individuals. The range of pathogenicity of the medically important mycobacteria that naturally produce tuberculosis and tuberculosis-like disease in man and certain animals is given in Table 29-1.

TABLE 29-1
Pathogenicity of M. tuberculosis and Related Mycobacteria

Animal	M. tuberculosis	M. bovis	M. avium	Atypical Mycobacteria
Man	+++*	+++	rare	− to +++
Guinea pig	++++	++++	−	− to +
Rabbit	+	++++	++	−
Mouse	+++	+++	−	− to +++
Cow	−	+++	−	?
Chicken	−	−	+++	?
Swine	+	++	++	?
Cat	++	++	−	?

* The degree of pathogenicity is designated by plus signs ranging from + to ++++ and is based on natural and/or experimental infections.

Guinea pigs and mice have been used most extensively in experimental tuberculosis. Whereas guinea pigs have the advantage of developing delayed sensitivity closely simulating that developed by man, virulence can be more easily quantitated in the more resistant mouse.

H. Infections in Man

Certain infectious diseases, characterized by chronicity and granuloma formation, are produced by facultative intracellular parasites that are not effectively destroyed by humoral factors in the extracellular environment or by neutrophils, but, instead, are phagocytized and grow within macrophages. Tuberculosis is the prototype of such diseases.

Man is highly susceptible to invasion by tubercle bacilli but is remarkably resistant to progression of the infection and the development of clinical disease. Although *M. tuberculosis* may infect many organs and tissues by many routes, the lung is by far the most common site of infection, evidently because of the high oxygen tensions that it provides, particularly anteriorly and in the lower lobes. For unknown reasons the parenchyma of a few organs, such as the pancreas, heart and thyroid gland, are extraordinarily resistant. *The only infection produced by M. tuberculosis that will be discussed in detail is pulmonary tuberculosis.*

Because of the great complexity and controversial nature of host-parasite relationships in tuberculosis, the *pathogenesis and immunology of the disease cannot be suitably dealt with as separate subjects.* They will be considered together in the discussion of the natural history of the disease and only summaries will be presented elsewhere.

It is notable that, *whereas primary infection during its early stages is characterized by essentially unrestricted growth and spread of organisms to local lymph nodes and blood, late primary, reactivation and reinfection tuberculosis are characterized by restricted growth of organisms and a tendency for the organisms to remain localized at the infection site* or to spread by contiguity, unless the tubercle ruptures into a bronchus or a vein. Another major point worthy of emphasis is that the nature and progress of the individual lesion appear to be related to the load of organisms in the lesion, and to the degree of hypersensitivity and cellular immunity possessed by the host. When hypersensitivity and cellular immune activities are strong and the load of bacilli is low, *proliferative healing lesions* dominate; when the load of bacilli is high, progressing exudative lesions dominate.

1. Primary Infection Tuberculosis

Primary infection is usually acquired by inhalation of droplet nuclei generated by individuals with active pulmonary disease who cough and thus discharge organisms into the air.* The droplet nuclei must have a diameter of < 10 μm in order to reach the alveoli where infection is initiated. Inhaled droplets of larger size are arrested short of the alveoli and removed by the mucociliary blanket and usually swallowed. The larger airways of the respiratory tract are highly resistant to infection. Studies on human necropsy material and experimental tuberculosis in animals suggest that the following events take place. Most of the inhaled bacilli reaching the alveoli are engulfed promptly by resident alveolar macrophages and grow readily in such cells for a week or more. Some of the inhaled bacilli may initially escape phagocytosis and grow unrestricted. Many of the macrophages initially parasitized are eventually killed, presumably as the result of growth and metabolic activities of the engulfed bacilli. Most of the organisms released by the macrophages are promptly engulfed by increasing numbers of infiltrating neutrophils and young macrophages, which either remain in the area or migrate to the local lymph nodes. Free organisms may also reach the local lymph nodes. Neutrophils cannot destroy bacilli, which are soon released on death of these short-lived phagocytes. Alternatively, neutrophils laden with bacilli may be engulfed by macrophages. A few bacilli usually escape from the nodes to the blood and lodge at distant sites. However, these few blood-borne organisms are usually destroyed by "immune macrophages" without leaving permanent evidence of a lesion. This is in contrast to the primary lesion that may be progressing, because organisms within areas of caseation are protected from macrophages. Alternatively, blood-borne organisms may lie dormant for many years and may sometimes serve to cause reactivation disease. Thus, during the initial phase of infection, essentially unrestricted local growth of organisms occurs both extracellularly and within "nonimmune macrophages," and lymph node and systemic blood-borne spread occurs before acquired immunity, with its localizing influences, develops. After about 2 to 3 weeks, when the first evidence of the immune response appears, all events become increasingly influenced by the developing forces of delayed hypersensitivity and cellular immunity. As tubercles form the intracellular growth of the organisms gradually slows, evidently in substantial measure because the macrophages become "activated." However, immunity does not become fully developed until host cells assemble in large numbers and form mature tubercles. If the developing immune forces are too weak or the number of infecting organisms is too large, the organisms are not restrained by tubercle formation and the disease may progress and spread. Indeed, if the infecting dose of bacilli is large enough and/or the immune response is sufficiently weak, the primary infection may progress and kill the patient rather than undergo spontaneous arrest, as occurs in the large majority of

* Bacilli survive for weeks in particles of dried sputum, which also constitute a potential source of infection.

cases. For example, primary infections often progress in the immunologically immature infant and the immunologically compromised adult.

The tubercle, a typical allergic granuloma, often presents centrally located giant cells (usually containing bacilli) immediately surrounded by epithelioid cells and a peripheral mantle of macrophages, lymphocytes and a few plasma cells (Figs. 29-1 and 29-2). The tubercle has long been recognized as the *sine qua non* of resistance to tuberculosis, but it is only recently that the relation between the composition and function of this "adaptive structure of immunologic defense" in immunity has become meaningful. Although the precise ways in which the various cells of the tubercle may contribute to immunity are unknown, B-lymphocytes and plasma cells could contribute by forming cytophilic Abs and those T-lymphocytes that develop sensitivity to Ags of the bacillus could react with locally released Ags to yield macrophage-activating lymphokines.

Epithelioid cells are elongated, nonmotile derivatives of macrophages. They have a reduced capacity to phagocytize but appear to have an increased capability to inhibit and kill microbes; they usually contain few if any tubercle bacilli. Epithelioid cells develop from macrophages present in the tubercle, but the factors that incite their development are unknown.

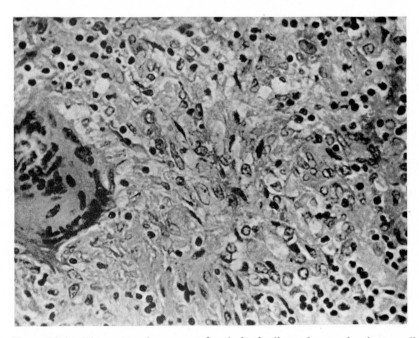

Figure 29-1. The center of a young tubercle in the liver of man, showing a well-marked epithelioid cell reaction, a giant cell and a peripheral zone of lymphocytes. The vesicular nuclei of the epithelioid cells and the cytoplasmic extensions of the giant cell are well shown. (From Florey, H.: General Pathology. Philadelphia, W. B. Saunders Co., 1970, p. 1193.)

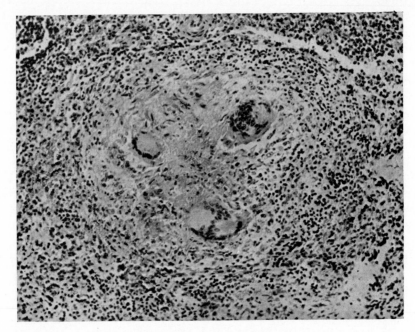

Figure 29-2. Microscopical tubercle in the spleen of man. At the center of the palely staining mass of epithelioid cells the earliest signs of necrosis can be seen. (From Florey, H.: General Pathology. Philadelphia, W. B. Saunders Co., 1970, p. 1193.)

One possibility is that the inciting agent is a lymphokine. It has been shown that monocytes attracted to the periphery of the tubercle by chemotaxis become activated, presumably under the stimulus of lymphokines, as they pass through the peripheral mantle of lymphocytes. It is also possible that, as macrophages move centrally, lymphokines exert additional effects on them, namely, immobilization and transformation into epithelioid cells. If a macrophage is to survive in the tubercle, transformation to an epithelioid cell with cessation of phagocytosis may be of advantage since otherwise the load of engulfed organisms might become so great that the cell would be killed. By interdigitation of their processes epithelioid cells literally form a solid multilayered wall around the center of the developing tubercle and may thus limit the spread of bacilli.

The Langhans-type giant cell of the tubercle, with its multiple nuclei distributed at the periphery of its cytoplasm, is the result of fusion of numerous macrophages. Giant cells occur in association with epithelioid cells; they often contain viable bacilli, and often occupy the centers of small tubercles undergoing caseation necrosis. Recent in vitro experiments indicate that lymphokines cause macrophages to fuse and form giant cells. However, lymphokines are evidently not the only stimulus for giant-cell production, and it is possible that giant cells are formed most readily under the combined influence of lymphokines and other factors, such as ingested bacteria.

With time, central caseation necrosis usually occurs in the primary tubercle, apparently as the result of death of epithelioid cells (Fig. 29-2). Whether death of other types of cells alone would provide the conditions necessary for the development of caseation necrosis is not known. The necrotic material consists of the partially digested remains of dead cells which lend to it a cheese-like consistency. Although the precise reason(s) for caseation necrosis remains an enigma, the probability that delayed sensitivity makes a major contribution to this event suggests that lymphokines, which are abundant in the tubercle, play a role. There is good evidence that lack of nutrition, due to the avascularity of the tubercle, does not serve as the sole basis of necrosis.

The growth of tubercle bacilli is markedly inhibited in areas of caseation necrosis, presumably because of lack of oxygen, the presence of toxic fatty acids, and possibly other factors such as lysozyme and other cationic cell components. Growth of bacilli is most favored in the outermost zone of necrosis near the periphery of the tubercle, where the organisms multiply extracellularly under favorable oxygen tensions and beyond the reach of macrophages. It is notable that, when softening (liquefaction) of caseous materials occurs, explosive growth of tubercle bacilli takes place, often leading to catastrophic spread of the organisms. Whatever the factors are that cause central necrosis of epithelioid cells, these factors evidently affect other cells as well, for fibroblasts at the periphery of such tubercles do not fare as well as in normal tissue and healing and vascularization of the necrotic area do not occur until the initiating cause of the whole process, the tubercle bacillus, disappears. Calcium deposits are sometimes laid down following caseation and are often present in healed primary lesions. Residual walled-off caseous materials and calcium deposits are of particular interest since bacilli remain alive in them for years and may serve as a source of organisms leading to reactivation disease.

The phenomenon of softening of the caseous material presents another enigma; although it invariably occurs when secondary infection with pyogenic bacteria takes place, which theoretically might result from enzymes liberated by dying neutrophils, it can also occur spontaneously, in certain tubercles but not others, in the absence of infection or infiltrating neutrophils. The softening of large caseous lesions usually is coincident with erosion and communication of such lesions to the airways of the lung. The liquefied caseous material plus increased availability of oxygen from the airways of the lung provide an environment favorable for an explosive multiplication of tubercle bacilli. Unfortunately, these events prompt extensive coughing and the highly infected caseous material is disseminated in the form of an aerosol. Evacuation of caseous material leads to the formation of a cavity harboring residual exudate and necrotic debris teeming with tubercle bacilli. The fibrous capsule lining the cavity provides a barrier to the normal cellular defense mechanisms as well as chemotherapy. The organisms can persist for an indefinite period in the residual caseous material lining a cavity, particularly if the cavity does not close and communicates with a bronchus. The above events also provide a mechanism to disseminate large numbers of tubercle bacilli to the blood stream if erosion into blood vessels occurs. *Cavities are the greatest deterrent to healing and the most difficult problem in clinical management.* Because of diffusion problems in cavities, chemotherapeutic agents lack effectiveness; obliteration by collapse therapy may fail and surgical extirpation is sometimes the only recourse.

Lymphokines undoubtedly influence cellular events within the tubercle, but their role is largely speculative and is based principally on information gained *in vitro* by exposing sensitive lymphocytes to bacillary Ags, particularly tuberculin. The supernatant fluids from such stimulated lymphocytes contain lymphokines that can produce delayed skin reactions resembling the cutaneous tuberculin reaction (Fundamentals of Immunology). The supernatant fluids of suspensions of cells obtained from the tuberculous lungs of animals are also rich in lymphokines that probably play a prominent role in determining cellular events within the tubercle.

It must be kept in mind that, subsequent to the initiation of the immune response, all lesions contain hypersensitive host cells and consequently differ from the earlier nonsensitive primary lesions in their character and dynamics of development. In the hypersensitive primary lesion, the mobilized and activated macrophages and lymphocytes proliferate; an exudate develops and caseation necrosis is prone to occur. The quantity of tubercle bacilli present at this point undoubtedly influences the magnitude and degree of caseation necrosis.

Two general types of lesions, *"exudative"* and *"productive,"* occur after the development of delayed hypersensitivity and cellular immunity. *In the exudative lesion the acute inflammatory component is pronounced;* fluid is abundant and many neutrophils as well as macrophages are present. The extent to which the neutrophils may contribute to the inflammation is not known.

The exudative lesion is common in the lung, a loose tissue, and appears to rest with the sudden escape of large numbers of organisms from the tubercle that presumably recruit to the site large numbers of sensitive lymphocytes from the circulation. If a tubercle ruptures into a bronchus a resultant massive delayed sensitivity reaction occurs, assuming the form of a tuberculous pneumonia. Depending on numbers of organisms and the degree of immunity and hypersensitivity, such bronchial spread may lead to either massive necrosis and cavity formation, transformation to a "productive-type" lesion, or healing by resolution.

The productive type of lesions consists of typical allergic granulomas, i.e., tubercles composed largely of epithelioid cells without escape of large numbers of organisms from the confines of the tubercle and without excessive exudate. Such lesions may heal or may caseate and progress. *Caseous tubercles often erode the walls of tubular structures,* such as bronchi and veins, or the integuments of body cavities, such as the subarachnoid space. Entrance of large numbers of bacilli into the blood leads to the widespread development of numerous small tubercles of millet-seed size (miliary tuberculosis). Unless the patient is treated, meningitis is invariably fatal and miliary tuberculosis is almost always fatal.

The primary tubercle is exudative in character and usually grows beyond microscopic size; bacilli often escape to set up satellite tubercles and to produce caseous lesions in the draining lymph nodes with resultant bacteremia. *The primary tubercle together with its affected draining lymph nodes is called the "primary complex" or "Ghon complex"; it contrasts sharply with typical lesions of subsequent disease (reactivation or reinfection tuberculosis) in which the draining lymph nodes are not substantially involved. Primary infections usually escape clinical notice, and the lesions commonly heal and remain quiescent throughout life.** Healing of the tubercle is attended by invasion of fibroblasts from the periphery. *Alternatively, primary lesions may sometimes progress and produce fatal disease,* especially in infants, debilitated individuals and individuals belonging to races with low innate resistance. The balance between host resistance and virulence of organisms is evidently a delicate one and is easily shifted by the size of the inoculum, the physiologic state of the host, or the fortuitous rupture of a tubercle into the blood stream, a tubular structure or a body cavity. *Small numbers of living bacilli commonly persist in healed primary lesions for many years*—indeed, usually for the lifetime of the individual, e.g., "once infected, always infected" is the general rule. Although such bacilli are virtually impossible to detect microscopically, they have been demonstrated by inoculating animals with necropsy material. Further evidence that bacilli persist in healed lesions is the observation that tuberculin sensitivity commonly persists for the lifetime of the individual. The lesions in which bacilli can persist are often minute areas of scar. The precise circumstances that permit the organisms to survive in healed lesions over long periods of time are an important but unsolved problem. Do they multiply slowly? Do they always remain in extracellular positions in old caseous residues or sometimes become incarcerated within long-lived but incompetent macrophages?

---

* As a rule, primary infection develops randomly at any site deep in the lung, whereas reinfection usually occurs in the apices of the lungs. Explanations proposed include (a) high oxygen level favors growth in the apices of the upper lobes and (b) a reduced blood circulation in the apices impedes expression of cellular immunity.

2. Reactivation and Reinfection Tuberculosis

In regions where the incidence of disease is low, most cases of clinical tuberculosis are the result of reactivation arising from the residual bacilli of primary infection (reactivation tuberculosis) rather than from exogenous bacilli (reinfection tuberculosis). Hence, in contrast to previous decades of high incidence of disease, when it was of advantage to bear healed primary lesions and be tuberculin positive and immune in order to meet the high risk of exogenous reinfection, it is currently disadvantageous to have experienced a primary infection because the risk of reactivation now outweighs the low risk of reinfection.

Obvious but unanswered questions are: Why do old healed, primary lesions sometimes reactivate in adulthood and why does reactivation disease in adults progress to severe clinical disease more often than does primary infection itself? Although the arguments on this question are many and varied, the explanation probably rests with the fact that most primary infections occur in children of ages of 3 to 12 years, a period in life when resistance is highest and progressive disease rarely occurs. There is strong evidence that reactivation in adulthood often occurs for physiologic reasons such as malnutrition (especially protein deficiency), overcrowding and stress. For example, after the release of inmates of Nazi concentration camps, the speed with which many of those with far-advanced tuberculosis recovered was astounding and indicated clearly that the conditions of imprisonment severely depressed resistance by some unknown mechanism.

The influence of age, sex and hormones on resistance to tuberculosis is well known, but the mechanisms involved are obscure. Whereas children between 3 and 12 years of age seldom develop progressive disease, infants are highly susceptible. Susceptibility increases substantially during adolescence, and tuberculosis among young adults is more frequent in females than males.

I. Mechanisms of Pathogenicity (a Recapitulation)

The mechanisms by which the tubercle bacillus invades and injures its host are not known. Despite many claims, the factor(s) that determines virulence has not been established. Although highly virulent strains tend to produce colonies with rougher surfaces than do less virulent strains, this property is not a consistent and reliable indicator of virulence. The best, but nevertheless imperfect, correlate of virulence is "cord formation" characterized by growth of the bacilli in serpentine aggregates with their long axes parallel. This manner of growth is associated with a high content of "cord factor" (trehalose-6-6'dimycolate), which is toxic for mice at high dose levels. Cord factor is reported to be granulomagenic; it may be important to virulence, but is not a key factor determining virulence since it is produced by some avirulent strains. Despite some claims that virulent bacilli and their products exert a primary toxic effect on phagocytes *in vitro,* no causative toxin has been identified. It is generally believed that the state of tuberculin sensitivity contributes significantly to tissue injury and caseation necrosis (Section H). It is possible that an exaggerated level of tuberculin sensitivity is harmful but that a low level is beneficial in terms of host defense.

J. Mechanisms of Immunity

In tuberculous tissues, tubercle bacilli exist largely either within macrophages or extracellularly. Consequently the factors of resistance, be they innate or acquired, that limit the growth of the organisms or kill them must operate in these two environments. *The experimental data available suggest that innate immunity may not be important and that immunity to tuberculosis is essentially all acquired during the infection.* Accordingly, resistant individuals or species have a better capability to acquire resistance than do susceptibles. Marked variation in this ability in human beings is exemplified by the Ludbeck disaster of 1930, in which 251 children were mistakenly given a large uniform dose of virulent bacilli instead of BCG vaccine; 77 died, 127 developed lesions that healed, but the remaining 47 never developed detectable lesions!

There is abundant evidence that, in the course of evolution, exposure to infection has played an important role in selecting individuals who have the capability of acquiring effective immunity to *M. tuberculosis.* Certain American Indians and Eskimos, who first experienced tuberculosis when contacted by Europeans, displayed greater genetic susceptibility to the disease than people of European stocks exhibit. Marked differences in immunity to tuberculosis have also been shown to exist among inbred strains of mice, guinea pigs and rabbits and among monozygotic human twins. To what degree such genetic resistance depends on constitutive factors unrelated to specific acquired immunity, as opposed to the constitutive capacity to respond with acquired immunity, is uncertain.

As compared to susceptible inbred rabbits, resistant inbred rabbits possess the genetic capacity to mount a more rapid and intense delayed hypersensitivity response, earlier caseation necrosis and stronger inhibition of growth of the organism.

Acquired immunity appears to be cellular. Intracellular suppression of bacilli rests on the activity of macrophages, and extracellular suppression depends on unfavorable environmental conditions within the tubercle. The tubercle itself is an allergic granuloma, and hence can be regarded to represent an adaptive immunologic structure of defense. Consequently, inquiry into the antibacterial events in acquired immunity should be directed at the tubercle. Bacilli seldom exist free of the tubercle for long periods, for tubercles always form readily as a response to free organisms, especially after delayed hypersensitivity and immunity have developed.

The first step in the formation of the tubercle starts with macrophages that are chemotactically attracted to the organisms and ingest them. Following this, it must be envisioned that Ags are released from the bacilli to reach immunocompetent lymphocytes in the developing lesion locally and/or in the draining lymph nodes. Evidently the resulting "sensitized T-lymphocytes" then accumulate around the clustered macrophages, and, meeting local Ag, respond with proliferation and release of lymphokines. Because of their many effects on lymphocytes and macrophages, lymphokines could bring about a cascade of reactions terminating in the mature tubercle with all its structural and functional metamorphoses and attributes, including caseation necrosis, which serves to suppress and kill tubercle bacilli. The fact that the *key effector cell* in acquired immunity to tuberculosis is the "activated macrophage" poses the question as to what force or forces are responsible for macrophage activation. Presumably the force or forces would have to act locally and continuously in the tubercle in order to activate newly arriving monocytes to replace macrophages that die or that transform to epithelioid cells and giant cells. *Any post-phagocytic activation of macrophages afforded by the organisms themselves is obviously insufficient, for otherwise the first organisms engulfed during primary infection would be destroyed.* The possibility that locally produced lymphokines (T-cells) and/or Abs (B-cells) cytophilic for macrophages could function in the tubercle to incite and maintain a high level of local activation of macrophages is the most attractive theory to account for macrophage activation in tuberculosis.

The controversy as to whether delayed sensitivity (allergy) to tuberculin is harmful or beneficial in tuberculosis has raged for decades. The original champions of the concept that allergy is harmful have claimed that the abolition of allergy in guinea pigs by "desensitization" with massive doses of tuberculin does not compromise immunity but assists it. However, neither this observation nor the observations that animals can be made tuberculin sensitive without at the same time becoming immune, or, alternatively, immune without becoming sensitive (as occurs with a vaccine of bacillary RNA-protein complex), establish for sure that delayed sensitivity makes no contribution to immunity. It is possible that the two phenomena, delayed sensitivity and cellular immunity, have certain components that are shared irregularly and that the expression of either phenomenon does not demand the simultaneous expression of all components. Moreover the measurement of delayed sensitivity by skin testing may not necessarily reflect the capacity of cells of the tubercle itself to mount a local delayed sensitivity response. For example, in animals that continue to remain tuberculin negative (dermal), tuberculous granulomas can be produced in the lungs which contain lymphocytes that are specifically sensitive to tuberculin by the macrophage migration-inhibition test. Moreover, such animals respond specifically to injected tubercle bacilli with an accelerated granulomatous reaction. *It is possible that delayed sensitivity is an exaggerated form of cellular immunity that is detrimental to the intended function of this form of immunity.* It is well known that rats are highly resistant to tuberculosis but develop weak delayed sensitivity, whereas guinea pigs develop high levels of delayed sensitivity but are highly susceptible to tuberculosis.

K. Laboratory Diagnosis

The diagnosis of pulmonary infections due to *M. tuberculosis* and related organisms is based largely on clinical, x-ray and bacteriologic findings. The tuberculin skin test is also helpful in certain cases.

Bacteriologic evidence is necessary to firmly establish a diagnosis of tuberculosis. The procedures used include culture, smears for detection of acid-fast bacilli, and animal inoculation. The materials examined are either fresh specimens or concentrates of specimens prepared by various physical and chemical procedures designed to selectively kill or inhibit contaminating bacteria and to concentrate tubercle bacilli. Specimens include such materials as sputum, gastric washings, spinal fluid, joint fluid, feces, lung aspirates and biopsied tissue.

The finding of typical acid-fast rods, even with strong clinical evidence of tuberculosis, constitutes only presumptive evidence that the disease is tuberculosis and further confirmatory tests should be performed. For example, on occasion, the nonpathogen *M. smegmatis,* a normal inhabitant of the genitalia, has been mistaken for *M. tuberculosis. In years past, numerous individuals with other diseases have been mistakenly sent to tuberculosis sanatoria because of faulty bacteriologic diagnosis based on smears alone!* However, it should be emphasized that the presence of typical acid-fast rods in stained smears of spinal fluid sediment is essentially diagnostic for tuberculous meningitis.

Cultural tests are usually sufficient to identify *M. tuberculosis* with reasonable certainty and animal inoculation is only resorted to under special circumstances. Niacin is produced by cultured *M. tuberculosis,* but not by other mycobacteria, and thus serves as a useful diagnostic aid. In some instances, finding the organism by any method may be difficult; *repeated and intense search is always recommended in suspected cases* since these bacilli are often shed intermittently and in small numbers.

The frequent occurrence of drug-resistant variants possessing altered pathogenicity for animals and the fact that atypical mycobacteria can produce lesions indistinguishable from those produced by *M. tuberculosis* have introduced complex and difficult problems in the diagnosis and therapy of mycobacterial diseases.

The cutaneous tuberculin test with various tuberculins (protein derivatives of bacilli) is becoming increasingly useful in the diagnosis of the mycobacterioses. Tuberculin elicits a delayed skin reaction (tuberculin reaction) in sensitive animals and man. "Old Tuberculin" (OT), a heated culture filtrate of *M. tuberculosis,* was first prepared by Koch in 1890. The tuberculin preparation "Purified Protein Derivative" (PPD) made from OT is commonly used for skin testing; it contains derivatives of low molecular weight (less than 10,000), of various proteins of the tubercle bacillus. Even though the proteins of various mycobacteria are related and cross hypersensitivity occurs among the mycobacterioses, skin tests, with proper concentrations of various tuberculins made from different species of mycobacteria, reveal marked differences in the size and intensity of reactions and can be of value in differential diagnosis. In infection due to *M. tuberculosis* (except for rare infections with *M. bovis* or photochromogens) a reaction of 10 mm or more in diameter to 5 tuberculin units (TU) of standard PPD is generally indicative of *M. tuberculosis* infection. Moreover, comparative skin tests with the various tuberculins are commonly confirmatory with respect to ruling out the possibility of infection due to nonmammalian mycobacteria.

The tuberculin test is of great value in the control of tuberculosis because of its diagnostic and case-finding usefulness. In interpreting the results of tuberculin testing *it must be kept clearly in mind that essentially all infected individuals give positive reactions regardless of whether their infection is clinically manifest or not.* Moreover, *whereas a negative reaction has a high exclusion value in diagnosis, a positive reaction only indicates the possibility of clinical tuberculosis.* As the rate of infection and clinical disease in a population decreases to low levels the value of the tuberculin test as a screening device for case finding and as a diagnostic tool rises. Since the reaction to the test converts from negative to positive soon after infection, the test has special value among groups of individuals who may experience frequent and heavy exposure, such as laboratory workers, doctors and nurses. The test is also useful for detecting new cases among "limited contacts" of tuberculous patients, especially children. Today, in most communities in the USA, a positive reaction in a child younger than 6 years old signifies that the source of infection is not far away.

Cutaneous tuberculin sensitivity may vary in intensity and temporarily may decrease or disappear during the course of high fever, in exanthematous disease, miliary tuberculosis, the terminal stages of pulmonary tuberculosis and during steroid treatment. Negative reactions in such cases may be specific for tuberculosis or may represent total anergy without response to any of the common skin test Ags such as mumps and histoplasmin. The intensity of the tuberculin reaction probably depends on the number of circulating T-lymphocytes sensitive to PPD. For unknown reasons an occasional individual may fail to react to tuberculin even after a natural infection or after BCG vaccination.

Although no reliable relationship exists between the level of tuberculin sensitivity and extent and severity of tuberculous infection, the intensity of the tuberculin reaction is not without significance. As a general rule, relatively high levels of sensitivity are found in persons with recently acquired infection, in those with caseous nonpulmonary tuberculosis (e.g., in lymph nodes and bones), and in those who are in continuous contact with open tuberculosis but who show no signs of active disease. Fluctuating levels of sensitivity to tuberculin are seen in patients with serous membrane tuberculosis (e.g., tuberculous pleuritis); these apparently reflect varying degrees of exudation and resorption of fluid. In persons with advanced tuberculosis and acute forms of the disease, sensitivity is usually low, and it appears to be a general truth that low levels of sensitivity in persons with active, progressive tuberculosis signal a poor prognosis.

L. Therapy

Older forms of therapy such as bedrest, lung collapse and surgical excision of infected tissue are limited in their effectiveness and have become, in large measure, unnecessary because of the marked success achieved with drug therapy. However, in accord with experience with other diseases, drug treatment of tuberculosis is not a perfect therapeutic measure; its limitations result because of the development of drug-resistant strains of organisms, because the drug fails to reach organisms within macrophages and necrotic tissue, and because maximal action of the drug is often blocked in these environments. Owing to the long periods of therapy involved and attending opportunity for multiplication of organisms, even in patients treated with the bactericidal agent *isoniazid (INH)*, drug-resistant mutants commonly arise unless a second drug is administered simultaneously (combined therapy). *Ethambutol (EMB)* has largely supplanted *para-aminosalicylic acid (PAS)* as a companion of INH because it is more active than PAS and causes fewer adverse effects. One of the most effective combinations is INH and EMB; another is *streptomycin (SM)* plus *ethionamide (ETA)*. However, the use of streptomycin has been limited because of its toxicity. A more recent and unusually promising agent is *rifampin (RM)*. A combination of INH and RM is said to be the least toxic and most highly effective combination of all. The only possible drawbacks to the use of rifampin are that it has immunosuppressive activity and it is expensive for long-term treatment. Although INH-resistant mutants retain their virulence for man and are transmitted from man to man, they have low virulence for the guinea pig, lack catalase and peroxidase activity, and grow more slowly than wild-type organisms. The impact that drug-resistant mutants may have on the future pattern of tuberculosis in human populations is unpredictable.

M.   Reservoirs of Infection

Man is the only important reservoir of M. tuberculosis. The disease is often contracted from tuberculous individuals who are unmindful or unaware of the nature of their disease, as well as from patients with recognized disease. On rare occasion the disease is contracted from experimental animals or from subhuman primates in close association with man (pets, animals in zoos, etc.). Bacteriophage typing has promise for epidemiologic studies.

N.   Control of Disease Transmission

Present-day efforts to prevent tuberculosis in the USA are largely directed at case finding and regulation of "shedders." Tuberculin screening tests, X-rays of contacts and high morbidity groups, and search for sources of infection, especially in families and among school children, have been the most effective means of discovering new cases. *Periodic tuberculin surveys are important for determining the effectiveness of community control of tuberculosis.* Infection with tubercle bacilli and tuberculin sensitivity commonly persist throughout life. Consequently the percentage of reactors is cumulative and increases with age. *Tuberculin testing carried out in sufficiently large test groups that are proportionately representative of the population with respect to age, sex, race and economic level furnishes the best available measure of the prevalence of tuberculous infection and has predictive value. For example, it has been found that when the infection rate in the age group under 14 years drops below 1%, tuberculosis in that population is on the way to virtual extinction.*

Prophylactic treatment with INH is used in special high-risk groups including recent "tuberculin converters," close contacts of known shedders and in high-mortality groups, such as infants who show positive reactions to tuberculin tests. Chemoprophylaxis with the combination INH-RM could prove to be even more successful. In rare instances, INH prophylaxis has been reported to cause hepatitis.

Prevention of tuberculosis by vaccination with the living attenuated bovine strain, called BCG, has definite but limited value. Whereas it has been widely used in various countries of Europe and other areas in the world, principally for vaccinating infants, its use in the USA has been largely experimental and has been restricted to "high exposure" groups. For such groups, chemoprophylaxis promises to replace BCG vaccination completely. The vaccine has the disadvantage of rendering the person tuberculin positive and thus destroys the value of the tuberculin test for mass screening, diagnosis and surveillance for "tuberculin converters" among contacts and in high-risk groups. The tuberculin test for surveillance studies is highly valuable and its use for this purpose should be encouraged.

Prompt initiation of chemoprophylaxis with INH of individuals who have recently converted from tuberculin negative to positive (i.e., have recently become infected), persons who are at high risk of reactivation, such as individuals with silicosis, and high-risk contacts, including infants, is highly effective for preventing the development of clinical disease.

With the highly effective drugs now available, it is conceivable that tuberculosis could be eliminated from a country such as the USA by mass chemoprophylaxis of populations representing focal reservoirs of infection.

Mycobacterium bovis

Mycobacterium bovis closely resembles *M. tuberculosis* and is highly pathogenic for man as well as for the cow, its natural host.

Human infections with *M. bovis* tend to involve lymph nodes and bone and are commonly contracted in childhood as the result of drinking milk from tuberculous cows. The principal means of shedding from cows is via the feces; on rare occasion, herdsmen acquire pulmonary infection by inhaling the dried feces and possibly pulmonary droplets of tuberculous cows. Ingested organisms are carried by macrophages either through the mucosa of the oropharynx to infect the cervical lymph nodes (a disease called scrofula) or through the mucosa of the intestine to infect the mesenteric lymph nodes. Organisms disseminating from the lymph nodes via the blood stream tend to localize selectively in joints and bones, particularly the vertebrae (Pott's disease). *The control of bovine tuberculosis stands among the greatest achievements in public health.* In the USA, tuberculosis due to *M. bovis* has been largely eliminated in both man and animals as the result of widespread pasteurization of milk and the legislated slaughter of animals giving positive reactions to tuberculin tests. In man, tuberculosis due to *M. bovis* stands as a classic example of how subtle the properties of an organism must be that determine its capacity to maintain itself in a natural host. Why does *M. bovis,* which is essentially identical with *M. tuberculosis* in its morphologic and biochemical properties and which is highly virulent for man as an accidental host, fail to adopt man as a natural host when the infection becomes pulmonary? Obviously, and for unknown reasons, the organism is incapable of establishing a permanent chain of communicability from one human being to another.

Mycobacterium avium

Mycobacterium avium has been claimed to infect man. A few of these claims appear to have been valid, but probably occurred because the patients involved were immunologically deficient; apparently, in other instances, the causative organism was one of the atypical mycobacteria that resemble *M. avium.*

Mycobacterium ulcerans

Although *M. ulcerans* rarely produces disease in man, the organism is of singular interest because infection is limited to low-temperature areas of the body, principally to the skin, where it produces ulcerating granulomatous lesions. This unusual temperature dependency evidently results from the inability of the organism to grow above 33°C, as can be demonstrated in culture. The lesions produced experimentally in mice occur selectively in the feet, ears and tail.

Since many saprophytic mycobacteria in soil and water have low-temperature growth ranges there is good reason to hypothesize that *M. ulcerans* represents a pathogen of "recent" evolutionary origin that still retains the growth-temperature characteristics of a saprophytic ancestor.

Mycobacterium marinum (M. balnei)

Infections with *M. marinum* were first reported in swimmers and the disease was termed "swimming-pool disease." The organism is a saprophyte that is facultatively parasitic and pathogenic for man as well as for frogs, fishes and other animals. It sometimes causes lesions on the hands and arms of fish fanciers as the result of contact with organisms shed into aquaria by infected fish. The ulcerous granulomas produced resemble the lesions of sporotrichosis. The infection tends to extend through superficial lymphatics to draining lymph nodes, but tubercles are not formed. Although the organism will grow at 33°C, its optimum temperature for growth is 30°C.

Other Mycobacteria That Produce Tuberculosis-Like Disease (Atypical Mycobacteria)

Mycobacterioses due to atypical species of the genus *Mycobacterium* have been recognized relatively recently; they are most frequent in white elderly males. The organisms are difficult to identify and misdiagnosis is common. They are presently classified among the so-called Runyon groups I, II, III, and IV; a few have been given species names. *Mycobacterium marinum* and *M. ulcerans* considered above are sometimes included among the atypical mycobacteria. In earlier years, *M. tuberculosis* and *M. bovis* were considered to be the only mycobacteria capable of producing lung infections in man. Other disease-producing mycobacteria isolated from patients were dismissed as "contaminants." Most of them are avirulent for laboratory animals; many are resistant to chemotherapeutic drugs and most have cultural characteristics different from those of *M. tuberculosis*. Atypical mycobacteria have received increasing attention in recent years, in part because, as tuberculosis wanes, they represent an increasing per-

TABLE 29-2

Some Properties of Representative "Atypical" Mycobacteria

Group	Representative Species	Growth		Pigment Produced	Sites of Human Disease			
		At 25°C	At 37°C		Lung	Lymph Nodes	Bones & Joints	Disseminated
I. (Photochromogens) Pigment only produced on exposure to light	M. kansasii	Slow*	Slow	Yellow	+	+	+	+
II. (Scotochromogens) Pigment production not light dependent	M. scrofulaceum	None	Slow	Yellow to orange	+	+	+	+
III. (Nonchromogens) Little or no pigment	M. intracellulare (Battey bacillus)	None	Slow	None or faint yellow	+	+	+	+
	M. xenopei	None	Slow†	Faint buff	+	−	−	−
IV.	M. fortuitum	Rapid	Rapid		+	−	−	−

* Rapid growers produce visible growth in a week or less. Slow growers produce visible growth only after 1 to 3 weeks or longer.
† Also grows slowly at 45°C.

centage of the organisms causing mycobacteriosis (as high as 10% of pulmonary cases) and, in part, because infection with "atypicals" is proving to be more widespread than was previously suspected. *Nevertheless, it should be emphasized that there is no evidence that an absolute increase in atypical disease is occurring.* Since the reservoirs of infection and the precise manner by which infections with atypicals are acquired are not known, control is difficult; consequently the relative importance of disease due to these organisms may continue to increase. However, even in areas such as the southeastern USA where the infection rate is highest, few clinical cases develop because infections with atypicals are generally milder and more self-limiting than classical tuberculosis; they seldom demand long hospitalization. The balance of factors that determine the production of clinical disease by these mycobacteria appears to be a delicate one. The most common sites of infection are the lung and cervical lymph nodes, the latter especially in children. Transmission from man to man is not known to occur. The frequent resistance of the atypicals to chemotherapy has made accurate bacteriologic diagnosis and drug-resistance testing highly important.

Various properties of some of the species of disease-producing atypical mycobacteria are given in Table 29-2. The reservoirs of atypical organisms of groups I, II and IV are probably soil and water. Organisms of group III closely resemble *M. avium;* soil, birds and possibly swine may serve as reservoirs of human infection. Most if not all of the atypical mycobacteria probably represent soil saprophytes, many of which often assume the role of facultative parasites for man and animals but seldom express pathogenicity. On occasion, certain atypicals have been isolated from the respiratory tract of healthy human subjects, possibly as members of the normal flora. Perhaps special circumstances including suitable exposure, genetic susceptibility and, more importantly, compromise of host defense are predisposing. In this respect the atypical mycobacteria appear to be similar to many of the opportunistic fungi.

Whether latent infection with atypical mycobacteria that are cross reactive with the pathogenic mycobacteria may serve to create a significant level of immunity to the latter or vice versa is unresolved but is a distinct possibility.

Because of the frequency of high drug resistance of the atypicals, a combined chemotherapeutic-surgical approach is favored for treatment. Lung resection is most commonly resorted to in patients with infection due to *M. intracellulare* (Battey bacillus).

Mycobacterium leprae

Leprosy (Hansen's disease) is a chronic debilitating disease that cripples, disfigures and blinds. However. it usually kills only after many years, principally as the result of secondary infection. It has a long incubation time that may range from many months to many years (average 3 to 5 years). Disfigurement of face and limbs is marked because nerves are destroyed leading to atrophy of muscle and bone; the anesthesia produced results in inadvertent injury due to lack of sensation to temperature and trauma.

A. Medical Perspectives

The origin of leprosy is shrouded in antiquity. Early evidence of the disease has been found in Asia.

It is a singular observation that among essentially every early civilization, especially the civilization of the early Christian era, fear of the disease was so intense that most every means of exterminating its victims were resorted to; this was done with the excuse that blame for the disease lay with the victim, who was being punished for some sin by a spiritual being. Early Christian beliefs fostered cruel treatment of lepers because suffering was generally accepted as divine punishment for sins both present and original. Isolation, torture and extermination of lepers were common practices for centuries. The Romans left lepers in the mountains without food or clothing. Lepraphobia became so intense in the 12th century that it was an easy matter to have one's creditor or enemy banished by simply initiating the gossip that "he has leprosy." Harsh treatment of lepers is by no means extinct today, and fear of the disease severely limits treatment and control. It is difficult to recruit doctors for research and patient care. In Nigeria, in 1967, only 3 physicians were available to treat half a million leprosy patients! *Only when leprosy is universally recognized simply as an unfortunate disease and not as a disgrace will injustices be terminated and treatment improved.*

The history of the spread of leprosy is of great interest. During the 12th and 13th centuries lepers became so numerous in Europe that strict isolation became necessary and some 19,000 "Lazar houses" (named after Lazarus of biblical times) were established for this purpose. Apparently leprosy spread from the Middle East to Greece in the centuries before the Christian era, thence to Rome with the returning armies of Gnaeus Pompey in 62 B.C. and was finally carried to most of Europe by the Romans. The second massive spread of leprosy in Europe occurred during the 6th and 7th centuries with the return of Christian crusaders from the Middle East. The disease assumed epidemic proportions beginning with the 11th century; its incidence peaked in the 15th century and declined sharply to near zero by the mid-16th century when the few remaining Lazar houses (which were really houses of isolation, neglect and death) were replaced by leprosy hospitals. Leprosy spread with the slave trade from Africa to South America, where it remains today. The few foci established in the USA by immigrants are now under control.

The reasons for the sudden decline of leprosy in Europe in the 16th century remain an unsolved mystery. Does this stand as an example of host-parasite evolution? Did loss of virulence of *M. leprae* or increase in immunity of the population play a part? To what extent did isolation practices, better living conditions or mortality due to other diseases play a part? One attractive hypothesis is that the waves of other highly lethal diseases such as bubonic plague (which in the first epidemic of the 14th century killed one fourth of the total population of Europe) and tuberculosis (which killed 1 of every 3 Europeans between 15 and 40 years of age) so completely decimated the highly susceptible leper population that the chain of communicability was not strong enough to maintain the disease. The possibilities for breaking the chain of communicability in leprosy are good since, in most populations, relatively few individuals (probably about 3 to 10%) apparently are innately susceptible to the disease.

Currently leprosy is largely restricted to underdeveloped tropical and subtropical regions and is rare in developed countries. For example, there are only about 3,000 leprosy patients in the USA, most of whom contracted their disease elsewhere. However, in the world at large the disease is still of major importance. The number of persons with active cases has been estimated to range between 10 to 20 million, only 2.8 million of these are under treatment. In some limited areas, 10% of the population is affected. Because no good test of inapparent infection is available the number of infected individuals cannot be accurately estimated.

Lack of suitable methods for in vitro culture and of experimental animal models has seriously hampered leprosy research. However, the Shepard mouse-footpad infection model is proving to be of great value for the screening of chemotherapeutic drugs and for immunologic studies. Although there is some evidence that leprosy may be on the increase in certain regions, the future outlook for control of leprosy in the world at large is encouraging. Current chemotherapy is moderately effective and new and improved antileprosy drugs are being developed. Experimental mass chemoprophylaxis over a period of 2 to 3 years on the Pacific island of Pingelapese has reduced the appearance of new cases to essentially zero and stands as a model for dampening or eradicating the disease. Since the chain of infection in leprosy is easily broken, ultimate eradication of the disease from large areas in the world by a combination of methods including mass chemoprophylaxis is clearly in the realm of possibility.

B. Physical and Chemical Structure

Hansen's discovery of *M. leprae* in the lesions of leprosy patients in 1878 provided the first reliable description of a bacterial agent as the cause of human disease. Although the organism has not been cultivated on bacteriologic media to this day, few investigators seriously dispute that

M. leprae is the sole etiologic agent of leprosy. Although it is often stated that *M. leprae* is an obligate intracellular parasite, it is by no means certain that the organism cannot grow extracellularly. Its usual intracellular position may be due to the readiness with which it is phagocytized. *Mycobacterium leprae* is a typical acid-fast rod resembling *M. tuberculosis*. It occurs in enormous numbers in the lesions of patients with the lepromatous form of leprosy; *the total estimated mass of organisms in the body exceeds that of any other microbial disease!* Certain strains of organisms grow more rapidly in the mouse footpad than others, but the meaning of this observation in terms of virulence is not evident. Some strains have become resistant to the sulfa drugs used for chemotherapy.

Studies on organisms isolated directly from tissues indicate that *M. leprae* is similar to *M. tuberculosis* in its chemical composition, being especially rich in lipids and waxes.

Little is known about the Ags of *M. leprae* except that certain polysaccharides stimulate high titers of Abs that cross-react with the Ags of certain saprophytic mycobacteria. Apparently, proteins stimulate delayed sensitivity as evidenced by the 48-hour Fernandez skin reaction, which resembles a tuberculin reaction. A protein that is alleged to elicit specific delayed skin reactions (Fernandez reactions) in patients with the tuberculoid form of leprosy has been isolated.

C. Genetics

Nothing is known about genetics and virulence of *M. leprae*.

D. Extracellular Products

No extracellular products of *M. leprae* are known.

E. Culture

The organism has never been cultured *in vitro* on nonliving media; reports of its growth in tissue culture remain to be confirmed. Its doubling time in the mouse footpad is about 12 days.

F. Resistance to Physical and Chemical Agents

Mycobacterium leprae is probably similar to *M. tuberculosis* with respect to most physical and chemical agents; however, lack of culture methods has made it difficult to test this directly.

G. Experimental Models

Man is the sole natural host of *M. leprae;* among animals only mice, rats, hamsters and armadillos have been infected experimentally. Most animals are highly resistant, the infections produced in most species being mild and self-limiting. By the use of mice crippled immunologically by thymectomy and x-irradiation and supported with bone marrow grafts, a more severe disease has been produced. The lesions in mice occur principally in low-temperature areas such as the feet and ears, a characteristic remarkably like *M. ulcerans* infections.

H. Infections in Man

Leprosy is a chronic systemic disease that involves primarily low-temperature areas of the body including the nose, ears, extremities and low-temperature areas of skin. The precise modes of transmission of leprosy are not known. The incubation period is long, averaging 2 to 3 years, but may be as long as 10 to 20 years.

Many cases of leprosy belong to one of two polar forms of the disease, lepromatous leprosy (LL) and tuberculoid leprosy (TL); other cases comprise intermediate and borderline forms of the disease that lie between the two polar forms. Although the reason for such diverse forms of the disease is an enigma, they are thought to be in large measure the outcome of variations in the immunologic response to the organism. *Essentially all of the organisms are within macrophages and the Schwann cells of nerves;* a few may invade muscle cells, particularly the erector-pili muscles. *The organism has a unique predilection for nerves.*

Lepromatous leprosy is presumed to reflect high susceptibility to the organism. The lesions of this form of the disease consist of masses of macrophages loaded with enormous numbers of bacilli and lipid-containing vacuoles; a continuous bacteremia exists. *It is notable that the macrophages of this form of the disease do not mature to form organized granulomas composed of epithelioid cells, and lymphocytes are few in numbers.*

Tuberculoid leprosy, in contrast, presents granulomas composed of cell collections resembling the tubercles of tuberculosis but without caseation. Bacilli are sparse and difficult to find and lymphocytes are abundant.

Intermediate forms of the disease may transform to either of the polar forms of the disease, but polar forms seldom if ever undergo change.

When heat-killed organisms isolated from biopsied tissue are injected into the skin, a local granuloma forms after 3 to 4 weeks in the majority of normal individuals. Except for infants, 90% or more of normal individuals respond to initial or repeated testing. *This reaction, the Mitsuda reaction,* is presumed to represent an "allergic granuloma," resulting from the development of delayed sensitivity to the injected organisms. Tuberculoid patients commonly develop the positive Mitsuda reaction but, in addition, show an earlier 48-hour reaction to the injected organisms, *"the Fernandez reaction,"* which is presumed to represent a delayed-type reaction due to sensitivity existing at the time of the test. The Fernandez reaction can also be elicited by leprolin, a protein-containing extract of *M. leprae.*

Lepromatous patients never show Fernandez or Mitsuda reactions. The reason for this is not known, but presumably is in some way related to the high susceptibility of the lepromatous patient to *M. leprae.* The immunologic deficiencies in LL are profound and appear to be of two kinds: *first, generalized deficiencies in lymphocyte function,* presumably T-cell function, demonstrable by such evidences as a partially depressed capacity of lymphocytes to support the mixed-lymphocyte reaction and of lepromatous patients to reject skin allografts; and *second, a complete depression of the specific immunologic capacity of T-lymphocytes of lepromatous patients,* as demonstrated by failure to yield positive macrophage-migration inhibition reactions in the presence of leprolin. The nonspecific lymphocyte deficiencies in TL are similar to those of LL but are manifested to a far lesser degree.

A notable feature of the histopathology of LL is that bacillus-laden macrophages accumulate in the paracortical areas of lymph nodes that become depleted of lymphocytes. This may contribute to the nonspecific immunologic deficiency seen in LL.

I. Mechanisms of Pathogenicity

Essentially nothing is known about mechanisms of pathogenicity. Leprosy bacilli are easily phagocytized by both neutrophils and macrophages but do not appear to be toxic for phagocytes, at least when the numbers of bacilli are not excessive. The organisms appear to be remarkably resistant to destruction by macrophages, especially lepromatous macrophages in which they multiply to reach enormous numbers. The ultimate destruction of lepromatous macrophages may, of course, result from the physical effects of the large accumulation of dividing organisms and the lipids that they produce. There is some evidence indicating that organisms may accumulate to "rupture" the phagosomes and exist as masses of bacilli, "globi," free in the cytoplasm. The lipids that accumulate to produce "foamy macrophages" appear to be largely bacterial lipids. Nerve damage is probably secondary to allergic inflammation. In fact, essentially all forms of tissue injury in leprosy may be on an immunologic basis.

J. Mechanisms of Immunity

Most human beings are evidently highly resistant to *M. leprae* and numerous individuals probably become infected without showing clinical evidence of leprosy. The major component of resistance is evidently cellular rather than humoral. Presumably resistance lies in macrophages activated somehow by specifically immune lymphocytes

Although it is possible that the specific immunologic defect in LL might be some acquired immunologic aberration, such as T-cell tolerance or immune deviation, identical twin studies strongly indicate that it is on a genetic basis. Whether the defect lies with the lymphocyte or the macrophage is not apparent. The macrophages of LL patients appear to have little if any capacity to digest *M. leprae* since organisms killed by drug treatment persist in the lesions for years. Whether the macrophages of TL patients have a greater capacity to digest killed *M. leprae* than lepromatous macrophages is not known. Whereas the two polar forms of leprosy do not shift, intermediate forms may shift; for example, a shift toward the tuberculoid form (i.e., toward increased resistance) may occur with an attending flareup of lesions (reversal reaction). This occurs spontaneously but sometimes appears to be precipitated by drug treatment. It may lead to severe nerve damage.

K.   Laboratory Diagnosis

Laboratory diagnosis is based on the finding of typical acid-fast rods in smears of scrapings from skin lesions or the nose or in sections made of affected skin or nerves. Nasal scrapings from leprosy patients often reveal the presence of acid-fast bacilli. However, the presence of acid-fast bacilli in nasal scrapings is not a reliable indicator of leprosy, since acid-fast organisms are sometimes present in nasal scrapings from normal persons. The organisms are often very sparse in patients with TL but may be found in sectioned tissues after careful search. Typical nerve lesions together with characteristic clinical findings usually permits accurate diagnosis.

L.   Therapy

The sulfones, DDS, DADDS and B663, are moderately effective for arresting and reversing the disease. However, treatment over many months or years is usually required and the development of drug-resistant organisms and drug reactions are frequent obstructions to treatment. A highly promising drug, rifampin, which renders the patient's organisms noninfective within 1 to 2 weeks, is now under clinical trial. "Reactions" characterized as "erythema nodosum leprosum" (ENL) appear to be due to the sudden liberation of Ags from dying organisms which unite with Ab to form Ag-Ab complexes that cause both local and systemic effects. However, ENL also occurs in a few untreated patients.

M.   Reservoirs of Infection

Patients with leprosy are the only known reservoirs of infection.

N. Control of Disease Transmission

Treatment of infectious patients and observation of proper sanitary practices when in contact with patients with infective disease are recommended prophylactic measures. The nasal mucosa of the untreated lepromatous patient is probably the chief "portal of exit" of the organisms. Although the usual route of infection is probably by way of the respiratory tract, the skin and other sites may serve as avenues; possible transmission by biting insects is being investigated. Drug treatment of close contacts to prevent development of disease could prove useful. The value of BCG vaccination from immunization against leprosy is highly questionable. Progress in the control of the disease has been slow and success is not in sight, principally due to overpopulation, poverty, ignorance, superstition and difficulties of recruiting trained personnel. Mass chemoprophylaxis may be a useful tool for controlling leprosy as indicated in Section A.

References

Bechelli, L. M., and Dominguez, V. M.: Further information on the leprosy problem in the world. WHO Bull. *46*:523, 1972.

Comstock, G. W., and Edwards, P. Q.: An American view of BCG vaccination. Scand. J. Resp. Dis. *53*:207, 1972.

Dahlgren, S. E., and Ekstrom, P.: Aspiration cytology in the diagnosis of pulmonary tuberculosis. Scand. J. Resp. Dis. *53*:196, 1972.

Dannenberg, A. M., Masayuki, A., and Shima, K.: Macrophage accumulation, division, maturation and digestive and microbicidal capacities in tuberculous lesions. J. Immunol. *109*:1109, 1972.

Florey, H.: General Pathology. Philadelphia, W. B. Saunders Co., 1970.

Gordon, J., and White, R. G.: Surface peptido-glycolipid filaments on *Mycobacterium leprae*. Clin. Exp. Immunol. *9*:539, 1971.

Lurie, M. B.: Resistance to Tuberculosis: Experimental Studies in Native and Acquired Defensive Mechanisms. Cambridge, Harvard University Press, 1964.

Mackaness, G. B.: The immunology of antituberculous immunity. Amer. Rev. Resp. Dis. *97*:337, 1968.

Neiburger, R. G., Youmans, G. P., and Youmans, A. S.: Relationship between tuberculin hypersensitivity and cellular immunity to infection in mice vaccinated with viable attenuated mycobacterial cells or with mycobacterial ribonucleic acid preparations. Infect. Immun. *8*:42, 1973.

Patterson, R. J., and Youmans, G. P.: Multiplication of *Mycobacterium tuberculosis* within normal and "immune" mouse macrophages cultivated with and without streptomycin. Infect. Immun. *1*:30, 1970.

Pearsall, N. N., and Weiser, R. S.: The Macrophage. Philadelphia, Lea & Febiger, 1970.

Rich, A. R.: The Pathogenesis of Tuberculosis. Springfield, Illinois, Charles C Thomas, 1951.

Stead, W. W., and Bates, J. H.: Evidence of "silent" bacillemia in primary tuberculosis. Ann. Intern. Med. *74*:559, 1971.

Youmans, G. P., and Youmans, A. S.: Recent studies on acquired immunity in tuberculosis. Current Topics in Microbiology and Immunology. New York: Springer-Verlag, *48*:129, 1969.

Chapter 30

Miscellaneous Pathogenic Bacteria

Spirillum minus, 368
Streptobacillus moniliformis, 369
Bartonella bacilliformis, 369
Erysipelothrix rhusiopathiae, 370
Veillonella sp., 371

A variety of organisms that cause infections rarely, or about which little is known, will be considered briefly in this chapter.

Spirillum minus

Spirillum minus is a member of the family *Spirillaceae* and the order *Pseudomonadales,* which indicates its relation to the pseudomonads and vibrios. Like most other members of this order it is gram-negative, bears polar flagella (bipolar tufts), and is aerobic. The cells are short and thick (0.5 × 3.0 μm), and usually present 2 or 3 spirals per cell.

Spirillum minus is the cause of the human disease *Soduku rat-bite fever.* The organism is widespread in rats and other rodents. The human disease occurs under circumstances in which man contacts rats. It can follow rodent bites or the bites of cats and other animals that ingest rodents. The disease is rare in the USA, but occurs more often in other regions of the world. After an incubation period of about 2 weeks an abrupt, febrile illness occurs, with an erythematous or purplish rash adjacent to the original wound. The fever may recur over a period of weeks to months and polyarthritis is common. A chancre-like lesion may develop at the wound site during the disease, and regional lymphadenitis is common. Mortality has been reported to range from about 5 to 10%. Either penicillin or streptomycin has been used successfully to treat Soduku rat-bite fever.

The spirilla of Soduku fever have not been cultured *in vitro;* however, they can be recovered from exudates of lesions, lymph node aspirates or blood by inoculation of these materials into spirillum-free laboratory rodents.

For diagnostic purposes, identification of the organism is usually made on the basis of typical morphologic appearance in wet mounts examined by darkfield or phase microscopy. If direct mounts are negative, animal inoculation should be performed.

Streptobacillus moniliformis

Streptobacillus moniliformis is indigenous to rodents and causes a form of *rat-bite fever* differing from that due to *Spirillum minus*. This form of the disease can be transmitted by the bites of rats or by drinking milk that has been contaminated by rats. The causative organism is a member of the family *Bacteroidaceae,* indicating its relationship to species of *Bacteroides* and *Fusobacterium;* however, unlike these obligate anaerobes, *Streptobacillus moniliformis* is a facultative anaerobe. Rat-bite fever following ingestion of contaminated milk is called *Haverhill fever* and has occurred in epidemics. Streptobacillus-induced rat-bite fever resembles Soduku, described above, in that it presents as a persistent febrile disease with polyarthritis; however, the rash in streptobacillus-induced disease is petechial, rubelliform, or morbilliform, rather than erythematous. There are reports of successful treatment with either penicillin, streptomycin, or tetracyclines.

Streptobacillus moniliformis is notable for its pleomorphism; representative organisms are usually gram-negative rods less than 1 μm wide, but may appear as filaments as long as 150 μm, coccoid forms as wide as 15 μm in diameter, or in other configurations.

An important characteristic of the organism is its ability to grow in either the bacterial phase with cell walls or in the wall-less L-form, in which the colonies are indistinguishable from mycoplasma colonies. In fact, much of the original work on L-forms was done with naturally occurring L-forms of streptobacilli.

Streptobacillus moniliformis is fastidious on culture; it requires rich media containing either blood, serum, or ascitic fluid and is favored by an increased CO_2 atmosphere. A rise in titer of specific serum agglutinins against the organism is useful in diagnosis.

Bartonella bacilliformis

The genus *Bartonella* (family *Bartonellaceae*) belongs to the order *Rickettsiales* and is related to the rickettsiae (Chapter 33) and chlamydiae (Chapter 34).

Infections with *Bartonella bacilliformis* are transmitted by the sandfly, *Phlebotomus,* and occur only in the Andes mountains of South America, where both the vectors and long-term human carriers are found. Infections may remain latent or may become clinically apparent. Two forms of clinical disease occur, often in succession: *Oroya fever,* which is a febrile, hemolytic anemia, and *verruga peruana* (Peruvian warts). Oroya fever is characterized by the growth of organisms on the surface of erythrocytes and within endothelial cells. As many as 90% of the red cells may be infected, and the mortality rate in untreated subjects is about 40%. Patients who survive the febrile disease often develop *verruga peruana,* a benign, generalized, granulomatous skin disease in which purplish papules and deep nodules occur, often in crops, during a period of several weeks to a year. Even if the patient is not treated, the mortality rate is less than 5%. Differences in host response undoubtedly contribute to the different disease processes.

In 1885, Carrion proved that Oroya fever and verruga peruana are caused by the same organism. He volunteered to be inoculated with material from verruga lesions, and died 39 days later of Oroya fever! In his honor, bartonellosis is often referred to as Carrion's disease. At present the disease is readily controlled by antibiotic therapy. In addition, insecticide control of sandflies has greatly decreased the incidence of bartonellosis.

The bartonellae are obligately aerobic, gram-negative, motile, nonsporing, pleomorphic organisms that usually assume the form of rods about 0.5×2.0 μm. They can be cultured *in vitro* in semisolid media containing fresh serum and hemoglobin. Growth becomes apparent after about 10 days' incubation at 28 to 37°C.

Several cases of a new disease characterized by hemolytic anemia and thrombocytopenic purpura have been reported in the USA; apparently the disease is caused by an unidentified but similar member of the family *Bartonellaceae.* The same organism was isolated from 3 patients and from mites collected in the environment of one of the patients.

Erysipelothrix rhusiopathiae

Being of the family *Corynebacteriaceae, Erysipelothrix rhusiopathiae* is related to members of the genera *Corynebacterium* and *Listeria.* The organism is parasitic for many animal species and may live as a saprophyte in dead organic materials. It causes erysipelas in swine and other animals and erysipeloid skin infections in man. The human disease develops in skin abrasions following contact with infected animals, and is most often seen in fish-handlers or others who work with animals. The lesions are painful, edematous, and erythematous. Penicillin therapy has proven to be effective. The organisms are gram-positive, facultatively anaerobic, nonsporing, nonmotile rods that tend to form long filaments. They can grow on a variety of rich media; their optimum growth temperature is about 37°C. It may be necessary to use a hand lens to see the colonies, which grow to a diameter of about 0.7 to 1.0 mm in 48 hours. Mice can be readily infected with the organism, and the mouse protection test with specific antiserum, along with cultural and biochemical characteristics, aids in identification.

Veillonella sp.

Members of the genus *Veillonella* are *gram-negative, anaerobic cocci* of the family *Neisseriaceae*. They occur among the normal flora of the mucous membranes of man and animals, but very rarely cause infections.

References

Hull, T. G., ed.: Diseases Transmitted from Animals to Man, 5th ed. Springfield, Ill., Charles C Thomas, 1963.

Mettler, N. E.: Isolation of a microtatobiote from patients with hemolytic-uremic syndrome and thrombocytopenic purpura and from mites in the United States. New Eng. J. Med. *281*:1023, 1969.

Weinman, D.: Infectious anemias due to *Bartonella* and related red cell parasites. Trans. Amer. Phil. Soc. *33*:243, 1944.

Wood, R. L.: Erysipelothrix. *In* Manual of Clinical Microbiology, J. E. Blair, E. H. Lennette, and J. P. Truant, eds. Bethesda, Md., American Society for Microbiology, 1970, pp. 101-105.

Mycoplasma and L-Forms

Mycoplasma

Near the end of the 19th century two French microbiologists, Nocard and Roux, discovered an unusual kind of microorganism that proved to be the cause of pleuropneumonia in cattle. This organism is unique because it lacks cell walls. It is small enough to pass through filters that retain most bacteria; however, it can be grown in cell-free media. Over the years, pleuropneumonia-like organisms (PPLO) were isolated from a variety of animal species, and in 1937 a human strain was discovered.

The taxonomy of PPLO organisms is controversial. It is agreed that they are members of the kingdom *Protista.* However, many investigators consider them to constitute a new class distinct from the *Schizomycetes,* which has been named *Mollicutes.* Other investigators group them with the bacteria, in a separate family, *Mycoplasmataceae.* Because of their fundamental similarities to the bacteria, they will be treated in this chapter as bacteria belonging to the genus *Mycoplasma.*

Lack of a cell wall accounts for many of the unusual properties of mycoplasmas. Other bacteria may exist temporarily without a cell wall, but members of the genus *Mycoplasma* are the only bacteria that normally lack the capacity to form cell walls.

The mycoplasmas are the smallest, free-living organisms known; indeed, their size is at the lower limits possible for self-sustaining cells. A smaller cell volume could not accommodate the ribosomes, enzymes and other cellular components essential for independent growth and reproduction.

Many species of *Mycoplasma* exist; many are parasitic for a wide range of animals and plants, and often cause disease. At least 5 species are parasites of man: *Myp. salivarius, Myp. orale* and *Myp. fermentans,* which are nonpathogenic; *Myp. hominis,* which may cause disease; and *Myp. pneumoniae,* which is often pathogenic.

Certain cell-wall-deficient forms of bacteria, L-forms, and mycoplasmas have similar properties. The L-forms will be discussed at the end of this chapter.

A. Medical Perspectives

The first mycoplasma shown to be pathogenic for man was *Myp. pneumoniae;* although it is one of the causes of primary atypical pneumonia (PAP), this was not discovered for many years because ordinary methods for culturing bacteria do not support the growth of mycoplasmas. The disease produced was classified as a "viral pneumonia" or "Eaton's agent pneumonia" because no bacteria were recovered from its victims. Serologic tests indicated that this form of PAP was caused by a single agent, and subsequent investigations proved that *Myp. pneumoniae* is the agent responsible for this disease. Other species of mycoplasmas are frequently isolated from patients with a wide range of diseases of unknown causes; however, it is difficult to prove a causal relationship to disease because these mycoplasmas are among the normal flora.

Experiments with human volunteers have fulfilled Koch's postulates for one, and possibly two species to date; *Myp. pneumoniae* produces disease when introduced into the human respiratory tract, and there are reports that *Myp. hominis* does also. It has been suggested that other mycoplasmas play a role in diseases such as nongonococcal urethritis and perhaps some cases of arthritis; however, this has not been proven.

Because mycoplasmas require special culture techniques and are difficult to work with, much remains to be learned about their relationships with human hosts. Substantial research effort is being expended to learn more about the basic biology of mycoplasmas and host-mycoplasma interactions. Studies in animal and plant models have provided information pertinent to the human host-mycoplasma relationship and it is likely that significant progress will soon be made in this area.

B.   Physical and Chemical Structure

Mycoplasmas are extremely pleomorphic because of their lack of a rigid wall. They vary in size from about 125 to 500 nm, and in shape from coccoid or stellate to branching, filamentous forms.

Mycoplasmas are rich in lipids, which account for 10 to 20% of the dry weight of the cells. Almost all of the lipids are part of the cell membrane and a large proportion is composed of sterols. Sterols stabilize and strengthen cell membranes and enable the cell to resist differences between external and internal osmotic pressures. This is a property generally characteristic of eucaryotic but not procaryotic cells. The organisms do not synthesize sterols, but, instead, assimilate them from the host or the culture medium. Consequently the sterols of mycoplasmal cell membranes are identical with the exogenous sterols present in the environment.

Both species-specific Ags and cross-reacting group Ags are demonstrable on the cell membranes.

The internal structure of mycoplasmas is typical of procaryotic cells. The DNA is found in a single membrane-free nuclear body, ribosomes are present, and mitochondria are lacking.

C.   Genetics

The genetics of mycoplasmas have been studied by means of species that infect animals, such as *Myp. gallisepticum,* and the free-living saprophytic species, *Myp. laidlawii.* The latter is commonly found in sewage, and differs from other mycoplasmas in that it does not require sterols for growth. Antibiotic-resistant mutants of these two species have been obtained; however, it is difficult to isolate biochemical mutants because the complex growth requirements of the mycoplasmas have not been defined, which precludes the use of defined isolation media.

Genetic mapping has not been successful because suitable genetic recombination systems for the mycoplasmas have not been found. The organisms have not been observed to undergo conjugation, transduction, or transformation to a significant extent. However, this may reflect a lack of adequate experimental methods, rather than failure of the mycoplasmas to recombine genetically.

The percent of the bases guanine and cytosine (GC) in the DNA of mycoplasmas ranges from 23 to 41. Many species have a GC content near the lower limits found in bacteria (the GC content of the DNA of bacteria ranges from about 25 to 75%); however, *Myp. pneumoniae* DNA contains about 40% GC.

Biochemical and antibiotic-resistant mutants of mycoplasmas have been studied. The recent discovery of viruses that parasitize mycoplasmas opens the possibility that transfer of genetic material may occur by transduction or other viral-associated transfer mechanisms.

D. Extracellular Products

The mycoplasmas are catalase-negative and some strains produce hydrogen peroxide, which acts as a beta hemolysin. Other strains produce alpha hemolysin. None of the human strains is known to produce toxins; however, some murine mycoplasmas elaborate neurotoxins and are lethal for mice.

E. Culture

Mycoplasmas can be grown aerobically, with or without 10% CO_2, in rich cell-free medium supplemented with 30% serum or ascitic fluid. After 2 to 3 days at 37°C in broth cultures, mycoplasmal growth is usually not visible to the naked eye, but the organisms can be seen in stained, centrifuged sediments. On agar-solidified media in sealed Petri dishes, small colonies form after 2 to 6 days' incubation at 37°C. The colonies are less than 0.5 mm in diameter and a lens must be used to see them. Typically, they have a "fried-egg" appearance, resulting from a dense, central, embedded core surrounded by a less dense surface growth. If a small piece of agar containing the colony is excised, streaked across a fresh plate of medium and incubated at 37°C more colonies will form. Alternatively, the colony can be subcultured by dropping it into a broth medium.

An unusual colony form consisting of tiny (T) colonies is characteristic of some mycoplasmas, especially those isolated from the urogenital tract. The central core of these colonies (corresponding to the "yolk" of the "fried-egg colony") is about ¼ the size of the central core of the colonies of other mycoplasmas. The T-strains differ from other mycoplasmas in that they have a pH optimum of 6.0, rather than 7.0 to 7.5, and produce urease.

F. Resistance to Physical and Chemical Agents

Mycoplasmas resist concentrations of thallium acetate that inhibit most other bacteria. Incorporation of 1:10,000 thallium acetate will prevent the growth of most contaminating bacteria in a specimen such as sputum, but permits the growth of most mycoplasmas. The T-strains, the only mycoplasmas sensitive to this agent, are completely inhibited by 1:500 thallium acetate.

All strains of mycoplasmas are resistant to penicillin and other antibiotics that act on bacterial cell walls. However, most strains are sensitive to tetracyclines, kanamycin and gold salts; they are rapidly destroyed by detergents.

G. Experimental Models

The widespread occurrence of mycoplasmas in the normal flora and as animal pathogens presents a variety of ready-made models. In addition,

13

mycoplasmas can infect chick embryos and many kinds of cell cultures. In fact, a majority of cultured cell lines harbor mycoplasmas, and primary cell cultures are often infected. Unfortunately the prevalence of mycoplasmal contamination of cell cultures has jeopardized or invalidated many experiments.

Swine have been used as models of human mycoplasmal diseases. Certain species of mycoplasmas native to swine cause an arthritis that is said to resemble human rheumatoid arthritis.

H. Infections in Man

The only naturally occurring human disease unequivocally shown to be caused by mycoplasma is PAP due to *Myp. pneumoniae*. The disease is an acute bronchopneumonia with fever, severe cough, headache, and pulmonary infiltration with neutrophils and mononuclear leukocytes. Transmission probably occurs principally by means of airborne droplets of respiratory secretions. The incubation period is about 2 to 4 weeks. The duration of symptoms depends on the severity of the infection, but in moderately severe cases is about 10 days to 2 weeks. In the more severe cases, cold agglutinins become demonstrable in the serum during the 2nd or 3rd week. Complications are rare and recovery is usually complete, even without treatment.

I. Mechanisms of Pathogenicity

The means by which mycoplasmas cause human disease are unknown. No toxins or virulence factors have been demonstrated. *The organisms generally do not invade cells, but live attached to the exterior of the host cell membrane.* In the inoculated chick embryo, *Myp. pneumoniae* localizes and grows in large numbers on the bronchial epithelial cells. This could be due to a tissue affinity of *Myp. pneumoniae* for its target cell in the respiratory tract.

J. Mechanisms of Immunity

Family studies have revealed a low attack rate among adults as compared with children in the family, suggesting that a long-lasting immunity develops to *Myp. pneumoniae*. However, neither the duration and degree of effectiveness nor the mechanisms of such immunity have been established. Second episodes of mycoplasmal pneumonia have been reported.

During infection, Abs are formed to species-specific Ags of *Myp. pneumoniae,* as may be shown by the immunofluorescence test. These Abs inhibit the growth of specific mycoplasmas *in vitro* by an unknown, C-independent mechanism.

Antibodies are also formed against a lipid-Ag complex found in other species of mycoplasmas. These Abs, which are measured by C-F tests, persist for 6 to 12 months after infection. They are useful in clinical diagnosis and epidemiologic studies, but do not indicate specific immunity.

Certain nonspecific factors of innate immunity have been shown to be active against mycoplasmas. The peroxidase-H_2O_2-halide ion system is mycoplasmacidal, and there is evidence suggesting that phagocytin (a heat-stable globulin of neutrophils) and perhaps some enzymes also kill or inhibit mycoplasmas.

K. Laboratory Diagnosis

For years before *Myp. pneumoniae* was discovered, "Eaton's agent PAP" was diagnosed on the basis of a rise in titer of cold hemagglutinins to human group O red blood cells and of agglutinins against a strain of streptococcus called MG. Apparently these Abs that are formed against antigenic determinants of *Myp. pneumoniae* fortuitously cross-react with the above Ags; they are present in most, but not all, patients following mycoplasmal pneumonia. These nonspecific tests are no longer used for diagnosis.

The C-F test for the lipid-Ag complex is useful as an indicator of recent infection with *Myp. pneumoniae.*

Sputum or pharyngeal secretions can be cultured directly in a medium containing thallium acetate and penicillin; however, demonstrable colonies may not appear before 2 to 3 weeks of incubation. Immunofluorescence or serologic methods are useful for final identification of species of mycoplasma.

L. Therapy

Mycoplasmas are sensitive to therapy with tetracyclines or erythromycin, which significantly decreases the duration of PAP.

M. Reservoirs of Infection

Infected human beings, often suffering from minor illness with cough, are the reservoir for *Myp. pneumoniae.* The organism has been shown to persist in the respiratory tract for at least a month, even when high titers of humoral Abs are present. The duration of the carrier state has not been established.

N. Control of Disease Transmission

Mycoplasmal pneumonia is endemic in most populations, but can become epidemic, especially in a crowded environment. Judging from serologic studies, only a small percentage of infected individuals develop pneumonia; whereas some may exhibit mild symptoms, others have no symptoms. Obviously, a degree of immunity is attained. Immunization with a vaccine should, therefore, be possible. However, if a vaccine were to be developed it is unlikely that it would be widely used, because of the low case rate, compared to the infection rate, and because of the very low mortality rate in active disease. A vaccine would be valuable for protecting military personnel who frequently experience epidemics of the disease.

L-Forms of Bacteria

Cell-wall-deficient forms of bacteria that grow in mycoplasma-like colonies are called L-forms because they were first studied at the Lister Institute in London. Like mycoplasmas, they are resistant to the action of penicillin. However, L-forms are derived from parental bacteria with cell walls, and most of them tend to revert to parental-type cells when environmental conditions are suitable.

Bacterial L-forms can be induced in the laboratory by treating growing bacteria with penicillin, antiserum and lysozyme. *They differ from protoplasts and spheroplasts, which require hypertonic media, in that they can multiply and form colonies on ordinary media.*

In vivo, L-forms may occur and could possibly account for persistence and recurrence of infection. For example, L-forms could readily survive for some time in the medulla of the kidney, after which they could regain their cell walls and pathogenic potential.

Several well-documented reports have established that L-forms can persist in the human host; for example, during bacterial infection of the urinary tract and in gonococcal arthritis. Nevertheless, it has been difficult to determine whether L-forms cause recurrent infections. The possible role of L-forms in infections and in causing hypersensitivity states is under investigation.

References

Boatman, E. S., and Kenny, G. E.: Morphology and ultrastructure of *Mycoplasma pneumoniae* spherules. J. Bact. *106*:1005, 1971.

Dienes, L.: Nomenclature of bacterial L-forms and cell-wall defective bacteria. J. Infect. Dis. *127*:476, 1973.

Foy, H. M., Kenny, G. E., McMahan, R., Kaiser, G., and Grayston, J. T.: *Mycoplasma pneumoniae* in the community. Amer. J. Epidemiol. *93*:55, 1971.

Hayflick, L., ed.: The Mycoplasmatales and the L-phase of Bacteria. New York: Appleton-Century Crofts, 1969.

Jacobs, A. A., Low, I. E., Paul, B. B., Strauss, R. R., and Sbarra, A. J.: Mycoplasma-cidal activity of peroxidase-H_2O_2-halide systems. Infect. Immun. *5*:127, 1972.

Maniloff, J., and Morowitz, H. J.: Cell biology of the mycoplasmas. Bact. Rev. *36*: 263, 1972.

McCormack, W. M., Braun, P., Lee, Y.-H., Klein, J. O., and Kass, E. H.: The genital mycoplasmas. New Engl. J. Med. *288*:78, 1973.

Thomas, L.: Mycoplasmas as infectious agents. Ann. Rev. Med. *21*:179, 1970.

Workshop on the Mycoplasmatales as Agents of Disease, NIH March 29-30, 1971. J. Infect. Dis. *127*: supplement, 1973.

Chapter 32

Treponema, Borrelia and Leptospira

Members of the family *Treponemataceae* are classified under 3 genera: *Treponema, Borrelia* and *Leptospira*. These organisms are helical-shaped and have the unique attribute of being highly flexible. They are characterized by sinuous flexing and rotary movements brought about by an axial filament that consists of a bundle of intertwined flagella-like contractile fibrils coiled in spiral fashion around the cell. Many species are parasitic for a wide range of animal hosts.

Treponema

The genus *Treponema* contains a number of pathogenic and nonpathogenic species; most if not all are anaerobes. Many of the nonpathogenic species belong to the normal flora of the alimentary tract and only appear to be able to exert pathogenic effects by participating as opportunists in mixed infections. *None of the pathogenic treponemes has been cultivated* in vitro *and the only known distinguishing characteristics of these organisms are the range of natural hosts that they attack, the experimental animals that they can infect and the nature of the diseases that they produce.* The prototype species of the pathogens of this genus is *Treponema pallidum,* the cause of human *syphilis.* Man is its only known natural host. Other human pathogens are *T. pertenue,* the cause of *yaws,* and *T. carateum,* the cause of *pinta.*

On a worldwide basis the treponematoses continue to be among the major afflictions of mankind despite the availability of highly effective therapeutic agents including penicillin, the "queen of antitreponemal drugs."

Treponema pallidum

A. Medical Perspectives

Syphilis is a serious, widespread, and often fatal disease encompassing all levels of society.* It is spawned by sexual promiscuity and thrives on ignorance and the social stigmas that it carries.

The origin of malignant syphilis is highly debated. *One theory* is that it was first introduced into Europe in 1493 by Columbus' sailors, who were alleged to have contracted the disease in the West Indies. Malignant syphilis was mentioned in an edict of the Diet of Worms issued in 1495 and treatment with mercury was introduced in 1497. Dr. Ruy Diaz de Isla treated several of Columbus' sailors, including the pilot, Pinzon of Palos, and later (1539) wrote a book about the "new disease," which stands as the first clear description of malignant syphilis. *An alternative theory* on origin is that the malignant form of the disease, first reported in 1494, resulted from a large-step mutation of some progenitor organism, then existent in the Old World, comparable to one of the present-day treponemes that cause the nonvenereal treponematoses of milder nature. In any event, some of the sailors of Columbus participated in the siege of Naples in 1495 where the first recorded epidemic of malignant syphilis ("the great pox") appeared and spread over Europe with the disbanding of troops. *The high malignancy of the disease at that time and the sweeping nature of the epidemic are expressions characteristic of a new infectious agent in a host population.* Many

---

* The name "syphilis" is derived from the principal character of the poem "Syphilis sive Morbus Gallicus," written by Fracastor in 1530, about an imaginary swineherd with the disease. Syphilis is sometimes called "lues," meaning plague or pestilence.

deaths occurred during the secondary stage of the disease, which is now less severe (deaths from secondary syphilis no longer occur). All attempts to control the original epidemic were unavailing and, in desperation, the Parliament of Paris of 1496 decreed that all persons with overt syphilis must leave the city within 24 hours. The disease spread rapidly to other parts of the world and persisted in Europe to become one of the great scourges of the 16th century.

Bell's observation (1793) that syphilis and gonorrhea are distinct entities was confirmed by Ricord in 1831, and Haensell (1881) infected the eyes of rabbits with exudates of human lesions. Discovery of the causative organism by Schaudinn and Hoffman in 1905 was quickly followed in 1906 by Wassermann's diagnostic serologic test. Ehrlich's discovery of arsphenamine (606) and neoarsphenamine was made a few years later. These therapeutic arsenicals, which replaced the highly toxic mercurials used earlier, marked the birth of modern antimicrobial chemotherapy. Wagner-Jauregg received the Nobel prize for his work on malarial fever treatment of neurosyphilis in 1927 and the Kettering electronic fever cabinet was introduced soon thereafter. *The sad addendum to the remarkably rapid advances made during the opening decades of this century is that little has been added to our understanding of* T. pallidum *or the pathogenesis of syphilis during subsequent years.*

In the Western World, syphilis was a major cause of death (mortality rate about 12% in untreated subjects) prior to the first widespread use of penicillin in about 1948. It is still a major killer on a worldwide basis and will always stand as a threat to public health whenever vigilance is relaxed. *In developed countries the case rate for syphilis showed a precipitous drop of some 85% after 1948;* the death rates due to late cardiovascular, CNS and congenital syphilis dropped even more dramatically than the overall case incidence.

The control of congenital syphilis by penicillin treatment has been especially successful because women seeking prenatal care are commonly required by law to undergo serologic tests for syphilis and, consequently, the diagnosis is made and treatment given if the reactions to the tests are positive. Because of common failure to report the disease the incidence of syphilis in pregnant women remains as the best available indicator for estimating the incidence of syphilis in the public at large.

In the USA the incidence of all forms of syphilis dropped from over 5% in 1943 to less than 1% in 1957. This sharp drop was probably due in substantial degree to the widespread general use of penicillin during that period, which undoubtedly effected cures in many cases of syphilis, both diagnosable and undiagnosed. *In the years since the low ebb in 1957 when 6,500 new cases were reported, the incidence of reported cases has fluctuated upward to reach 24,000 in 1972.* The actual number of new cases can be presumed to have been 5 to 10 times the number of cases reported.

Because of the great therapeutic effectiveness of penicillin, high hopes were initially held that syphilis might be essentially eradicated from large populations by mass penicillin treatment. An example was provided by the control of endemic nonvenereal syphilis of childhood achieved by the WHO in Bosnia, Yugoslavia, a small area with a highly stable resident population. The trial began in about 1950. An incidence of clinical disease of 0.4% among a population of a million people was reduced to zero within 2 years and no new cases have subsequently appeared in the course of 20 years. Officers of WHO initially expressed the view that, with proper cooperation, yaws, the sister disease of syphilis, might be eradicated from large areas within 5 to 10 years by mass penicillin treatment. Since then, mass antitreponemal programs of the WHO have involved the treatment of 50 million persons with various treponematoses. Although these programs have greatly reduced the incidence of disease, they have not served to eradicate any of the treponematoses in any large area.

The most disappointing aspect of the history of syphilis is that, despite the discovery of a highly effective therapeutic tool, which was so fervently hoped for in the past, a shocking rise in the incidence of new cases has occurred in many countries in recent years. The current indifference and lack of knowledge about venereal diseases are appalling. Increasing promiscuity resulting from changing moral attitudes on sex behavior, the introduction of modern contraceptives, and public trust in penicillin as a cure, together with a slowdown in fundamental research on the biology of venereal diseases, are matters of rising interest and serious concern. The following comments of Stokes and Beerman are pertinent:

> "Great advances in the therapeusis of a disease have an unfortunate tendency to discourage fundamental research, and to create an impression, even among critical minds, that the disease in question being now "in the bag" there is no further occasion for hunting. In the case of syphilis, and indeed of all the venereal group of infections, such a reaction is particularly unfortunate; for these diseases carry in their own biology and clinical course the means of their indefinite perpetuation . . . Before the venereal diseases are conquered an immunizing procedure must be developed, a vaccine of high if not absolute effectiveness, to protect the originally uninfected person through long periods if not through life; and to prevent reinfection, which is now suspected of being a loophole through which magnificent cure possibilities leak away to relatively unsatisfactory epidemiologic results."

Needless to say, the future outlook for the control of syphilis will only be good so long as effective therapy persists, and major efforts are sustained in the areas of research and medical education, and full cooperation is achieved between the public, the physician and public health authorities.

*Under present circumstances, eradication of syphilis from any large popu-
lation will only be possible providing physicians report all cases of the disease that they encounter to public health authorities.*

B. Physical and Chemical Structure

The morphology of *T. pallidum* is singularly deserving of attention because of its importance in identification of the organism and its bearing
on invasiveness, pathogenicity and immunity. *Treponema pallidum* is a
slender, pleomorphic, helical-shaped organism with tapered ends terminating in a nosepiece; it averages about 0.18 μm in diameter and varies in
length from about 5 to 20 μm. The organism possesses a cell wall, albeit
delicate and lacking in rigidity; muramic acid is present, and lysozyme
enhances lysis by Ab and C. The organism is encased in a special semi-
permeable outer envelope (periplast) surrounded by a mucoid slime layer.
The envelope, which is 70 to 90 Å thick, is presumed to be of lipoprotein
nature and to protect the organism against osmotic stress. Three contractile fibrils (Nichols' strain) arise from each end of the cell, each attached
to a basal cytoplasmic granule in the protoplasmic cylinder. The fibrils lie
between the cytoplasmic membrane and the cell wall. Each fibril is
attached to one or the other end of the cell and has a free end. The fibrils,
which may exceed the length of the cell, overlap and entwine to form
the axial filament; on contraction they force the cell to assume its helical
shape (Fig. 32-1).

The coils of the body of the organism are about 0.3 μm deep and are
spaced at intervals of about 1.0 μm. The organism is highly motile and
exhibits rapid rotary corkscrew-like movements, interrupted by marked
flexing, around its long axis. Since it has no anteroposterior polarity, movement may be either forward or backward. The unique motility, flexibility
and slender shape of *T. pallidum* probably contribute to its great power to
pass bacterial filters and to invade tissues and spread rapidly throughout
the body.

Contrary to general belief, *T. pallidum* stains readily with basic dyes and
is regarded to be gram-negative. However, because of its small diameter,
the organism cannot be observed readily by ordinary light microscopy unless stained by some special method such as "silver staining" which leads
to the deposition of silver on the cell surface. The organism can be observed by darkfield illumination, phase contrast microscopy and negative
staining.

Little is known about Ags of *T. pallidum* because the organism has not
been grown *in vitro;* obtaining pure suspensions of organisms from infected
tissues is essentially impossible. Although group-specific proteins and
polysaccharides have been reported, no treponemal Ags have been identified as being responsible for virulence, immunity or induction of the Abs

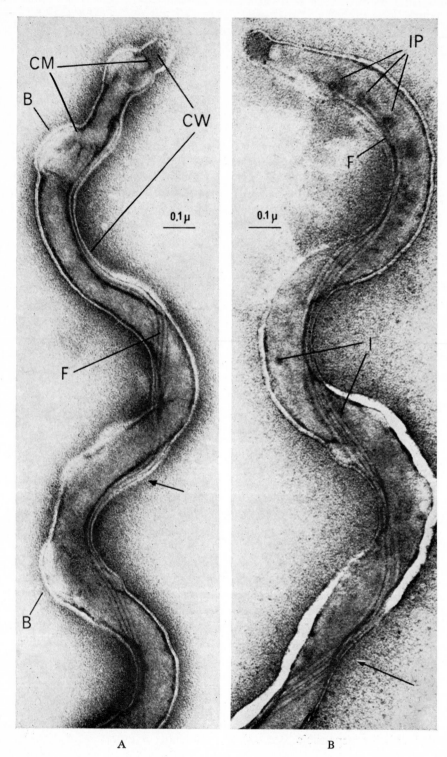

Figure 32-1. Legend on opposite page.

measured in serologic tests (Section J). The Ag(s) responsible for the
C-activating Ab (*Treponema pallidum* immobilizing Ab or TPI Ab) and
for immunity is presumed to be highly labile. It has been claimed that one
immunogen is a heat-labile envelope protein.

Treponema pallidum is rich in lipids and is coated with a mucoid material rich in a hyaluronic acid-like substance (Section J). It has been suggested that the mucoid material may protect the organism against TPI Ab,
presumably by masking Ag; it may also protect the organism against
phagocytosis and could represent a virulence factor.

Freshly isolated organisms, which are initially resistant to immobilizing
Ab and C, become immobilized by this system after a few hours of incubation *in vitro,* which presumably leads to loss of integrity of the surface
coat material and unmasking of Ag.

C. Genetics

Organisms from different patients have varying degrees of immunogenicity and virulence for the rabbit, but whether rabbit virulence parallels human virulence is not known. Isolates that are mildly virulent for the rabbit
can be made more virulent by rabbit passage.

D. Extracellular Products

No extracellular products have been identified.

E. Culture

Treponema pallidum *and related pathogenic treponemes have probably
never been cultured* in vitro, *even in the chick embryo or tissue culture.*
Many nonpathogenic species have been cultured anaerobically, and it is
probable that *T. pallidum* is a microaerophile or anaerobe. Maintenance
media can support its continued motility for 10 days or longer in an atmosphere of 95% N_2 and 5% CO_2.

Figure 32-1. A, The cytoplasmic membrane (CM) is seen as a borderline between zones 1 and 2 of the organism. Beyond CM is cell-wall material only (CW).
CW is seen in close contact with CM except in the regions of lower electron density,
blebs (B), and the part of the cell where the fibrillar bundle (F) passes straight
along the cytoplasmic body (arrow). Formalin fixation; negative staining; 1% ammonium molybdate. Magnification 90,000 ×. B, The three zones at the tip of the
organism are clearly illustrated. Three fibrils (F) with insertion points (IP) are seen
in zone 3, whereas 5 fibrils are seen more centrally. Two thin fibrils are present
(arrow) and dense inclusions (I) are seen. Formalin fixation; negative staining; 1%
phosphotungstic acid. Magnification 90,000 ×. (From Jepsen, O. B., Hougen, K. H.,
and Birch-Andersen, A.: Acta Path. Microbiol. Scand. *74*:247, 1968.)

The shortest generation time of *T. pallidum* in the rabbit is between 24 and 33 hours. This slow growth rate probably contributes to the long incubation time of 2 to 10 weeks observed in human syphilis and the slow therapeutic action of penicillin.

F. Resistance to Physical and Chemical Agents

Treponema pallidum is extremely sensitive to drying, osmotic stress and aerobic conditions. *Because of this, transmission of syphilis is limited largely to direct contact between moist integuments of infected and uninfected individuals rather than agents such as fomites and aerosol droplets.*

The organism remains alive for 1 to 3 days in blood stored at 4°C; consequently, on rare occasions the transmission of syphilis has followed transfusion of relatively fresh blood. *Treponema pallidum* can be stored in the virulent state for many years at the temperatures of solid CO_2, or preferably liquid N_2, especially if suspending media containing 15% glycerol are used. However, the organism does not withstand lyophilization, presumably because of the drying involved. Maintenance of motility outside the body does not ensure retention of rabbit infectivity, which, for unknown reasons, is usually lost within hours.

The *in vivo* temperature growth range of *T. pallidum* in the rabbit is 30 to 39°C (optimum 35 to 37°C); at temperatures of 40°C or above the organism does not survive for extended periods. In *in vitro* environments it is killed by 1 hour of exposure at 41.5°C. This temperature susceptibility evidently accounts for the occasional benefits of fever therapy formerly employed in man and for the elective distribution of experimental lesions in the testes and cool regions of the skin and extremities of rabbits (body temperature 38 to 39°C).

The organism is very sensitive to many chemical agents, including iodides, bismuth, mercury salts, arsenicals, and certain antibiotics.

G. Experimental Models

Although natural infection with *T. pallidum* is limited to man, many animals, including guinea pigs, mice, rats, rabbits, hamsters and subhuman primates, are mildly susceptible to experimental infection. In most of these animals, tissue responses to the presence of the organism are mild or absent and in many the growth of the organism is severely limited; however, infection can persist for months to years. Only primates regularly develop the late lesions of tertiary syphilis. Certain Abs, called reagins, that are produced in man do not develop in small laboratory animals, presumably because of lack of tissue destruction necessary to their production (Section J).*

---

* The term "reagin" is unfortunate and confusing because it is also used to designate the IgE Ab of immediate sensitivities such as hay fever.

In the commonly employed experimental animal, the rabbit, a mild chronic infection can be produced by inoculating the cool skin, eye, extremities or the favored site, the testes. The standard laboratory organism is the Nichols' strain of *T. pallidum* and the site used to produce organisms for laboratory use is the testicle.

Only one or a few organisms are required to infect the testicle of the rabbit, and it is probable that man is as susceptible to infection as the rabbit. Although the organisms spread readily from the injection site and remain alive, their growth is apparently restricted at most sites, and metastatic lesions only occur in abundance in the nose and cool areas of the skin and bones of the extremities where the temperature is 1 to 3 degrees lower than the internal body temperature. Immunity to superinfection is characterized by a strong tendency of the organisms to remain *localized* at the injection site.

Apparently, passage of *T. pallidum* in the rabbit does not reduce its virulence for man since both accidental and intentional human infections have resulted from organisms maintained for some 40 years by rabbit passage.

H.   Infections in Man

Syphilis, "the great imitator," is a systemic disease in which essentially every organ may become infected. So many and varied are its manifestations that Osler wrote, "to know syphilis is to know medicine."

In man, one of the most notable characteristics of syphilis, and other treponematoses as well, is that the disease commonly progresses in stages with intervening periods of quiescence, each stage presenting lesions of different morphologic characteristics.

Infection commonly results from contact of mucous membranes, and some 90% of cases of noncongenital syphilis in man are contracted during sexual intercourse. Most of the remaining 10%, including those in infants and children, are acquired by kissing, with resulting primary lesions (chancres) on the lips or in the oral cavity (Colle in 1631 was the first to prove that syphilis could be transmitted by common drinking cups and kissing). "Local epidemics" due to unusual modes of nonvenereal transmission have been reported, including wet nursing, common use of razors or public cigar cutters, carriage by means of surgical or musical instruments, and tattooing and glassblowing.

The organisms readily penetrate breaks in the skin or mucosa, no matter how miniscule, and possibly transgress intact mucosa as well; approximately 50% of those exposed become infected.

After breaching mucosa or skin the organisms quickly invade the local perivascular lymph spaces, pass to the local lymph nodes and may reach the blood stream within a matter of minutes or a few hours at most. Bacteremia, which can be demonstrated readily by injecting defibrinated blood of the patient into the rabbit testicle, is a constant feature in the large majority of persons having primary syphilis and can occur sporadically in any stage of the disease.

Within 3 months (usually 2 to 4 weeks) after exposure the treponemes multiply and reach large numbers in the local lymphatics and the draining lymph nodes, as well as at the site of entrance where the chancre develops. The chancre is often solitary and is commonly the size of a pea. The time of its appearance probably bears an inverse relation to the size of the infecting dose of organisms. Since the chancre is commonly painless, unless it is extragenital or becomes secondarily infected, and is frequently in a concealed position, the patient is often unaware or unmindful of its presence. *Forty to 60% of patients (especially women) pass through the primary and secondary stages of syphilis without knowing that they have the disease.* The chancre originates in the corium; early infiltrating PMNs are soon followed by other leukocytes. The fully developed chancre is indurated (hard) and contains large numbers of lymphocytes, macrophages and plasma cells; in fact, plasma cells are singularly prominent in the lesions of all stages of syphilis. Endothelial proliferation and obstructive endarteritis of infected blood vessels cause necrosis and attending ulceration of the overlying epidermis. The ulcerated lesion yields a serous exudate rich in treponemes and the draining lymph nodes, which are swollen, hard and painless, yield treponemes on aspiration. Healing of the chancre, which occurs within a few weeks, is accompanied by the local disappearance of organisms.

The secondary stage is a generalized infection; it usually appears after a quiescent period of about 6 to 12 weeks, but can occur before the chancre heals. During this period the organisms slowly multiply and invade widely, often involving the skin, mucous membranes, eyes, lymph nodes, bones, the CNS and the walls of major vessels. *The lesions and symptoms of secondary syphilis are legion. Although the secondary lesions are histologically similar to primary lesions and contain enormous numbers of treponemes, they usually do not lead to extensive and life-threatening tissue destruction and commonly heal spontaneously, without scarring, within a few weeks or months, a situation quite in contrast to the highly destructive lesions of tertiary syphilis.* In some patients several alternating relapses and remissions of the secondary stage or even the primary stage may occur within 1 to 2 years, apparently because of a weak and vacillating immune response. Relapses are more common than is generally believed; they range from 15 to 20% and include late latent as well as early syphilis. The term "early syphilis" includes primary, secondary, early relapsing and early latent forms of the disease as contrasted with later stages.* During the secondary stage, the saliva, semen and the uterine secretions (particularly

*Latent disease of less than 4 years' duration is defined as *early latent* syphilis and of more than 4 years' duration as *late latent syphilis.*

at the time of menstruation) commonly contain enormous numbers of treponemes. In contrast, patients with late syphilis are usually noninfectious except during pregnancy. Among patients with secondary syphilis who are not treated the *majority progress* to the *tertiary* stages either insensibly or after a latent period that may be brief or may extend for 2 to 20 years.

The severity of tertiary syphilis bears an inverse relation to the severity of secondary syphilis (law of inverse relation of Brown and Pearce). In about 30 to 50% of persons with early untreated syphilis the disease progresses steadily and usually positive reactions to serologic tests for *specific Abs* are continually obtained; about 20 to 30% of this group eventually die of the disease. The overall mortality due directly to syphilis is about 12%; however, the disease also contributes to death attributed to other causes. In another 25% of untreated subjects, infection remains latent for long periods (*late latent syphilis*); the specific serologic reactions remain positive and reactivation occasionally occurs. In the remaining 25% of those untreated the lesions and symptoms subside completely and reactions to serologic tests become negative. (*However, despite spontaneous clinical cures it can be seriously questioned whether spontaneous bacteriologic cures take place simultaneously.*)

The *late stages of syphilis progress slowly, but are nevertheless the most destructive;* they are characterized by the *focal lesion, the gumma,* a painless lesion with central coagulation necrosis, which is of gum-like consistency, and the *diffuse lesion,* involving principally the walls of blood vessels and the CNS. *Patients in whom diffuse lesions prevail present the most tragic cases, for during long years of apparent good health the treponemes continue with their tardy but terrible acts of destruction that are only too familiar to the pathologist.*

The development of the gumma of syphilis is sometimes precipitated by trauma. Gummas produce symptoms readily; they are often solitary and usually develop in skin, bones, testes, liver and in the brain where they cause the symptoms of tumor. They vary greatly in size and are composed of epithelioid cells and a few foreign-body giant cells and Langhans' giant cells surrounded by macrophages and enormous numbers of lymphocytes and plasma cells. The tissue destruction involved is presumed to be largely on a hypersensitivity basis with vascular occlusion accounting for some of the necrosis. Gummas contain relatively few organisms, but reactions to serologic tests are usually strongly positive. Large gummas tend to heal centrally and progress peripherally. They are readily arrested by penicillin therapy and heal rapidly. Individuals who develop gummas often fail to develop late CNS and cardiovascular syphilis due to diffuse lesions, presumably because immunologic mechanisms concerned in the formation of gummas are associated with strong immunity. Syphilis involving gummas is sometimes termed "benign syphilis." This is unfortunate because if the gumma is in a vital spot such as the heart or brain it can be highly lethal.

In contrast to *gummas, diffuse lesions* are characterized by slow, insidious destruction of blood vessels and other tissues, such as those of the CNS. They often progress asymptomatically for many years until irreparable damage of the entire vessel wall has occurred. In diffuse lesions, as in most lesions of the disease, the organisms show a predilection for perivascular lymph spaces. *Perivascular infiltration with lymphocytes, plasma cells and macrophages is the hallmark of the diffuse lesion.* Destruction of the valvular endocardium and walls of small vessels, such as the supporting vasa vasorum of the walls of large vessels, often occurs. Small and medium-sized arteries, such as cerebral and coronary arteries, may suffer obliterative endarteritis, which restricts the circulation and leads to severe disturbances in the function of many tissues and organs. Cerebral hemorrhage, aortic valvular disease and aneurysm of the thoracic aorta are common results of such lesions (Fig. 32-2).

Late CNS syphilis commonly becomes symptomatic earlier than syphilis of the aorta; it involves the meninges (*syphilitic meningitis*) and parenchymal tissues of the brain (*general paresis*) and the spinal cord (*tabes dorsalis*). In some cases, destruction of the optic nerve occurs and leads to blindness.

Congenital syphilis results from the passage of the highly invasive treponeme from mother to fetus *in utero,* an uncommon occurrence among bacterial diseases. *Pregnancy* markedly *suppresses the symptoms of syphilis* in the mother, probably, in part at least, as a result of estrogenic hormone effects. *However, a mobilization of treponemes in the blood is favored by pregnancy and bacteremia often occurs in the pregnant female with late syphilis; thus the opportunities for infection of the fetus are great during*

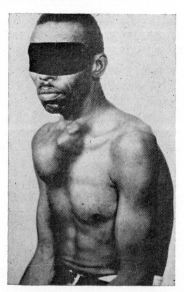

Figure 32-2. Aneurysm of the ascending arch of the aorta with erosion of the clavicle and ribs. Loss of elasticity of the damaged aorta has allowed the pulsating pressure of the expanding aorta to beat its way through muscle and bone; early fatal hemorrhage is the usual outcome in such patients. (Adapted from Kampmeier, R. H.: Essentials of Syphilology. Philadelphia, J. B. Lippincott Co., 1943.)

pregnancy. Infection of the fetus is seldom manifest before about the 5th month of gestation, allegedly because of the barrier against treponemal invasion afforded by Langhans' cell layer of the early placenta and/or because immune responses are lacking.

Maternal anti-treponemal Abs afford little or no protection to the fetus; the organisms may reach tremendous numbers and cause great damage, especially in the viscera. The infected fetus may be born dead, either at term or prematurely, born alive with clinical evidence of syphilis or born in apparent good health and subsequently develop clinical disease.

The hallmarks of congenital syphilis are based on arrests of embryonic development. The lesions, which are evident both early and late after birth, are numerous and may resemble those of the secondary and tertiary stages of noncongenital syphilis in adults. *The stigmas of late congenital syphilis,* e.g., the telltale indicators that accompany late lesions in the maturing individual, usually include at least two of "Hutchinson's triad," notched permanent incisors, and interstitial keratitis of the cornea leading to corneal opacity and blindness. Since these are developmental conditions resulting from injury of embryonic tissues, they are not helped by penicillin treatment.

Prevention of congenital syphilis can be readily accomplished by penicillin treatment initiated early in pregnancy to suppress maternal bacteremia. In such cases the newborn infant, although uninfected, may show a positive reaction to serologic tests (due to maternal IgG Abs); this reactivity steadily lessens in early postnatal life. When syphilis is acquired by the mother late in pregnancy the infected newborn can be apparently healthy and serologically negative.

I. Mechanisms of Pathogenicity

The pathogenesis of syphilis is an enigma. There is no evidence that *T. pallidum* forms a toxin that could account for the lesions seen in syphilis. The generally accepted alternative possibility is that tissue injury rests largely on immediate and/or delayed hypersensitivity reactions. However, it is difficult to envision how immunologic events alone could account for the extensive destruction of tissue often seen in the immunologically deficient syphilitic fetus, even with the participation of maternal IgG Abs.

J. Mechanisms of Immunity

Less is known about the nature of immunity to syphilis than of immunity to most any other bacterial disease; only the theoretical aspects of the topic will be emphasized in this section.

Levels of total serum globulins are usually high and the Abs produced are of two kinds: (1) *reagins,* which are autoantibodies against tissue Ags, and (2) *treponemal Abs* specific for treponemal Ags. Reagins are chiefly of the 19S class, especially early in the disease, and functionally may be either "complete" or "incomplete." They are measured by either complement fixation (Wassermann type) tests or flocculation (Kahn type) tests using tissue-derived Ags. They are not specific for syphilis and appear sporadically in certain unrelated infectious and noninfectious diseases.

Tissue Ags, which are presumed to represent structural cellular Ags released from injured host cells, evidently engender *reagins* of 2 classes. Reagins of one class react with tissue Ags only, whereas those of the other class react with both Ags of *T. pallidum* and tissue Ags. *The level of reagins in the serum of syphilitics correlates well with the rate of tissue destruction and is the best guide for assessing the effectiveness of therapy.* Tests for reagins frequently yield either *false positive* or *false negative* reactions, the latter being especially frequent in early primary syphilis, latent syphilis or in tertiary syphilis in which tissue destruction is limited. Cold autoantibodies specific for the Tj^a antigen of human red cells often arise in late and congenital syphilis; following chilling of the extremities they act with C to destroy RBC and cause paroxysmal cold hemoglobinuria.

The second general category of Abs, the *treponemal Abs,* consists, on the one hand, of *"specific Abs" that react only with* T. pallidum *and closely related pathogenic treponemes* and, on the other hand, of *"group Abs" directed against cross-reacting Ags present in a wide variety of distantly related treponemes* as well as *T. pallidum.* Treponemal Abs are principally of the class IgG (7S), but include IgM (19S) and occasionally IgA Abs as well. Specific Abs cause agglutination and some belonging to the class IgG are cytotoxic for the organism in the presence of C, causing loss of motility detectable by the TPI test. Specific treponemal Abs can also be detected by a number of other tests, including the fluorescent treponemal Ab test (FTA test), an indirect fluorescent Ab test. This test is conducted by applying suspected serum to known dried *T. pallidum* on a slide, followed by washing, adding fluorescein-tagged anti-human globulin serum and examining with the fluorescence microscope. The specificity of the FTA test can be improved by properly absorbing the suspected serum with Ags of the nonpathogenic Reiter strain treponeme to remove many of the cross-reactive "group Abs" (FTA-ABS test). *Of the current routine tests for syphilis and closely related treponematoses, the FTA-ABS test is the most specific, reliable and sensitive.* Treponemes of the normal flora, especially when they participate in opportunistic infections, may incite "treponemal Abs" that are not absorbable by Reiter Ag and thus abrogate the specificity of the FTA-ABS test. The highly specific TPI test is used occasionally to detect false positive reactions to FTA-ABS tests. Despite their shortcomings, the tests for treponemal Abs have been of great value in diagnosis, positivity being largely limited to syphilis and closely related treponematoses. They have been especially useful for detecting the false positive reactions encountered in reagin screening tests for syphilis.

Treponemal Abs tend to appear somewhat earlier in the course of the disease than reagins and often persist indefinitely after spontaneous or therapy-induced clinical cure. Consequently, a *positive reaction to the FTA-ABS test provides no certain evidence of clinical activity or necessity of treatment. It simply indicates that the subject has or has had one of the treponemal diseases.* In a minority of untreated patients with late CNS or cardiovascular syphilis, especially those with tabes dorsalis or long-standing congenital disease, the reaction may be negative.

The formation and distribution of Abs in CNS syphilis and congenital syphilis deserve special consideration. In CNS syphilis, Abs are produced locally by infiltrating cells. Since Abs do not readily pass the blood-brain barrier in either direction unless this barrier is severely damaged, syphilis limited to the CNS may be accompanied by Abs in spinal fluid alone, or, if not so limited, by Abs in both serum and spinal fluid. For example, in 40% of persons with tabes dorsalis, positive reactions are limited to tests on the spinal fluid.

Since 7S as well as 19S Abs are represented among reagin and treponemal Abs, the newborn infant of a syphilitic mother with positive serologic reactions may show positive reactions for both reagin and treponemal Abs as the result of maternal transfer of 7S Abs on the one hand and the formation of 19S Abs by the fetus on the other.* Demonstration of treponemal IgM Abs in fetal blood by use of anti-H chain serum constitutes presumptive evidence of congenital syphilis. In some instances, maternal IgM Abs may reach the fetus through a "leaky" placenta. Such leakage can be detected by comparing the ceruloplasmin concentration in the serum of the mother and child. If the infant has active disease, the serologic reaction will remain positive, but, if free of infection, it will become negative in a matter of weeks to 3 to 4 months owing to metabolic decay of maternally derived Abs. If the mother contracts the disease late in pregnancy the serologic reaction of both the mother and infant may be negative at birth and become positive later.

Apparently man possesses little or no innate immunity to syphilis and all individuals are susceptible (although not necessarily equally so) to primary infection. *A substantial level of acquired immunity develops in most infected individuals,* albeit insufficient in the majority to accomplish early arrest of the disease. Acquired immunity is manifested by marked resistance to natural superinfection, occasional spontaneous permanent arrest of disease following the secondary stage (some 25% or more of untreated individuals), a paucity of tissue treponemes in late lesions, slowly progressing disease, and evidence of an anamnestic response on reinfection. *However, acquired immunity is not absolute* and heavy inocula of organisms into the skin of syphilitic patients will often produce lesions charac-

---

* Antibodies responsible for false positive maternal serologic reactions can also be transferred to the fetus.

teristic of the stage of existing disease. *Immunity sufficient to prevent the development of clinically evident lesions on natural reexposure does not necessarily protect against tissue invasion by superinfecting organisms.*

A strong stimulus by the treponemes appears to be necessary for the initiation and maintenance of immunity, as indicated by the following observations: (1) immunity to superinfection does not arise until after the development of the primary lesion, (2) an inverse relation exists between the severity of the secondary lesion and the extent of tertiary lesions and (3) immunity to reinfection wanes following cure with therapeutic agents, being especially rapid following cure effected in the early stages of the disease. *The alleged need for living organisms to maintain high immunity has led to the term "infection immunity."* It is notable that maximum immunity to either reinfection or superinfection is not gained earlier than about 3 months in the rabbit and possibly 2 or more years in man. In rabbits, measurable immunity can persist for substantial periods after the organisms have been eliminated with drugs. *Total immunity could result from one or a combination of 2 or more of 3 general mechanisms,* namely, humoral Abs of immobilizing and lytic nature, cellular immunity (possibly of an unusual kind) and nonantibody humoral factors of immunity such as lysozyme.

Past investigations have not provided convincing evidence that humoral immunity plays an important role in acquired immunity to experimental syphilis in animals. Neither is there good correlative evidence to indicate that humoral Abs contribute to immunity against human syphilis. How-

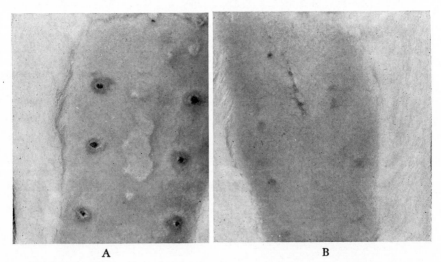

A   B

Figure 32-3. The influence of immune serum on the development of cutaneous syphilitic chancres in rabbits. Syphilitic skin chancres on the shaved backs of 2 rabbits. Control rabbit A presents 6 ulcerated chancres 4 weeks after inoculation of 10^6 *T. pallidum* at each site. Rabbit B treated with specific immune serum 80 Ml/Kg on the 5th day after inoculation with *T. pallidum* presents 6 small arrested lesions. (From Perine, P. L., Weiser, R. S., and Klebanoff, S. J.: Infect. Immun. *8*:787, 1973.)

ever, it has recently been demonstrated that large volumes of immune serum can passively transfer limited protection against skin infection in rabbits (Fig. 32-3). The observations that the human fetus receives little or no protection from maternal IgG Ab, even though the mother displays immunity to superinfection, together with the fact that the fetus forms IgM, are also compatible with the concept that cellular rather than humoral forces play the dominant role in immunity to human syphilis. If, as claimed, live, intact treponemes are seldom, if ever, engulfed by professional phagocytes, the opsonizing action of humoral Ab should not contribute to acquired immunity. The observation that TPI Ab and C can kill treponemes *in vitro* only after they have "aged" for a matter of many hours and presumably have lost their protective mucoid coat appears to be inconsistent with the concept that humoral Ab conveys substantial immunity. However, it is possible that treponemes are susceptible to Ab and C *in vivo* because their protective coat is interrupted during division and that only non-multiplying treponemes, or perhaps treponemes sequestered in sites where Abs and C may be at low levels, escape *in vivo* killing by Ab and C.

The concept that *specific cellular immunity* may be the principal component of total immunity can also be challenged. If living treponemes are completely resistant to phagocytosis by macrophages, conventional cellular immunity involving intracellular events within macrophages would be ruled out. A possible alternative mechanism of cellular immunity is that lymphokines released from immune lymphocytes under the stimulus of treponemal Ag might be directly toxic to the organisms or could convey protection indirectly by inciting inflammation.

Hypersensitivity reactions may play a role in acquired immunity to syphilis. Positive skin test reactions to killed *T. pallidum* or its extracts, characteristic of immediate-type hypersensitivity, have been reported in early preserologic syphilis; in late syphilis they are of the delayed type.

K. Laboratory Diagnosis

The laboratory diagnosis of syphilis is commonly based on the direct demonstration of *T. pallidum* in material from the lesions or draining lymph nodes and/or serologic tests for Abs in serum and cerebrospinal fluid. *Since Abs do not arise until some 1 to 3 or more weeks after the chancre first appears, the only available test for judging early primary lesions involves detection of the organism.* Under darkfield illumination, *T. pallidum* is easily confused with nonpathogenic treponemes, and the examination is only reliable when it is conducted by experts and is repeated if necessary. A highly promising modified darkfield test has recently been developed in which a known absorbed fluorescein-tagged syphilitic serum specific for the organism is used (FADF test).* *The physician should be mindful of the fact*

---

*Fluorescent antibody darkfield (FADF) test.

that atypical lesions due to mixed infections sometimes occur and that the frequent dominance of organisms other than T. pallidum can be misleading. Failure to find the organisms by darkfield examination is not certain evidence that the disease is not syphilis.

Since treponemes are usually very scarce in the lesions of late syphilis and can only be demonstrated directly by painstaking examination of biopsy material, which is usually unavailable, *the only useful routine methods for laboratory diagnosis of tertiary syphilis are serologic tests.* Serologic tests, which are legion (over 200 have been proposed), are concerned (1) with the detection of *reagins* by testing the patient's serum and spinal fluid with tissue Ag preparations* and (2) with the detection of *treponemal Abs* by tests with a laboratory strain of *T. pallidum.* The use of different tests by different laboratories has led to much confusion in reporting and interpretation of results. Consequently it is advisable for the physician to make a concerted effort to become thoroughly acquainted with the tests used in local laboratories. Tests in current use in most laboratories include the Venereal Disease Research Laboratory test (VDRL test), a flocculation type of slide test for reagin, and the FTA and FTA-ABS tests for treponemal Abs. *Serologic tests for syphilis are not as reliable as has been generally believed and proper interpretation of results demands keen judgment by experienced personnel,* taking into consideration the clinical aspects of the case as well as the limitations of the tests themselves.

L. Therapy

Although the development of arsenicals for the treatment of syphilis was one of the greatest achievements in the history of medicine, penicillin and certain other antibiotics have much greater treponemicidal activity and much lower toxicity.

Penicillin kills T. pallidum *slowly* because the organism grows slowly. Treatment is usually effective within about 2 to 6 weeks. Late syphilis is the least responsive, presumably because the organisms are multiplying less rapidly than during early disease and because tissues destroyed prior to treatment do not regenerate. If the patient is sensitive to penicillin other antibiotics, including tetracyclines, carbomycin, synnematin, and especially erythromycin, may prove useful.

In past years, fever induced by the malarial organism (malarial therapy) or by physical means was occasionally used with some success in late syphilis.

Serologic tests for reagin are highly useful in therapeutic management because they correlate best with the rate and extent of tissue destruction.

---

* Apparently the tissue component specific for reagin is diphosphatidylglycerol. A lipid extract of beef heart serves as a good source of the Ag. Cerebrospinal fluid tests should be included in the management of all cases of syphilis because of their prognostic and diagnostic value in CNS disease.

The VDRL test should be run at 3-month intervals for 1 to 2 years or longer as a measure of the adequacy of treatment. A persisting or rising VDRL titer implies continued disease or possibly reinfection.

The life-threatening systemic "Herxheimer" or "Jarisch-Herxheimer" reaction with accompanying exacerbation of local lesions and associated destruction of liver, which was a troublesome problem in the days of arsenical treatment, particularly in the therapy of paretics and patients with secondary syphilis or congenital syphilis, is an even greater problem with penicillin treatment. For example, penicillin treatment of infants with congenital syphilis is attended by the Herxheimer reaction in 30% of these patients, evidently because of the enormous numbers of organisms in the lesions. It is presumed to represent an allergic or, possibly, a toxic reaction caused by the sudden release of treponemal components following initiation of treatment. Reactions usually begin about 4 hours after initiation of treatment and persist for 10 to 15 hours. They are accompanied by fever and heavy infiltration of neutrophils in local lesions and can be fatal in patients with late cardiovascular or CNS syphilis.

Since early treatment of primary infections with penicillin destroys the organisms before immunity can develop, the patient often remains fully susceptible to exogenous reinfection following cure with penicillin.

Although it is the consensus that permanent clinical and serologic cures can often be effected with arsenicals and antibiotics, especially in early syphilis, the concept that, following such cures, the body is always completely ridded of the organisms has always been seriously challenged. There is now substantial evidence that an occasional patient cured clinically and serologically with penicillin harbors live *T. pallidum* in the inner ear, the CNS, and most notably in the anterior chamber of the eye. These are sheltered sites where penetration of immune forces and penicillin is limited, especially in the absence of inflammation. Although the status of *T. pallidum* in possible sites of sequestration will only be settled by further investigation, present evidence suggests that great care should be exercised to ensure that the treatment of late syphilis is rigorous and adequate.

M. Reservoirs of Infection

Infected human beings are the only natural reservoirs of infection. Experimental laboratory animals have been a source of accidental human infection on rare occasion.

N. Control of Disease Transmission

Inasmuch as syphilis is acquired chiefly by sexual intercourse, effective measures of control consist of education, early detection and adequate treatment of cases and contacts. Since early syphilis is readily cured with penicillin and late syphilis is seldom infectious, it should be possible to eradicate the disease from a population. *However, this can never be achieved unless essentially all persons with early disease and contacts of individuals with infectious syphilis are detected and treated with a sense of immediacy.* Unfortunately, in recent years indifference on the part of patients, the public and even the medical profession has made control of syphilis far less effective than it could be. Abandonment of the hospital practice of conducting routine serologic tests for syphilis on all patients has aggravated the problem. *The weakest links in control are case reporting and detection of contacts. It is a sad commentary that for every case reported to public health authorities at least 5 to 10 additional cases known to the physician go unreported.* Also, because of the social stigmas involved, the detection of cases and contacts is exceedingly difficult, especially among teenagers and sexually perverted individuals; the hunted are like a will-o'-the-wisp. The detection and management of contacts are best conducted by public health experts; the trails are long and may even extend to foreign countries. Moreover, the fact that many individuals, especially females, remain unaware that they have contracted the disease is a great deterrent to case finding and frequently a great tragedy since the disease may reach the late destructive stages before it is recognized. Another deterrent to case and contact detection is secretive self-treatment which, being frequently inadequate, often leads to false cures and the development of late disease.

Military experience has shown that no local prophylactic measure has more than limited value, in part because of faulty use of such measures and in part because the measures are inadequate. For example, the infecting treponemes often invade tissues beyond the reach of such agents as topical ointments within minutes to a few hours after exposure. Inadequate prophylactic measures often mask infection by suppressing the early lesions, leaving the individual unaware of any need for further treatment. Moreover, inadequate suppression of early infection depresses the specific immune response and predisposes to the development of severe tertiary lesions. Chemoprophylaxis is only effective when it meets the minimum requirements for curative treatment. In instances of known exposure, especially of the pregnant female, chemoprophylaxis is justified but should always be supervised by a physician.

No suitable vaccine for syphilis has been developed to date; if such were available it should be highly useful for immunizing patients after completing drug treatment and especially for preventing infection among prostitutes. This is supported by the observation that venereal syphilis is rare in areas of endemic yaws.

Treponema pertenue

Although yaws can be distinguished from syphilis on epidemiologic and clinical grounds and by infection in rabbits, the causative organism, *T.*

pertenue, is serologically and morphologically indistinguishable from *T. pallidum.* Since organisms closely resembling *T. pertenue* have been isolated from African baboons, man may not be the only natural host of this species.

Unlike syphilis, yaws is not a venereal disease and is probably contracted largely by skin contact and by insect bites. Infection tends to occur early in life and the majority of a population often become infected. Yaws is most prevalent in moist tropical regions where little clothing is worn. Indeed it is thought that clothing greatly limits infection and breaks the chain of transmission. High humidity favors the persistence of open skin lesions and disease transmission.

The course of yaws is similar to the course of syphilis. During the first few years, early relapses involving skin may occur; late latent disease with relapses is common. Many of the late lesions of yaws closely resemble those of syphilis but are largely confined to skin and bones. Mutilating deformities of the face and feet are common. Immunity is weak and superinfection often occurs. Singular characteristics are that the cardiovascular and nervous systems are rarely involved and congenital disease is rare. Penicillin is highly effective and has been used widely in WHO campaigns to control yaws. However, eradication of yaws has posed a new problem, namely, that of creating a population lacking the protection against syphilis naturally conferred by yaws.

In 1954 the number of cases of yaws in the world was estimated to be 50 million. The numbers today are fewer.

Treponema carateum

Pinta due to *T. carateum* is another nonvenereal treponemal disease. It is endemic in Mexico, Cuba and Central and South America. The organism is indistinguishable from *T. pallidum* and *T. pertenue* by present methods. In the skin, the only apparent site of attack, the organism is almost exclusively in the lower malpighian layers of the epidermis. It produces chronic, scaly, pigmented lesions that sometimes result in atrophy, scarring, and depigmentation. In common with yaws, infection usually occurs in childhood, presumably as the result of skin contact. Mass chemotherapy with penicillin has been effective, and at present only about one million cases are known to exist. It is doubtful whether the rabbit can be infected with *T. carateum.*

Other Treponemes

Diseases that probably represented nonvenereal syphilis have been recorded from time to time from the 17th century onward.

Bejel is a modern example of nonvenereal syphilis; it is endemic among the Arabs of the Upper Euphrates Valley. Owing largely to unsanitary conditions, the majority of individuals in endemic areas become infected in childhood, probably in such ways as by the use of common drinking utensils; essentially all individuals in endemic areas are infected by the time they are adults. Skin, bones, and especially mucous membranes of the URT are often involved; gummas are common but congenital disease and lesions of the cardiovascular and nervous systems seldom occur. Mutilating deformities of the face and limbs often develop. Reactions to serologic tests are positive. Penicillin treatment is effective. Immunity is weak and superinfection can occur. The organism is infectious for the rabbit.

Interrelations of the Treponematoses

Interrelationships between the treponematoses is a subject of great interest and speculation. Although cross immunity exists, especially between syphilis and yaws, its nature is not understood.

It has been suggested that differences in disease patterns and organ tropisms of species of treponemes may have resulted from evolution involving both ecologic and geographic separation of groups of human beings. For example, whereas yaws, which is characterized by skin-to-skin transmission, is favored by warm, humid climates where little clothing is worn, the disease can also exist in temperate climates where personal hygiene is poor and numerous members of the family sleep together because of overcrowding. It has been proposed that in the evolution of civilized man the advent of improved clothing and living conditions restricted the opportunity for skin-to-skin transmission and introduced selective pressures leading to the emergence of new mutant strains of treponemes best fitted to accomplish mucosa-to-mucosa transmission, especially by venery, for their maintenance in the host population. Selection may subsequently have led to changes that endowed the organism with increased capabilities for invading internal organs, the CNS and the fetus.

Borrelia

Members of the genus *Borrelia* have a coarser spiral structure than the treponemes and are large enough to be seen in stained smears by phase and darkfield microscopy. The only species of known pathogenic significance for man is *Borr. recurrentis,* the cause of relapsing fever. Other species such as *Borr. vincenti* are occasionally present among the flora of mixed infections, such as ulcerative lesions of the mouth and skin and lung abscesses, but their possible contributions to these infections are not known.

During relapsing fever, *Borr. recurrentis* is abundant in blood; it was first observed by Obermeier (1873), in the blood of a patient, as a highly motile, spiral, thread-like rod with dimensions averaging about 8 to 30 μm $\times$ 0.3 to 0.5 μm. A wide range of animals, principally rodents and their insect parasites, serve as natural hosts; man and certain animals are usually accidental hosts.

Relapsing fever in the USA (principally in the West and Southwest) is of limited medical importance. However, from the time of Hippocrates it has been documented as a disease of major medical importance in Europe, Asia and Africa. It continues to be a disease of great importance in Northern Africa and Central Asia.

Borrelia recurrentis is closely related to *T. pallidum,* but unlike the latter is not sensitive to O_2; it has an outer slime-like coat and exhibits marked instability in antigenic composition in the face of host immunity. Because of this, residence in different mammalian and insect hosts has led to great heterogeneity of strains and difficulty in classification. *Some investigators have given the variants species status (usually named after the region where isolated), whereas others regard the variants to be strains within a species.* The species name *Borr. recurrentis* is sometimes used to designate the organism responsible for *louse-borne disease* but not *tick-borne disease.* Louse-borne strains probably do not adapt to become tick-borne strains or vice versa.

Relapsing fever in man consists of (1) tick-borne disease contracted from ticks as biologic vectors that parasitize rodents and (2) louse-borne disease passed from person to person by the louse *Pediculus humanus* and sometimes the bedbug. *Borrelia recurrentis* grows on egg embryos. Culture has recently been achieved on nonliving media with tick-borne strains but not with louse-borne strains.

Tick-borne relapsing fever is essentially a worldwide disease. The natural reservoirs for man are wild rodents and other small animals and their insect parasites, principally ticks of the genus *Ornithodoros.* The causative organism is passed transovarially in the tick. The ticks infect man primarily by shedding contaminated coxal gland fluid into the bite wound while feeding. Tick-borne disease is seldom fatal.

Louse-borne relapsing fever is often mistaken for typhus. The causative organism apparently has man and certain other primates as its only natural hosts. Organisms released from feeding lice crushed by scratching invade through the bite wound. Many large epidemics of louse-borne disease have occurred in the past with mortalities ranging from 5 to 70%. During the 1942 to 1944 epidemic in the Eastern Mediterranean region, one million cases and 50,000 deaths occurred. A pandemic in the early 1900s involved 50 million cases and 5 million deaths.

The disease begins abruptly, usually within a few days after exposure. The symptoms are many; they often include high fever, nausea, photophobia, prostration, splenic enlargement, cough, thirst, epistaxis, delirium, jaundice and leukocytosis and sometimes petechiae appear in the skin. The organisms invade widely and grow freely in the blood stream. Live organisms are not phagocytized, but on rare occasion have been seen within endothelial cells.

The most singular aspect of relapsing fever, either tick-borne or louse-borne, is the relapsing nature of the fever. The initial fever, which lasts for 3 to 10 days, is followed by a remission of a few days before the second attack occurs. This cycle of recurrent fever and relapse may be repeated on as many as 4 or more occasions, each relapse being due to a new and antigenically distinct variant. During each remission the organisms disappear from the blood, allegedly because of newly formed bactericidal Abs specific for the Ag unique to the new variant that caused the attack.

In animal work it has been shown that serum taken after each attack protects again the organism(s) responsible for the preceding attack(s) but not succeeding attacks. Apparently any given strain of *Borr. recurrentis* is genetically capable of expressing certain antigenic phase variations that determine the number of relapses that can occur in an animal it infects.

Little is known about immunity to the organism except that cross immunity between strains is limited, and that specific immunity has been passively transferred in the rabbit and in man on an experimental basis. The protective Abs are probably directed at a number of surface Ags. One of the 2 Abs of greatest importance in immunity achieves immobilization of organisms without C participation and the other achieves lysis with C participation; none promotes phagocytosis of living organisms. To what extent these various Ab activities contribute to immunity is not known.

A formalized vaccine has been shown to be effective in the rabbit. However, the development of a useful vaccine for man is difficult because of the bewildering number of antigenically different strains present in any area of endemic disease.

Relapsing fever activates latent kala-azar but the mechanism involved is not known.

Diagnosis of relapsing fever is easily established by observing typical organisms in routine or thick blood smears specially stained with Giemsa stain, or in darkfield preparations of fresh blood. Infection with some pathogenic strains can also be established in mice by injection of blood. Therapy with penicillin, tetracyclines and chloramphenicol is effective but is sometimes complicated by the Jarish-Herxheimer reaction.

Preventive measures of importance are rodent and insect control and avoidance of insect bites. Practical vaccines and antisera have not been developed.

Leptospira

A new classification has been suggested for organisms of the genus *Leptospira* in which the basic taxon is the serotype. Two species would be recognized, *L. interrogans,* to represent the pathogenic strains, and *L. biflexa,* to represent the nonpathogens (largely saprophytes). According to the new classification the prototype member of the pathogens (over 100 have been described), formerly called *L. icterohemorrhagiae,* would be designated *L. interrogans* serotype *icterohemorrhagiae.* The leptospira have a wide range of natural hosts, principally rodents and other small animals, in which they commonly produce mild or asymptomatic infection. Each serologic type tends to have one or a few natural hosts. Man and some domesticated animals serve as accidental and terminal hosts. In these hosts the disease can be serious and often fatal. Infections, known by many different names, have been described in numerous species of animals.

Leptospirosis is a broad term applied to any of the similar infections in different hosts due to the various leptospires. *The organisms produce systemic disease and reach the kidney tubules where they colonize* in large numbers. Since such colonization occurs in unnatural as well as natural hosts, both types can serve as chronic urinary carriers. For example, the Norway rat, a common natural host of serotype *icterohemorrhagiae,* can remain a carrier for its lifetime.

Although many thousands of cases of human leptospirosis occur annually throughout the world the disease is not of great importance in the USA where the average number of hospitalized leptospirosis patients seldom exceeds 100. However, because the disease is often mild, the total number of cases far exceeds this number.

Members of the genus Leptospira are thin, enveloped, flexible, thread-like organisms 7 to 20 μm $\times$ 0.1 to 0.2 μm. They possess some 12 to 18 tightly coiled spirals and in most strains the terminal third of one end of the cell body is bent in the form of a hook. Motility depends on an axial structure called the axistyle. The leptospiras possess strain-specific surface Ags and a genus-specific somatic Ag. However, their role in determining serologic interrelationships between strains and immunity has not been elucidated. The organism is highly mutable and mutants can be selected with immune serum.

The organism grows slowly under *aerobic conditions* at 30°C on serum-containing media (pH 7.2), on synthetic media and in the chick embryo, which it kills within a few days. Pathogens do not grow below about 15°C and do not multiply in natural waters. They survive freezing but are destroyed at 50 to 55°C. Among laboratory animals, young guinea pigs, hamsters and chicks are the most susceptible; jaundice and hemorrhage are prominent features of disease.

Human leptospirosis is commonly contracted by contact with organisms present in the urine of infected animals. *The organisms can remain alive for months in contaminated neutral or alkaline waters and wet soils to infect man through skin abrasions or mucous membranes, particularly of the URT.* Infection can also result from direct contact with urine or tissues of infected animals. For example, herdsmen in close contact with infected swine often contract the disease, hence the alternative term "swineherd's disease." *The disease in man is largely an occupational one,* being common among individuals working in water or damp surroundings where rats exist, such as in rice fields, around docks, in mines and in abattoirs. Epidemics have resulted from swimming in waters polluted with urine of infected livestock. In the USA, dogs are a more frequent source of human infection than has been generally realized.

Human leptospirosis is a biphasic systemic disease; its acute phases are characterized by bacteremia and organisms in the cerebrospinal fluid. The disease appears abruptly, after an incubation period of 3 to 30 days, with numerous symptoms, often including severe headache, chills, fever, muscle pain, cough, nausea and vomiting, conjunctival suffusion, cutaneous hyperesthesia and stiff neck. After 4 to 9 days the organisms disappear from the blood and CSF and a remission of 1 to 3 days ensues before the CNS symptoms and Abs characteristic of the second "immune phase" of 1 to 3 days' duration appear. The second phase is often diagnosed as "aseptic meningitis." In rare instances a second relapse occurs during convalescence.

A clinically severe form of the disease with jaundice was described by Weil in 1886 (*Weil's disease*) and later identified as leptospirosis by Inada and Ido (1915), who discovered the etiologic agent. It is seen in about 25% of leptospirosis patients. It appears on about the 3rd to the 6th day of illness and does not peak until the 2nd stage is reached. Hepatic involvement, together with necrosis of renal tubules and serious renal dysfunction, occurs. Widespread hemorrhage from capillaries is observed in various sites including the skin, GI tract, adrenals and lung. Endocarditis and iridocyclitis are sometimes present. *Pretibial fever* (Fort Bragg fever), due to serotype *autumnalis,* was described in 1942. Its distinctive features are splenomegaly and a pretibial rash on about the 4th day of illness. Serum Abs appear after about 1 to 2 weeks of illness and persist for many years. They can be measured by several procedures including agglutination. The immune adherence *phenomenon of Rieckenberg* is of particular interest; when leptospires are sensitized with Ab and C they adhere to RBCs for some unknown reason.

Mortality in leptospirosis, which usually results from renal failure, varies widely with the subject's age, being some 10% in patients under 50 years of age and about 55% in older patients. In jaundiced patients the mortality ranges from 15 to 40%.

Pathogenetic mechanisms in leptospirosis are largely obscure. Although no endotoxin has been described, a cytotoxic protein is produced; this has been reported to be present in greater abundance in culture fluids from virulent than from avirulent strains. A leptospiral *hemolysin* is evidently responsible for intravascular hemolysis and severe anemia. The agents and events responsible for jaundice, azotemia, thrombocytopenia, hypoprothrombinemia and hemorrhage have not been defined.

The mechanisms of acquired immunity to leptospirosis are poorly understood. However, immunity to infection is largely serotype specific and little cross immunity between serotypes occurs. Convalescent serum protects guinea pigs against experimental infection even though the organisms are not readily killed *in vitro* by specific Ab and C. However, there is evidence that neutralizing Abs for the hemolysins of leptospires are formed; these may protect against invasion as well as against other pathologic effects of the organisms, including excessive red cell destruction and anemia. Although phagocytosis has been observed, its possible role in immunity has not been elucidated nor has cellular immunity been evaluated.

Laboratory diagnosis during the first week is based principally on daily blood culture and, if indicated, spinal fluid culture; thereafter urine should be cultured on selective media. Leptospires tend to be present in the blood in small numbers during the first week of disease and subsequently in the urine. Multiplication *in vitro* is slow and several days are required before growth appears. Because of the small numbers of leptospires in blood and their frequent confusion with blood debris, neither the direct smear nor the darkfield procedure is recommended. Providing suitable formalized serotype antigens are available, a demonstrated rise in specific Ab titer late in the course of the disease and during convalescence is of diagnostic significance retrospectively. Animal inoculation is a necessary and useful adjunct or substitute for culture in some instances.

Therapy includes administration of antimicrobial drugs as early as possible in the course of the disease. Unfortunately, early diagnosis is seldom made and treatment after the 5th day is of doubtful value. The agents used include penicillin G and tetracycline congeners. Supportive treatment is highly important. Peritoneal dialysis has been suggested when azotemia develops. No effective antiserum is available.

Prevention of disease rests largely on sanitary measures. Protective vaccination has been proposed for individuals with a high risk of infection.

References

Bryceson, A. D. M., Parry, E. H. O., Perine, P. L., Warrell, D. A., Vukotich, D., and Leithead, C. S.: Louse-borne relapsing fever. Quart. J. Med. New Series *XXXIX*:129, 1969.

Cannefox, G. R.: Immunity to syphilis. Brit. J. Vener. Dis. *41*:260, 1965.

Cockburn, T. A.: Origin of treponematoses. WHO Bull. *24*:221, 1961.

Collart, P., Borel, L. J., and Durel, P.: Spiral organisms persisting after therapy. Brit. J. Vener. Dis. *40*:81, 1964.

Felsenfeld, O.: Borreliae, human relapsing fever and parasite-vector host relationships. Bact. Rev. *29*:46, 1965.

Guthe, T., Ridet, J., Vorst, F., D'Costa, J., and Grab, B.: Methods for surveillance of endemic treponematoses and sero-immunological investigations of "disappearing" disease. WHO Bull. *46*:1, 1972.

Kelley, R.: Cultivation of *Borrelia hermsi*. Science *173*:143, 1971.

Perine, P. L., Weiser, R. S., and Klebanoff, S. J.: Immunity to syphilis. I. Passive transfer in rabbits with hyperimmune serum. Infect. Immun. *8*:787, 1973.

Rice, N. S., Dunlop, E. M., Jones, B. R., Hare, M. J., King, A. J., Rodin, P., Mushin, A., and Wilkinson, A. E.: Demonstration of treponeme-like forms in cases of treated and untreated syphilis. Brit. J. Vener. Dis. 46:1, 1970.

Stokes, J. H., and Beerman, H.: Dermatology and syphilology. Am. J. Med. Sci. 215:461, 1948.

Turner, L. H.: Leptospirosis. Brit. Med. J. 1:199, 1969.

Turner, T. B.: In Infectious Agents and Host Reactions, p. 346, Edited by Stuart Mudd. Philadelphia, W. B. Saunders Co., 1970.

Turner, T. B., Hardy, P., and Newman, B.: Infectivity tests in syphilis. Brit. J. Vener. Dis. 45:183, 1969.

Turner, T. B., and Hollander, D.: Biology of treponematoses. WHO Monograph Series 35, 1957.

Wallace, A. L., and Norins, L. C.: Progress in Clinical Pathology, Vol. II. Edited by Mario Stefanini. New York: Grune & Stratton, Inc., 1969.

WHO Bull. No. 455. Treponematoses Research, 1970.

Wiegand, S. E., Strobel, P. L., and Glassman, L. H.: Electron microscopic anatomy of pathogenic Treponema pallidum. J. Invest. Dermat. 58:186, 1972.

Willcox, R. R.: A world-look at the venereal diseases. Med. Clin. N. Amer. 56:1057, 1972.

Willcox, R. R.: The treponemal evolution. St. John's Hospital Dermatological Society 58:21, 1972.

Willcox, R. R., and Guthe, T.: Treponema pallidum. WHO Bull. Suppl., Vol. 35, 1966.

Wilson, G. S., and Miles, A. A.: Topley and Wilson's Principles of Bacteriology and Immunity, 5th ed. Baltimore: Williams & Wilkins Co., 1964.

Yam, P. A., Miller, N. G., and White, R. J.: A leptospiral factor producing a cytopathic effect on L cells. J. Infect. Dis. 122:310, 1970.

Rickettsia and Coxiella

Members of the genera *Rickettsia* and *Coxiella,* of the family *Rickettsiaceae* (order *Rickettsiales*), are obligate intracellular parasites that usually have arthropods as their natural hosts. Some of them are highly pathogenic for man, an accidental host. The major rickettsial diseases of man and their etiologic agents are listed in Table 33-1. *Coxiella burneti,* an organism closely related to members of the genus *Rickettsia,* is included in the table. It has been classified in a separate genus because, in contrast to the rickettsiae, *Cox. burneti* can survive extracellularly for long periods, and hence is usually transmitted via inhalation of contaminated dusts and not by an arthropod vector.

14

TABLE 33-1
Some Characteristics of the Major Diseases Caused by Rickettsiae

Disease	Etiologic Agent	Transmission to man via:	Reservoir	Symptoms	Case Mortality Rate Untreated	Case Mortality Rate Treated
Epidemic typhus	Rickettsia prowazekii	Body lice	Man	High fever (104°F or more); rash beginning on trunk and spreading peripherally	20% to 70%	Unknown
Endemic murine typhus	R. mooseri	Rats to rat fleas to man	Rat Rat flea	Fever and rash as above; usually less severe than epidemic typhus	5%	< 5%
Rocky Mountain spotted fever (RMSF)	R. rickettsii	Wood ticks or dog ticks to man	Rodents Dogs Dog tick Wood tick	High fever; rash beginning peripherally and spreading to the trunk	5% to 90%	< than untreated
Boutonneuse* disease (Marseilles fever)	R. conori	Dogs to dog ticks to man	Dog Dog tick	Similar to RMSF; characterized by indurated, necrotic lesion at site of infected tick bite and enlarged regional lymph nodes	1%	< 1%
Rickettsial pox	R. akari	House mice to mites to man	House mouse	Vaccinia-like lesion at site of infection by mite; fever, vesicular rash resembling chickenpox	No fatalities reported	No fatalities reported
Tsutsugamushi disease (scrub typhus)	R. orientalis (R. tsutsugamushi)	Wild rodents to mites to man	Wild rodents Mites	Indurated lesion at site of infection by mite; fever, rash, and pneumonitis	1% to 35%	< than untreated
Q Fever	Coxiella burneti	Inhalation of contaminated dusts	Marsupial rats Ticks	Pneumonitis, without a rash	Rarely fatal	Rarely fatal

* An example of a group of tick fevers.

It is apparent from Table 33-1 that the pathogenic members of the genus *Rickettsia* share many characteristics; for example, each of them is transmitted to man by an arthropod vector (lice, fleas, ticks, or mites), and each causes a febrile disease attended with a rash and headache. However, the rickettsioses differ in their severity and in both the type and the distribution of the rash. The cycle of transmission of some of the pathogenic members of the genus *Rickettsia* is also indicated in the table.

In this chapter, *R. prowazekii* will be discussed in greatest detail. Many of its properties apply to the other rickettsiae and to *Cox. burneti*.

Rickettsia
Rickettsia prowazekii and Rickettsia mooseri
(Typhus Fever Group)

A. Medical Perspectives

Rickettsia prowazekii causes epidemic typhus and *R. mooseri* causes endemic typhus. Typhus fever, like certain other infectious diseases, has played a larger part in shaping the history of the world than has any single ruler or even any nation. Epidemics of typhus have been responsible for deciding many battles and campaigns. It is probable that typhus fever was introduced into Spain around 1490. Ferdinand and Isabella, while battling the Moors for possession of Granada, fought a far greater battle with typhus; in one campaign during that war, 3,000 soldiers were killed by the Moors whereas 17,000 died of typhus fever! The disease followed armies of that time, spreading across Europe to the East, and gradually to the North.

One of the most violent epidemics of typhus in all history occurred in Serbia near the start of World War I. This epidemic may well have been a crucial factor in deciding the ultimate outcome of the war. In less than 6 months, over 150,000 people died of typhus, including about a third of all the physicians of Serbia. The attacking Austrians, although in an excellent position to sweep through Serbia and establish a battleline against Russia, knew better than to enter the area and were delayed for 6 crucial months until the epidemic subsided.

Russia bore the brunt of epidemics of typhus and a number of other infectious diseases during the turbulent years of World War I. At least 25 million cases of typhus fever occurred in Russia during the years 1917 to 1921, resulting in 2.5 to 3 million deaths. Although subsequent outbreaks of typhus have occurred, they have not been of such magnitude.

The striking coincidence of wars and typhus epidemics is not accidental, but is simply due to the fact that *the rickettsiae of epidemic typhus are transmitted via the bite of the body louse,* the bane of military personnel in the field. Whenever conditions of crowding and poor hygiene (lack of opportunity to bathe and launder clothing) permit body lice to proliferate on man, typhus is liable to appear. Typhus occurs frequently in certain parts of the world, being endemic in some countries; however, it occurs only rarely in the USA.

B. Physical and Chemical Structure

Rickettsiae are tiny (about 0.3 to 0.6 μm), gram-negative coccobacilli. They are pleomorphic and may also take the form of rods or filaments; they occur singly, in pairs, or short chains. The rickettsiae lack flagella and are nonmotile. Giemsa or Macchiavello stains are commonly used to demonstrate them; the organisms appear blue with Giemsa and red with the Macchiavello stain. Their typical gram-negative bacterial cell walls contain muramic acid and endotoxin-like materials. Both group-specific and type-specific Ags are demonstrable by the CF test.

C. Genetics

It is probable that these obligate intracellular parasites have evolved from free-living bacteria that gradually lost certain metabolic capabilities essential for an independent existence. Although they share antigenic determinants with some strains of the genus *Proteus,* there is no evidence to indicate that the two organisms are genetically related.

D. Extracellular Products

Hemolysins are produced by some rickettsiae; however, they lyse sheep and rabbit but not human erythrocytes.

E. Culture

Rickettsiae grow readily in the yolk sac of embryonated chicken eggs. They can also be propagated in rapidly growing cultures of cells. *Rickettsia quintana* (the cause of trench fever) can be grown on blood agar in the absence of host cells. Under optimal conditions the generation time of rickettsiae is about 18 hours.

Although rickettsiae have lost some of their metabolic capabilities, they have retained the capacity to carry out certain energy-yielding reactions (e.g., oxidative phosphorylation), and to synthesize proteins from amino acids. It has been postulated that *they possess an extremely permeable cytoplasmic membrane that permits them to utilize essential preformed nutrients from the host cell;* however, it is possible that this apparent "leakiness" may be an artifact caused by laboratory manipulation of the organisms.

F. Resistance to Physical and Chemical Agents

The rickettsiae are moderately susceptible to drying, heat and most common disinfectants. However, they can survive in dried arthropod feces for months.

G. Experimental Models

Guinea pigs and mice can be infected with rickettsiae, but at present the trend is toward utilizing *in vitro* models, or infected embryonated chicken eggs, to study the interaction of rickettsiae with host cells. Development of these organisms within arthropod hosts is also the subject of investigation.

H. Infections in Man

Man is the only natural host of R. prowazekii, the etiologic agent of epidemic typhus fever. The body louse, *Pediculus corporis,* is the usual vector, although other species of *Pediculus* (especially *P. capitis*) can sometimes transmit the infection from man to man. The body louse lives in clothing, kept warm by body heat. Several times a day it takes a meal of blood from its human host. While feeding, the louse defecates; because the bite is irritating, the host usually scratches and rubs louse feces into the open wound. If the louse is infected with *R. prowazekii,* the host readily becomes infected. Conversely, if the host is infected the feeding louse becomes infected. *The rickettsiae multiply within cells of the intestinal tract of the louse,* and huge numbers are excreted in the feces. As Zinsser has pointed out in his erudite account of typhus fever, "Rats, Lice and History," the louse fares worse than man. In fact, *R. prowazekii* infections are invariably fatal for lice within 1 to 2 weeks; this is in contrast to most rickettsial infections of arthropods, which do not lead to disease of the vector.

A latent form of *R. prowazekii* infection exists in man known as *Brill's disease.* This mild form of typhus fever does not produce the characteristic rash, but leads to a specific IgG Ab response of the anamnestic type. The patient with Brill's disease represents activation of an inapparent infection with *R. prowazekii* that may have been latent for many years. Obviously, patients with Brill's disease may initiate new epidemics of typhus fever if they become louse-infested.

Typhus fever is often fatal, and lice feeding on patients who die of typhus are heavily infected. Soon after death, as the body temperature decreases, these lice leave the corpse and seek a new host to provide warmth and nourishment. Conditions of crowding favor the spread of typhus, because crowding provides ideal opportunities for new hosts to become infested, and subsequently infected, before the lice succumb to the rickettsiae.

The symptoms of epidemic typhus fever appear 5 days to 3 weeks after exposure to infected lice. For several days the disease resembles influenza, with high fever (103° to 104°F or higher), chills, severe headache, and depression. On the 4th or 5th day after onset, the *characteristic rash appears on the trunk and gradually extends peripherally.* The original pink spots become purplish and finally brown as the rash fades. The face is usually free of rash, and no spots are seen on the mucous membranes. Cough and CNS manifestations are not uncommon. The name "typhus" is derived from a Greek word meaning "hazy," because of the frequent mental haziness and delirium that occur.

Endemic typhus, or murine typhus, has many of the characteristics of epidemic typhus, but is generally less severe. The causative organism, *R. mooseri,* produces only inapparent latent infections in *the natural rat host and in the fleas that are vectors* for its transmission from rat to rat, and from rat to man.

I. Mechanisms of Pathogenicity

The rickettsiae contain endotoxin-like substances that, in large doses, kill laboratory animals within a few hours. However, rickettsial toxins differ from most endotoxins in that they incite the production of protective antiserum. The fever, rash and intravascular coagulation produced during the rickettsioses suggest that rickettsial endotoxins are important in the pathogenesis of these diseases.

The usual site of rickettsial proliferation in infected hosts is *within endothelial cells of small blood vessels. In vitro* experiments have shown that the organisms of some species are pinocytosed or phagocytized. The rickettsiae must be viable in order to penetrate endothelial cells. After penetration of the host cell, they *cause the disruption of phagosomal membranes* and thereafter multiply within the cytoplasm.

J. Mechanisms of Immunity

The results of both clinical experience and animal studies suggest that 7S IgG Abs protect against rickettsial infection. Perhaps they inhibit the entrance of organisms into host endothelial cells. Specific Abs of the class IgG that protect guinea pigs against challenge with *R. prowazekii* are, at least in part, directed against soluble Ags associated with cell-wall endotoxins.

Peritoneal macrophages of immunized animals phagocytize the specific organisms more rapidly than do normal macrophages, even in the absence of immune serum. It is possible that more efficient uptake of rickettsiae by "immune phagocytes," plus Ab-mediated inhibition of penetration into endothelial cells, may lead to destruction of the organisms, by macrophages and/or by humoral factors.

In typhus, as in most infectious diseases, early Abs are predominately of the IgM class and late Abs are of the class IgG. During latent infection, the Ab response is evidently maintained to some extent, as shown by the prompt production of 7S but not 19S Abs during Brill's disease. The location of rickettsiae during latent disease and the means by which they persist and evade host defenses have not been determined. The observation that physiologic resting forms remain unchanged within cultured cells over a period of days to months suggests that similar inactive, resting organisms may persist within host cells *in vivo*.

K. Laboratory Diagnosis

Although rickettsiae can often be cultured from clinical specimens from infected patients and animals or from vectors, laboratory personnel run high risk of becoming infected in the course of carrying out the procedures involved. The hazards of working with rickettsiae in the laboratory are emphasized by the designation, *Rickettsia prowazekii,* so named for Howard Ricketts and Stanislaus von Prowazek, two investigators who died from infections contracted while working with these organisms. Consequently, serologic testing of the patient's serum is commonly used for laboratory diagnosis, rather than the isolation of rickettsiae.

Rising titers of Abs against various strains of *Proteus vulgaris* in the Weil-Felix reaction serve as indicators of the nature of the infecting agent (Table 33-2). Specific C-F or agglutination tests with suspensions of Ags prepared from yolk-sac cultures of rickettsia are also useful procedures. A rise in titer of specific Abs in the patient's serum during the course of the disease serves to identify the infecting species of rickettsiae with reasonable certainty.

TABLE 33-2
The Weil-Felix Reaction

Serum from Patient with:	OX-19	OX-2	OX-K
Epidemic typhus	++++	+	0
Brill-Zinnser disease	0*	0*	0
Murine typhus	++++	+	0
Scrub typhus	0	0	+++
Spotted fever group	{ ++++ { +	{ + { ++++	0
Q fever	0	0	0
Rickettsial pox	0	0	0

* Variable, often negative.
From "Manual of Clinical Microbiology," Blair, J. E., Lennette, E. H., and Truant, J. P.: American Society of Microbiology, Bethesda, 1970, p. 606.

L. Therapy

Tetracyclines and chloramphenicol are therapeutically effective against all of the rickettsiae. Since the organisms are inhibited but not killed, treatment should be continued for 4 to 5 days after the fever subsides.

Sulfonamides should not be used for treating the rickettsioses because they enhance growth of the organisms and promote the disease process.

M. Reservoirs of Infection

The reservoirs of rickettsial disease are indicated by Table 33-1.

N. Control of Disease Transmission

Rickettsial diseases are best prevented by interrupting the cycle of infection. Epidemic typhus depends on transmission by lice; therefore elimination of lice prevents its spread. Endemic murine typhus requires rats and rat fleas for its transmission from rat to rat and rat to man; hence the elimination of either the rat or the flea, or both, will prevent transmission of the disease to man. In areas where infected rats are known to exist, insecticides should first be used to get rid of the flea vectors in the environment before using rat poisons. If rats are killed first, their infected fleas will quickly seek man as a source of nourishment and will thus intensify spread of the infection.

Vaccines of formalin-killed rickettsiae prepared from cultures in yolk sacs of chick embryos are available for immunization against typhus and certain other rickettsioses. The typhus vaccine contains both *R. prowazekii* and *R. mooseri*. It lessens the severity and mortality of typhus fevers, but does not decrease their incidence. Rickettsial vaccines are recommended only for those at high risk of contracting the rickettsioses.

Rickettsia rickettsii, Rickettsia conori and *Rickettsia akari* (Spotted Fever Group)

Rocky Mountain spotted fever caused by *R. rickettsii* is not uncommon in the USA. About 200 to 500 cases are reported annually to the USPHS. The disease may occur wherever the species of *Dermacentor* ticks that serve as the vectors for *R. rickettsii* are found. Although numerous cases are reported from the Rocky Mountain area, Figure 33-1 shows that the disease is most prevalent in the eastern USA.

Various rodents, dogs, and other mammals can serve as reservoirs of the spotted fevers—Rocky Mountain spotted fever and boutonneuse fever. Ticks feeding on contaminated blood become systemically infected; their ovaries permit rickettsial growth and infected ova transmit the organisms from one generation of ticks to another. Growth of rickettsiae in the sali-

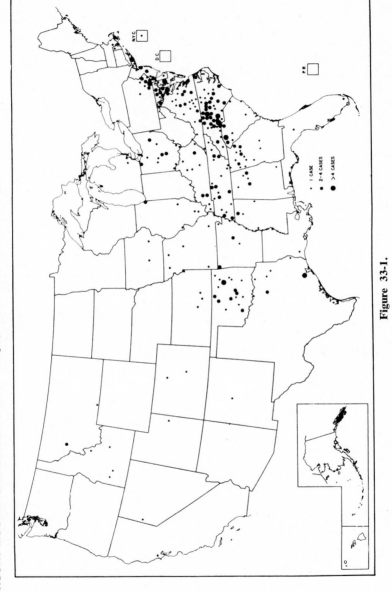

ROCKY MOUNTAIN SPOTTED FEVER – Geographic Distribution, United States, 1971

Figure 33-1.

vary glands of the tick and excretion of the organisms in saliva permit the injection of large doses of rickettsiae into the skin of the human host when the tick feeds.

The *spotted fevers* have a relatively short incubation period of 3 to 12 days, and an onset similar to that of typhus fever or influenza, with high fever and chills. The rash appears earlier than in typhus, becoming apparent on the 2nd to 5th day of illness. *The eruption begins peripherally, on the feet, hands, or forehead, and spreads to the trunk.* The fever usually lasts for 2 to 3 weeks and subsides gradually. In fatal cases, death most often occurs during the 2nd week of illness. Major symptoms of the spotted fevers and the related rickettsial pox are briefly described in Table 33-1.

It has been shown that avirulent strains of *R. rickettsii* fail to attach to human host cells, and thus cannot infect.

Studies on the virulence of *R. rickettsii* in guinea pigs have shown that organisms growing in tick hosts are avirulent until after a blood meal is taken. The change from avirulence to virulence has also been studied *in vitro*. It depends on utilization of factors from host RBCs, and occurs at 35°C but not at low temperatures.

Control of infection by these organisms includes clearing brush where ticks and mites propagate; in addition, the use of insecticides and rodent control are excellent measures for preventing the transmission of some of these rickettsioses. Ticks should be watched for and promptly removed from the body. A period of several hours is required after attachment of the tick before virulent rickettsiae are passed to the host; thus, prompt removal of ticks may prevent transmission of infection.

Rickettsia orientalis (Scrub typhus)

Rickettsia orientalis (*R. tsutsugamushi*) is the cause of a typhus-like disease known either as tsutsugamushi fever or scrub typhus. The disease is transmitted by the bite of a mite. It differs from epidemic typhus fever in that a punched-out eschar is commonly present at the location of the bite. A black scab marks the site of the eschar. Transovarial transmission of the rickettsiae occurs in certain mites and allows them to serve as reservoirs of scrub typhus. Tsutsugamushi fever occurs over a wide area in the Asiatic Pacific region, including Japan, Korea, Formosa, Malaya, Burma, New Guinea and the Philippines.

Coxiella

Coxiella burneti is the cause of Q fever, which differs from the rickettsial diseases in several ways. Originally described in Australia, the disease results from infection with *Cox. burneti,* which has the marsupial rat as a natural host. Ticks, which can also serve as reservoirs for *Cox. burneti,* are the vectors responsible for transmitting the organisms among cattle and sheep. Infected domestic animals disseminate huge numbers of the organisms in secretions and excreta; these organisms are much more resistant to adverse conditions than are most of the rickettsiae. The organism not only survives drying but also is more resistant to heat than most pathogens. Therefore, the recommended times and temperatures for pasteurization of milk have been increased to 71.5°C (161°F) for 15 seconds to assure killing of coxiellae.

Human Q fever is usually contracted via inhaled contaminated dusts, often from barns or animal sheds. The disease presents as a *febrile pneumonitis, but, in contrast to most rickettsial diseases, a rash is not usually seen and the disease is rarely fatal.* It has been shown that Abs may persist for as long as 7 years after an attack of Q fever, suggesting that *Cox. burneti* may become latent within immunized hosts.

Coxiella burneti is morphologically identical to the rickettsiae. In nature, the organism possesses a surface polysaccharide coat (Phase I) that is antiphagocytic. Following adaptation to growth in the chick embryo, this surface Ag is lost; these organisms are known as Phase II strains.

Following entrance into cells by pinocytosis or phagocytosis, *Cox. burneti* organisms may not disrupt the phagosomal membrane, but, instead, multiply within the phagosome as do most intracellular bacteria. There is evidence that coxiellae interfere with the regulation of energy metabolism by host cells.

References

Cohn, Z. A., Bozeman, F. M., Campbell, J. M., Humphries, J. W., and Sawyer, T. K.: Study on growth of rickettsiae. V. Penetration of *Rickettsia tsutsugamushi* into mammalian cells *in vitro.* J. Exp. Med. *109*:271, 1959.

Downs, C. M.: Phagocytosis of *Coxiella burneti,* Phase I and Phase II by peritoneal monocytes from normal and immune guinea pigs and mice. Zentralbl. Bakteriol. *206*:329, 1968.

Fiset, P., and Ormsbee, R. A.: The antibody response to antigens of *Coxiella burneti.* Zentralbl. Bakteriol. *206*:321, 1968.

Gilford, J. H., and Price, W. H.: Virulent-avirulent conversions of *Rickettsia rickettsii in vitro.* Proc. Nat. Acad. Sci. *41*:870, 1955.

Murphy, A. M., and Field, P. R.: The persistence of complement-fixing antibodies to Q fever (*Coxiella burneti*) after infection. Med. J. Aust. *1*:1148, 1970.

Musher, D. M.: Q fever: A common treatable cause of endemic non-bacterial pneumonia. JAMA *204*:863, 1968.

Paretsky, D.: Biochemistry of rickettsiae and their infected hosts, with special reference to *Coxiella burneti.* Zentralbl. Bakteriol. *206*:283, 1968.

Paretsky, D., and Stueckemann, J.: Chemical and biochemical changes in sub-cellular fractions of guinea pig liver during infection with *Coxiella burneti.* J. Bact. *102*: 334, 1970.

Wisseman, C. L.: Some biological properties of rickettsiae pathogenic for man. Zentralbl. Bakteriol. *206*:299, 1968.

Chlamydia

The etiologic agents of trachoma and inclusion conjunctivitis (the TRIC agents) and of psittacosis and lymphogranuloma venereum (the PLGV agents) are members of the family *Chlamydiaceae* and the order *Rickettsiales*. They are gram-negative, nonmotile, obligately intracellular bacteria that in some ways resemble organisms of the genus *Rickettsia*. However, rickettsiae are generally transmitted by arthropods and chlamydiae are not.

For many years the chlamydiae were considered to be viruses because they are small enough to pass through bacterial filters, are obligate intracellular parasites, and appear as inclusion bodies within the host cell. Nevertheless, it is now well established that *the chlamydiae are bacteria and not viruses*. They contain DNA, RNA and muramic acid, are susceptible to certain antibacterial agents and have many of the metabolic characteristics of other bacteria. These tiny, coccoid organisms are thought to be derived from more complex bacteria that, in the course of evolution, became adapted to obligate parasitism by losing metabolic capabilities that are not essential for an intracellular existence.

Many chlamydiae are important animal pathogens; however, the following discussion will be limited principally to those that are pathogenic for man.

Although it has been proposed that the family *Chlamydiaceae* be divided into 5 genera, the current consensus is that differences between the 5 groups are small. Therefore, at present they are all included within the genus *Chlamydia,* formerly called *Bedsonia,* and the diseases that they cause are referred to as chlamydioses. Although species designations are subject to change, there is general agreement that the chlamydiae can be classified into 2 subgroups: A and B. Group A includes the agents of trachoma, inclusion conjunctivitis (IC), lymphogranuloma venereum (LGV) and some others. These organisms induce the formation of compact, glycogen-containing inclusions in the cytoplasm of infected cells. All of the members of Group A are inhibited by sulfadiazine. The agents that cause psittacosis (or ornithosis), and certain organisms of little medical importance, comprise Group B.

Group A Chlamydiae
TRIC Agents

A. Medical Perspectives

Trachoma is seen only occasionally in the USA, principally among the Indians of the Southwest. On a worldwide scale, however, the WHO estimates that at least 400 million people currently have trachoma, and 20 million of these have been left blind. *Inclusion conjunctivitis* is also common, but is of less consequence since it does not lead to blindness.

Tremendous research efforts are being made to learn more about the TRIC agents, commonly called *Ch. trachomatis*. High priority has been given to efforts to develop effective vaccines, particularly one that protects against trachoma. Until such a vaccine becomes available, or until adequate sanitation and hygiene are universal, trachoma will probably remain the most common cause of blindness.

B. Physical and Chemical Structure

The infectious forms of chlamydiae are spherical cells as small as some of the larger viruses, ranging from 0.2 to 0.3 μm in diameter. They are gram-negative or gram-variable, but are more readily visible when stained with basic dyes, such as Giemsa or Macchiavello stains.

Once within an appropriate host cell the infectious forms enlarge to produce round or irregular-shaped *initial bodies* or *reticulate bodies* varying from approximately 0.5 to 1.0 μm in diameter. Experimental evidence suggests that typical bacterial cell-wall mucopeptide is either absent or defective in the reticulate bodies.

Chlamydial cells contain heat-stable, group-specific Ags common to all chlamydiae. These Ags appear to be lipopolysaccharides, and can be detected by C-F or other tests. Species-specific, heat-stable, protein Ags are also present on the cell-wall surface and are associated with toxic activities of the organisms. A single strain may contain more than one specific Ag. Antibodies against species-specific Ags neutralize the infectivity of the chlamydiae and their toxicity for mice.

C. Genetics

Antibiotic-resistant mutant strains of chlamydiae have been selected in the laboratory.

D. Extracellular Products

Hemagglutinins (HA) are secreted into the medium during chlamydial growth. They are group-specific and appear to consist of a complex of lecithin, DNA and protein. Hemagglutinins clump erythrocytes of mice, hamsters and chickens. Hemagglutination is inhibited by specific Abs against HA.

E. Culture

All of the chlamydiae share a unique life cycle (Fig. 34-1). The small spherical *infectious particles* (*elementary bodies*) enter host cells by phagocytosis. Infectious particles stain purple with Giemsa and red with Macchiavello stain. After a lag period of about 20 hours, the engulfed infectious particles begin to reorganize and to change to the larger, much less infectious initial bodies. These bodies stain blue with Giemsa stain. During the logarithmic phase of growth, extending from 20 to 25 hours after infection of the host cell, the initial bodies divide repeatedly by binary fission to yield numerous small *infectious particles*. Although the reasons for changes from small to large to small forms of chlamydiae are not understood, it is possible that metabolic activities necessary for cellular multiplication demand the larger, more active cell form. At the end of the logarithmic phase, infected cells contain a mixture of the large *initial bodies* and numerous small *infectious particles* in a membrane-bound *inclusion body* that stains dark purple with Giemsa stain. A stationary phase follows, during which more of the bacteria assume the smaller, more infectious form. Finally, by 48 hours or earlier, the host cell lyses, liberating *infectious particles* to begin the cycle again.

One of the major reasons that the chlamydiae are obligate intracellular parasites is that they have little or no ability to generate energy, but must depend on the host cell for energy. During their intracellular existence the organisms possess unusually permeable cytoplasmic membranes that allow the uptake of many host cell metabolites, including ATP.

Most of the chlamydiae can be cultured readily in the yolk sac of the embryonated egg, in cell cultures, or in experimental animals. Currently *Ch. trachomatis* can be grown in large quantities only in embryonated chicken eggs.

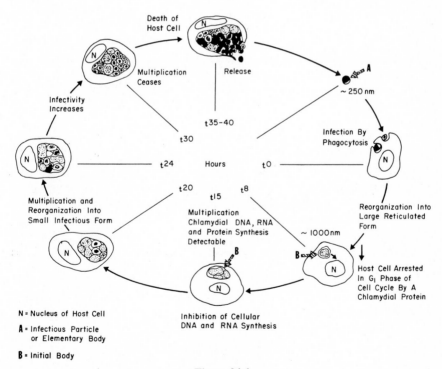

Figure 34-1.

F.   Resistance to Physical and Chemical Agents

Extracellular chlamydiae are readily inactivated. At room temperature or above, most strains lose infectivity within 8 hours to several days, depending on the strain and the nature of the suspending medium. Many strains are inactivated within 5 to 10 minutes at 56°C; however, they are resistant to freezing and remain viable indefinitely at −70°C.

Exposure to high and low pH, 0.1% formalin, 0.5% phenol and other disinfectants rapidly inactivates chlamydiae. For example, *Ch. trachomatis* is killed after 1 to 30 minutes of contact with appropriate concentrations of alcohols, ether, chlorine, iodine, permanganate, formalin, acids or bases. Nevertheless, it remains infective for 2 to 3 days at room temperature in unchlorinated tap water.

G.   Experimental Models

Only man and subhuman primates are susceptible to natural infection with *Ch. trachomatis;* a variety of monkeys and apes are used as experimental animal models.

H.   Infections in Man

Trachoma is usually transmitted by direct human contact, and most often occurs under crowded conditions with associated poor sanitation and personal hygiene. The organisms live only *within epithelial cells of the conjunctivae.* The lesions consist of hyperplastic nodules on the inner aspects of the eyelids. Conjunctivae infected with the organism readily become secondarily infected. Vascularization and scarring of the cornea, leading to blindness, can occur unless treatment is started early.

Inclusion conjunctivitis is much less severe than trachoma; it rarely leads to blindness. Although the organism can cause venereal disease in adults, asymptomatic infections of the genital tract probably are the usual reservoir of the IC agent. Man is the only natural host of the organism of IC. The disease may occur in newborn infants who acquire the organisms at birth from the infected genital tract of the mother. This form of the disease resembles gonorrheal conjunctivitis (*ophthalmia neonatorum*). In the newborn, IC becomes apparent 5 to 12 days after birth. In all age groups the infection is self-limiting, usually within several weeks; however, it may be months before it clears completely.

I.   Mechanisms of Pathogenicity

The mechanisms of pathogenicity of *Ch. trachomatis* are shared by other chlamydiae. Host cells die as a result of chlamydial infection. The phagocytized intracellular organisms multiply over a period of about 2 days before the host cell ruptures and the bacteria are released. Host cell death would appear to result from "energy parasitism" by the chlamydiae, which usurp and utilize substances that the cell needs for survival.

Strains of chlamydiae vary greatly in their virulence, but the basis for this variation is also not understood.

The disease process often depends in part on the host response to the infection. For example, trachoma seems to be, at least in part, a hypersensitivity disease, with pannus formation representing an allergic response to chlamydial Ags. In addition, secondary infection in tissues damaged by chlamydial growth may account for part of the disease process.

The cell walls of chlamydiae have toxic properties; injection of cell-wall material is lethal for mice. The contribution of this toxin to human disease has not been determined.

J. Mechanisms of Immunity

Immunity following human infections with *Ch. trachomatis* or other chlamydiae is relative and probably represents an "infection immunity"; cellular immunity may be of primary importance. Although humoral Abs are sometimes demonstrable for many years following recovery from disease, there is no clear correlation between the presence or titer of Abs and protection against disease.

Recurrences of chlamydial diseases are common, suggesting that immunity is easily overcome by minor changes in the host-parasite balance that permit the persisting organisms or newly encountered ones to escape the restraints imposed by the immune response.

Age is an important factor in resistance to the chlamydioses of certain animals. The young of most species appear to be more susceptible than older subjects. For example, mice are most susceptible to infection at about 3 weeks of age and become increasingly resistant with age. It could be postulated that infection with avirulent chlamydiae that share group-specific Ags with virulent strains affords some degree of cross-protection; however, this is mere speculation.

In recent years, extensive attempts have been under way to develop an immunization procedure that will protect against trachoma, but these have been attended with only moderate success. A vaccine prepared with large numbers of formalin-inactivated chlamydial elementary bodies in an adjuvant emulsion protects monkeys against experimental infection, and the protection is strain-specific. Killed vaccines prepared with aluminum hydroxide adjuvant were given field trials in preschool children in Taiwan; the incidence of trachoma was reduced by 60% for about 2 years, but by 6 years the incidence was the same in the immunized and control groups.

Efforts to develop a safe and effective vaccine are continuing. It would seem that eventual success will depend on a better understanding of the relative roles that cellular, humoral and hypersensitivity responses play in overall immunity.

K. Laboratory Diagnosis

Epithelial cells from conjunctivae of patients infected with TRIC agents usually contain the bacteria, which can be demonstrated by fluorescent Ab techniques, or grown either in the yolk sac of embryonated eggs or in cell cultures. Serologic methods are commonly used to identify chlamydiae that grow in embryonated eggs or in mice.

Antibodies may be present in the sera of infected patients, and a *rise in titer* is demonstrable during the course of the disease. Strain-specific Abs against protein-cell wall Ags are associated with protection against infection, as can be shown in a mouse-protection test. Antibodies against both common Ags and strain-specific Ags are useful in diagnosis.

L. Therapy

Infections with chlamydiae respond to treatment with various antibacterial agents. As a rule, infections with the TRIC agents usually respond to either sulfonamides or tetracyclines.

Antibiotic therapy may overcome the disease but may allow the persistence of some chlamydiae within cells, thus leading to a *carrier state* that can last for years. Carriers are also frequent among untreated persons who have developed enough immunity to suppress growth of the organisms, but not enough to destroy all of the intracellular bacteria completely.

M. Reservoirs of Infection

Man is the principal reservoir for the TRIC agents that are parasitic for primates only.

N. Control of Disease Transmission

Trachoma and IC can be prevented, in part, by good hygiene. At present, immunization procedures remain in the experimental stages. Venereal infections with the agent of IC depend on avoidance of sexual contact with infected individuals.

LGV Agent

Lymphogranuloma venereum is endemic in the southern USA; although it occurs worldwide, its incidence is greatest in tropical and subtropical climates. It ranks 3rd in incidence among the venereal diseases. Many of the characteristics of the LGV agent are shared with the TRIC agents (see appropriate sections above).

The disease LGV is transmitted by venereal contact and may pass unnoticed in the early stages of infection. After an incubation period of 1 to 2 weeks, a *painless herpes-like lesion appears at the site of infection,* usually in the genital tract. This lesion is self-limiting and soon heals. Enlarged and tender lymph nodes become apparent from 1 week to 2 months after the initial lesion heals. These so-called *"venereal buboes" represent a granulomatous response* to the infecting organisms, which frequently results in scarring and consequent obstruction of lymphatic vessels. The scarring, in turn, leads to various symptoms, depending on the site of the draining lymph nodes. For example, obstruction of the genital tract or rectum may occur.

Although the mechanisms of pathogenicity have not been fully elucidated, it is known that the granulomatous response of the host and consequent formation of scar tissue are responsible for some of the more serious complications of the disease, such as obstructions.

Cell-culture methods are used to isolate the LGV agent from clinical specimens. A rise in Ab titer during the disease is also useful in diagnosis.

The *Frei reaction* (a skin test), which measures delayed sensitivity to the infecting chlamydiae, becomes demonstrable about 6 weeks after infection and usually remains positive for life, indicating that latent infection persists.

Either sulfonamides or tetracyclines are usually effective for treating LGV.

Group B Chlamydiae

Psittacosis Agent

A.   Medical Perspectives

Diseases caused by the psittacosis agent are widespread. Psittacosis, also known as ornithosis (when transmitted by other than psittacine birds) and as parrot fever, occurs in many parts of the world. Cases occur in the USA, especially among workers in the poultry industry and others exposed to infected birds. Even with laws designed to prevent importation of infected animals, the disease will undoubtedly continue to occur in the USA because it is impossible to eliminate avian carriers.

B through G.

Many of the characteristics of the psittacosis agents are shared with the TRIC agents and reference should be made to the corresponding sections above.

H. Infections in Man

Psittacosis-ornithosis organisms, often called *Ch. psittaci,* are natural parasites of parrots and many other kinds of birds; *they infect man as an accidental host.* The organisms can persist within the cells of healthy birds or man to cause a carrier state for years. *Chlamydia psittaci* is shed in excretions such as bird droppings and respiratory secretions of man. Infection is transmitted by the inhalation of dried bird droppings, or, in direct man-to-man infection, by respiratory secretion droplets. Consequently, human psittacosis is chiefly a lung disease. The causative organisms enter the respiratory tract directly and grow there during the incubation period of 1 to 3 weeks. Although the human disease is often mild, it can be severe and fatalities are not infrequent. Chills, fever and headache are common; atypical pneumonia is often revealed by x-ray examination even in asymptomatic patients. *Chlamydia psittaci has a predilection for reticuloendothelial cells of the host,* and may often be found in Kupffer cells and splenic macrophages of infected animals.

I. Mechanisms of Pathogenicity

The mechanisms of pathogenicity of *Ch. psittaci* resemble those of the TRIC agents. In infections with *Ch. psittaci,* host responses also influence the disease process.

J. Mechanisms of Immunity

See Section J, page 423.

K. Laboratory Diagnosis

See Section K, page 424.

L. Therapy

Psittacosis is most successfully treated with the tetracyclines; sulfonamides and streptomycin are usually not effective.

M. Reservoirs of Infection

The psittacosis-ornithosis agents have a broad host range and are able to infect many kinds of birds and mammals that constitute the reservoirs of infection.

N. Control of Disease Transmission

Psittacosis was infrequent in this country and many other parts of the world before 1929 and 1930, when a pandemic of some 300 cases was reported in the USA and 11 other countries. Parrots and other birds from tropical countries were identified as the source of the pandemic; since then their importation has been strictly regulated. Many kinds of birds carry *Ch. psittaci* throughout their lifetimes, hence it is virtually impossible to eliminate avian carriers. For example, turkeys are a frequent source of infection. Birds that are obviously ill with ornithosis should be destroyed.

References

Chlamydial infection. Brit. J. Vener. Dis. *48*:416, 1972.

Editorial: Chlamydiae and genital infections. Lancet *1*:703, 1973.

Ford, D. K., and McCandlish, L.: Isolation of humoral genital TRIC agents in non-gonococcal urethritis and Reiter's disease by an irradiated cell culture method. Brit. J. Vener. Dis. *47*:196, 1971.

Gordon, F. B., and Quan, A. L.: Isolation of *Chlamydia trachomatis* from the human genital tract by cell culture: a summary. *In* Trachoma and Allied Diseases. Edited by R. L. Nichols. Amsterdam and New York, Excerpta Medica, 1970.

Grayston, J. T.: Immunization against trachoma. *In* First International Conference on Vaccine against Viral and Rickettsial Diseases of Man. PAHO Publication *147*:546, 1967.

Jones, B. R.: Advances and prospects in the study of certain diseases due to infections by subgroup A *Chlamydia*. Brit. J. Vener. Dis. *48*:13, 1972.

Schacter, J., Rose, L., and Meyer, K. F.: The venereal nature of inclusion conjunctivitis. Amer. J. Epidemiol. *85*:445, 1966.

Stortz, J.: Chlamydia and Chlamydia-induced Diseases. Springfield, Illinois, Charles C Thomas, 1971.

Woolridge, R. L., Grayston, J. T., Chang, I. H., Wang, C. Y., and Cheng, K. H.: Long-term follow-up of the initial (1959-1960) trachoma vaccine field trial on Taiwan. Amer. J. Ophthalmol. *63*:1650, 1967.

The Actinomycetes

A few species of the genera *Actinomyces* and *Nocardia,* of the order *Actinomycetales,* are pathogenic for man. The taxonomic relationship of these and some other medically important members of the order *Actinomycetales* is indicated in Table 35-1. Species of the genus *Streptomyces* rarely cause disease but are of medical importance because several important antibiotics are produced by various members of this genus. Members of all of these genera share many properties with the mycobacteria, which belong to the same order. A common form of pustular dermatitis of cattle, sheep, horses and certain other animals, called *streptotrichosis,* is caused by another member of this order, namely, *Dermatophilus congolensis.* Aside from its importance as an animal pathogen, *Dermatophilus congolensis* has been occasionally implicated as the cause of a similar disease in man. Because the disease resembles a staphylococcal infection, and responds to the antibiotics used to treat staphylococcosis, it is possible that streptotrichosis may, in fact, be more common in man than is presently realized.

Traditionally, actinomycetes have been referred to as fungi, because they bear some resemblance to mycotic agents and often cause diseases resembling the mycoses. However, it is clearly established that the actinomycetes are bacteria. Consequently, they are known as *pseudomycetes,* in distinction to the true fungi or *eumycetes.*

TABLE 35-1

Taxonomic Relationship of Medically Important Genera of the Order *Actinomycetales*

Family	Genus
Actinomycetaceae	*Actinomyces*
	Nocardia
Streptomycetaceae	*Streptomyces*
Mycobacteriaceae	*Mycobacterium*
Dermatophilaceae	*Dermatophilus*

Three major diseases are caused by actinomycetes. One of these, *mycetoma,* is also produced by a variety of species of eumycetes, and will be discussed in Chapter 38. The other two, *actinomycosis* and *nocardiosis,* will be considered in this chapter.

Actinomyces israelii

A. Medical Perspectives

Actinomycosis was first described in 1877 in cattle and was given the aptly descriptive name of "lumpy jaw." *Actinomyces bovis* was found to be the causative agent. Soon it was discovered that a similar disease in man results from infection with *Actinomyces israelii*. This organism is part of the *anaerobic normal flora* of man and has not been isolated from other sources. Thus, human actinomycosis may occur in any geographic location. Infection usually follows an abrogation of normal defenses, particularly by trauma, that allows the bacteria to become established in tissues. It is probable that actinomycosis will continue to occur with the same low frequency as it has in the past; alternatively, increased use of immunosuppressive therapy could conceivably result in an increase in its incidence.

B. Physical and Chemical Structure

Actinomyces israelii is pleomorphic. It may appear as slender, branching filaments 0.5 to 1.0 μm in diameter, as diphtheroid-like rods, or as bacillary or coccoid forms. The organisms are gram-positive, non-acid-fast, nonsporing, nonencapsulated and nonmotile.

When growing in pus, *A. israelii* often forms small colonies of radiating filaments surrounded with eosinophilic material of host origin. The yellowish color of these colonies prompted the name *sulfur granules.* The name *actinomycetes* was derived from the ray-like appearance of the filaments in the granules.

Actinomycetes possess bacterial mucopeptide in their cell walls. In addition, they have all the other properties of procaryotic cells (Chapter 2). The formation of hyphal-like filaments is responsible for their being confused with true fungi; however, the filaments of actinomycetes are more slender than typical hyphae of eumycetes.

Actinomyces israelii is difficult to maintain through repeated subcultures; the Ags of cultured organisms may differ from the Ags of organisms grown *in vivo*.

C. Extracellular Products

Although actinomycetes produce many extracellular products, there is little evidence available concerning these substances or the roles that they may possibly play in pathogenesis and immunity.

D. Culture

Clinical specimens often contain "sulfur" granules, which should be separated from surrounding material and crushed before being added to culture media. Since the organism is anaerobic, a good culture medium is thioglycollate broth in which growth occurs in the form of small "cotton balls." Cultures on solid media, such as brain heart infusion agar (with or without added blood), must be incubated under anaerobic conditions (e.g., in a Brewer anaerobic jar). Optimal growth occurs at 30° to 37°C. Compared with many bacteria, growth is slow, and colonies do not appear before 2 to 5 days of incubation. Other anaerobic bacteria almost invariably are found in lesions associated with *A. israelii*. Consequently, the actinomycetes must be isolated from mixed cultures.

E. Experimental Models

There is no good animal model for human actinomycosis. Hamsters and suckling mice can be infected and have been used for experimental studies.

F. Infections in Man

The course of actinomycosis in man depends on the site of primary infection. The disease occurs chiefly in one of 3 patterns: cervicofacial, thoracic, or abdominal. Although hematogenous spread may occur, the disease is usually limited to the general area of initial infection.

Cervicofacial actinomycosis results from invasion of A. israelii of the normal oral flora, usually following tooth extraction, periodontal abscess, jaw fracture, or other trauma. Chronic lesions that often involve bone occur; sinus tracts, which open and discharge pus and necrotic material to the outside, develop. The firm, indurated lesions may be mistaken for malignant tumors, and, indeed, unnecessary surgical procedures may be performed to remove a supposed cancer when the lesion could have been treated successfully with antibacterial agents.

Thoracic actinomycosis, a chronic lung disease, is characterized by consolidation and by extension of the primary infection through the pleura and chest wall. Multiple draining sinus tracts are common. There may be fever, cough and production of bloody, purulent sputum. The source of the infection is thought to be indigenous *A. israelii* from the tonsils or oral cavity.

Abdominal actinomycosis probably results from organisms that colonize the oral cavity or throat and are swallowed; apparently they invade through any sort of perforation or break in the intestinal tract. Extension occurs from the primary site of infection and may involve any adjacent organ.

Of these 3 kinds of infection, the cervicofacial form occurs most often.

G. Mechanisms of Pathogenicity

The ability to persist and produce a chronic response is the principal pathogenic attribute of *A. israelii;* however, the factors or mechanisms that enable the organism to resist host defenses and produce a persistent infection are not known. The course of actinomycosis, which is much like a tuberculous infection, probably rests on similarities between actinomycetes and mycobacteria.

Although other anaerobic bacteria are commonly present in the lesions, their contributions to the disease process are unknown.

H. Mechanisms of Immunity

Little is known about immunity to the actinomycetes. However, there must certainly be close parallels to the mechanisms of immunity to the mycobacteria. The similarities between actinomycosis and certain of the mycobacterioses suggest that the principal forces of acquired immunity are cellular in nature. It is possible that subtle cellular immune deficiencies predispose to infections with various actinomycetes.

I. Laboratory Diagnosis

Pus or other clinical materials contain hyphal fragments, or "sulfur" granules. Wet mounts examined with reduced light often reveal tangled hyphae or hyphal fragments. Sulfur granules, when present, are characteristic.

Direct culture of clinical specimens (Section D) often yields colonies after a few days of incubation.

J.   Therapy

Long-term (6 to 18 months) therapy with penicillin, in conjunction with surgical drainage of lesions, has proven successful. Tetracyclines or erythromycin can be used for treating patients allergic to penicillin.

K.   Reservoirs of Infection

Man is the only known reservoir of *A. israelii*.

L.   Control of Disease Transmission

Actinomycosis results from endogenous organisms, with no evidence to suggest that it is contracted in any other way. Prevention of infection depends on preventing tissue trauma that would allow endogenous organisms to invade.

Nocardia asteroides

A.   Medical Perspectives

Nocardiosis, like actinomycosis, was first recognized in cattle. The causative organism was isolated by Nocard from cattle with farcy, and was subsequently named *Nocardia farcinica*. Soon thereafter it was discovered that human nocardiosis results from infection with a similar species, *Noc. asteroides*.

Either *Noc. asteroides, Noc. brasiliensis,* or *Noc. caviae* can cause a mycetoma, indistinguishable from that caused by eumycetes (Chapter 38). Of the 3 species, *Noc. brasiliensis* is the most common cause of mycetoma. Although all species of *Nocardia* are soil saprophytes, only a few are known to cause disease in man or animals.

Because of the ubiquitous distribution of nocardiae, it is possible to predict that the incidence of nocardiosis will not decrease. In fact, increasing use of immunosuppressive agents may lead to an appreciable increase in nocardial infection. Even now, nocardiae are recognized as common agents of infection in immunosuppressed patients.

B.   Physical and Chemical Structure

Nocardia sp. are similar in appearance and structure to *A. israelii*. They form filamentous, branching hyphae, less than 1 μm in diameter, and some species fragment to bacillary and coccoid forms. The nocardiae are grampositive and may present a beaded appearance. Their property of acid-

TABLE 35-2
Acid-fast Actinomycetes*

Genus and Species	Principal Disease Produced
Nocardia asteroides	Pulmonary or disseminated nocardiosis in man
Noc. brasiliensis	Mycetoma in man
Noc. caviae	Mycetoma in man
Noc. farcinica	Bovine farcy (a lymphatic disease)

* Ziehl-Neelsen stain with an acid-alcohol decolorization period not longer than 5 to 10 seconds. Even under these conditions, acid-fastness is a variable property of these species of actinomycetes.

fastness emphasizes their relationship to the mycobacteria; however, only certain species of nocardiae are acid-fast, and these only weakly so (Table 35-2).

C. Extracellular Products

See *A. israelli*, above.

D. Culture

A major difference between the various actinomycetes is that Nocardia *sp. are aerobic, whereas* Actinomyces *sp. are anaerobic.* Nocardiae grow well on Sabouraud's glucose agar, blood agar, Lowenstein-Jensen medium, and other media, providing antibacterial agents are not added. Colonies grow slowly and do not become visible before 3 days to 1 week of incubation at the optimal temperature range of 30 to 37°C. Various species of *Nocardia* can grow over temperature ranges from 10 to 50°C.

E. Experimental Models

There is no established model for human nocardiosis; however, mice, guinea pigs and rabbits can be infected intraperitoneally. Cattle, dogs and other domestic animals are subject to natural infections with this organism.

F. Infections in Man

Abscess formation is the rule in nocardiosis. Human nocardiosis often begins as a pulmonary infection; it may range from mild to severe and from transient to chronic. Lung lesions may be solitary or diffuse, and extensive cavity formation can occur. The symptoms are similar to those of pulmonary tuberculosis or actinomycosis. As in the latter disease, sinus tracts frequently form and discharge pus to the exterior through the chest wall, or into abdominal viscera. Hematogenous spread often occurs, with dissemination of organisms to the brain or other organs. In the brain, small lesions tend to coalesce to form a large brain abscess. Infections of kidney, liver, spleen and adrenals also occur, secondary to lung involvement; however, it is of interest that bone is seldom infected in this form of nocardiosis. In mycetoma caused by nocardiae, as well as by other agents, bone involvement is frequently observed.

Cutaneous and subcutaneous lesions of nocardiosis occasionally result from invasion of the organisms directly through a break in the skin, the organisms possibly having been transported on thorns or splinters. There is also evidence that subcutaneous lesions may be initiated by hematogenous spread from a primary focus in the lungs.

G. Mechanisms of Pathogenicity

Little is known about the manner in which nocardiae cause disease; however, their similarities to species of the genera *Actinomyces* and *Mycobacterium* suggest that similar pathogenetic mechanisms characterize all of these organisms.

H. Mechanisms of Immunity

See *A. israelii,* above.

I. Laboratory Diagnosis

Direct examination of pus, either in a wet mount under reduced light or in a gram-stained preparation, usually reveals characteristic hyphae. Clinical specimens should be crushed between 2 glass slides, to break up clusters or masses of hyphae, and then spread on the slides. Acid-fast staining, involving a brief period (5 to 10 seconds) of decolorization with acid-alcohol or careful destaining with 0.5% aqueous sulfuric acid instead of acid-alcohol, is of value. Periods of exposure to acid-alcohol longer than 5 to 10 seconds will completely decolorize the nocardiae.

Tissue sections may contain visible radial colonies or scattered, branching hyphae. Because the hyphae are quite narrow, a routine hematoxylin and eosin (H and E) stain will usually not suffice, and either methenamine-silver or gram staining is preferable. In tissue sections from mycetoma patients, however, granules of nocardiae may be seen on H and E-stained slides.

Cultures should be prepared as described in Section D, and examined for colony formation at intervals ranging from 2 days to 2 weeks. Biochemical tests in media incubated at 27°C help to differentiate nocardiae from similar species of *Streptomyces*. Immunofluorescence with specific antisera has been used to distinguish the various species of *Nocardia*.

J. Therapy

Although antibiotics are effective in nocardiosis, about half of all cases have been fatal, chiefly because the disease is not diagnosed until after dissemination to the brain or other vital organs has occurred. Surgical drainage of abscesses and other lesions is an essential adjunct to antimicrobial therapy.

Treatment with large doses of sulfonamides given over a long period, extending for at least 6 weeks after the disease has apparently cleared, has given the best results. *In vitro* studies have indicated that ampicillin and capreomycin may have greater antinocardial activity than other antimicrobial agents; however, *in vivo* data are not thus far available.

K. Reservoirs of Infection

Nocardiae are present in soil worldwide, and man is continually exposed. The infrequency of clinical nocardiosis suggests that normal human beings possess a high degree of resistance to these ubiquitous organisms.

L. Control of Disease Transmission

The prevalence of primary pulmonary nocardiosis indicates that inhalation is the major mechanism of infection. Because the nocardiae are widespread in nature, it is reasonable to assume that subclinical pulmonary infections result in the development of protective immunity, analogous to the responses seen in histoplasmosis, coccidioidomycosis, and a number of other diseases that result from inhalation of soil organisms. However, proof for this is lacking. In any event, nocardiae would appear to have much lower pathogenic potential than the causative organisms of histoplasmosis and coccidioidomycosis (Chapter 37). It is probable that development of disease depends more on the immunologic status of the host than on exposure to the nocardiae; consequently, no measures are available for control of nocardiosis.

References

Dementjeva, G. R.: Studies on a case of actinomycetoma pedis in Queensland. Sabouraudia *8*:81-92, 1970.

Emmons, C. W., Binford, C. H., and Utz, J. P.: Medical Mycology. Philadelphia, Lea & Febiger, 1970.

Gordon, M. A.: Aerobic pathogenic actinomycetes. *In* Manual of Clinical Microbiology, pp. 137-150, edited by J. E. Blair, E. H. Lennette, and J. P. Truant. Bethesda, Md. American Society for Microbiology, 1970.

Grueber, H. L. E., and Kumar, T. M.: Mycetoma caused by *Streptomyces somalien-sis* in north India. Sabouraudia *8*:108-111, 1970.
Ortiz-Ortiz, L., Contreras, M. F., and Bojalil, L. F.: The assay of delayed hyper-sensitivity to ribosomal proteins from *Nocardia*. Sabouraudia *10*:147-151, 1970.
Thammayya, A., Basu, N., Sur-Roy-Chowdhury, D., Banerjee, A. K., and Sanyal, M.: Actinomycetoma pedis caused by *Nocardia caviae* in India. Sabouraudia *10*:19-23, 1972.
Wilson, J. W., and Plunkett, O. A.: The Fungous Diseases of Man. Berkeley, Uni-versity of California Press, 1967.

Chapter 36

An Introduction to Medical Mycology

Mycology is the study of fungi, a diverse group that includes molds, yeasts, mushrooms, and related organisms. Although hundreds of thousands of species of fungi are recognized, fewer than 50 species are responsible for most of the fungal infections of man. The fungi of medical importance are the subjects of study in medical mycology. Other fungi may be harmful or even lethal by virtue of forming hallucinogens or toxins such as aflatoxin and mushroom poisons, and some may incite allergic reactions. However, this discussion will be limited principally to the fungi that produce clinical infections in man.

A. Characteristics of Fungi

The fungi are eucaryotic protists that differ from bacteria and other procaryotic protists in many ways. Some of the important differences between fungi and bacteria are presented in Table 36-1.

The fungi have several *distinguishing characteristics*. They possess *unique, rigid cell walls* that differ considerably from the cell walls of bacteria. The basic units of fungal cell walls are certain large polysaccharides, such as chitin and mannan, which are present in a thatched arrangement in the wall. The cytoplasmic membranes of fungi contain *sterols*, a property that distinguishes them from virtually all bacteria except the mycoplasmas. All fungi reproduce asexually and most can also reproduce sexually. In fact, asexual reproduction may be so efficient that the sexual forms seldom if ever occur and are never observed; this is true of most of the fungi of medical importance.

Fungi may be unicellular or multicellular. From a single mold spore, extension of the cell wall and an increase in cytoplasmic content cause the formation of a tubular structure, called a hypha. Hyphae can branch and extend, as diagrammed in Figure 36-1, to form an intertwined filamentous mass known as a mycelium. The cottony mass of bread mold represents a familiar example of a mycelium.

Even though the hyphae of molds are long and complex, they are not truly multicellular. Rather, each hypha represents a communicating hollow-tube system that is coenocytic, i.e., has many nuclei enclosed in the cytoplasm within a single cell wall. The hyphae may be *nonseptate* or *septate,* having incomplete septa through which cell contents can move.

Yeasts, in contrast to the molds, are single-celled fungi that reproduce by budding. Some species of fungi are *dimorphic,* meaning that they can exist in either the yeast or the mold form, depending on environmental influences. *Many of the pathogenic fungi are dimorphic,* existing in nature in the mycelial form and in the human host in the yeast form.

TABLE 36-1
Some Important Differences between Fungi and Bacteria

Property	Fungi	Bacteria
Cell structure	Eucaryotic	Procaryotic
Diameter of representative species	> 5 μm	< 2 μm
Cell wall composition	Contains chitin, mannan, other polysaccharides	Contains murein
Cytoplasmic membranes	Sterols present	Lack sterols (except for mycoplasmas)
Cytoplasmic contents	Include mitochondria, endoplasmic reticulum; cytoplasmic streaming	Lack mitochondria, endoplasmic reticulum; no cytoplasmic streaming
Nucleus	True nucleus with nuclear membrane: chromosomes, in pairs	Nuclear body equivalent to a single chromosome, without nuclear membrane
Mode of reproduction	Either sexual or asexual, with spore formation	Binary fission

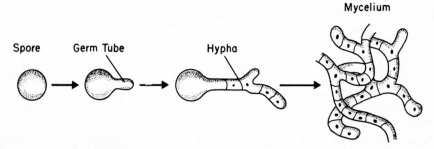

Figure 36-1. Development of fungal mycelium.

Soil is especially suited for supporting mycelial growth and is the natural habitat of many fungi. Because of their rigid cell walls, fungi must acquire nutrients in soluble form, either by absorption or by pinocytosis. It is of interest that some fungi growing in nature possess means for trapping amebae or worms, which die and serve as a source of nutrients for the fungi. Others, notably those of medical importance, can lead an exclusive parasitic existence and derive their nourishment from the host. In either case, the fungi secrete a variety of extracellular enzymes that aid in the degradation of substances of large molecular weight to small molecules that can be transported into the fungal cell.

B. Classes of Fungi

The fungi comprise 4 classes. The lower fungi make up the class called *Phycomycetes*. The root of this word, phyco, means seaweed or algae, and the phycomycetes are sometimes called the algal fungi; some of them are aquatic and some are terrestrial. A familiar example of a terrestrial phycomycete is black bread mold, which is a member of the genus *Rhizopus*. Phycomycetes differ from higher fungi in that they have endogenous asexual spores formed in sac-like structures called sporangia, and that they have nonseptate mycelia.

The other 3 classes, the higher fungi, are characterized by exogenous asexual spores, called conidia, which are formed outside of the hyphae, and by the presence of septate mycelia with pores that permit the passage of nuclei and cytoplasm from one part of the mycelium to another.

The class *Ascomycetes* includes yeasts, morels, truffles, and many of the common molds. The word "ascus" means a bag or sac-like structure, and the ascomycetes were so named because they bear their sexual spores in an ascus. The ascomycetes include many fungi of practical importance to man, such as the yeasts of the genus *Saccharomyces* that leaven bread and ferment alcoholic beverages.

The class *Basidiomycetes* consists of higher fungi that produce sexual spores on a basidium or base. This class includes the mushrooms.

Most of the fungi of medical importance belong to the class *Deuteromycetes (Fungi Imperfecti)*. These fungi cannot be classified on the basis of their mode of sexual reproduction, because their sexual stages are unknown. They are probably members of other classes but are included in the so-called "taxonomic dump-heap," *Deuteromycetes,* because they cannot be properly identified.

C. Characteristics That Aid in Identification of Fungi

The *asexual spores* of the higher fungi *aid in the identification* of some species (Fig. 36-2). These spores may be small, single-celled microconidia,

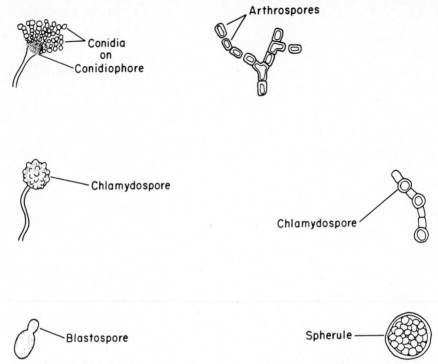

Figure 36-2. Asexual spores produced by medically important fungi.

or large, single or multi-celled macroconidia. Some fungi have both micro-conidia and macroconidia; other species have one or the other. The shapes and arrangement of the conidia are characteristic for a given species of fungus.

Other asexual reproductive structures that are useful in the identifica-tion of medically important fungi include blastospores, arthrospores, and chlamydospores (Fig. 36-2). The blastospores of yeasts are formed by budding. Arthrospores are formed by the segmentation of a mycelium; the segments disarticulate to yield spores, each of which is capable of giving rise to a new mycelium. Chlamydospores are thick-walled resting spores, formed by rounding-up and thickening of a segment of a hypha. Like the endospores of bacteria, chlamydospores have the ability to resist adverse conditions and to germinate when placed in a favorable environment. Arthrospores and other conidia promote the aerial dissemination of fungi, because they break away from the mycelium and are dispersed in air.

Non-morphologic characteristics of fungi also are exploited in common laboratory tests and aid in identification (Table 36-2). Fungal cell walls are resistant to strong alkali (10% KOH or NaOH) which will degrade tissue and mucus; consequently, fungi can be observed more readily in

TABLE 36-2

Common Laboratory Procedures Used to Identify Fungi of Medical Importance

Procedure	Advantage
Wet mount of tissue or mucus-containing specimens in 10% KOH	Strong alkali degrades tissue and mucus and permits visualization of fungi
Wet mount of portions teased from fungal colonies and mounted in lacto-phenol blue	Permits observation of fungal morphology and presence of spores
Fixed slides stained with periodic-acid-Schiff (PAS) or methenamine silver stains	Both PAS and silver stain fungal cell walls to give good contrast with background in tissue sections or other clinical materials
Sabouraud's glucose agar for culture; incubation at room temperature (RT) for up to 6 weeks, or at 37°C for days	Low pH of the medium and RT incubation favor growth of fungi over bacteria Antibiotics may also be added to discourage bacterial growth
Slide cultures, with inoculated blocks of Sabouraud's glucose agar (about 1 cm square and 2 or 3 mm deep) on a glass slide covered with a coverslip and incubated in a moist chamber at RT; when spores form, the coverslip is carefully removed and examined in a lactophenol-blue wet mount	Permits observation of relatively undisturbed fungal growth

many specimens following alkali treatment than without such treatment. The cell wall also can be stained with periodic-acid-Schiff (PAS) or methenamine silver stains. Fungi are not affected by penicillin because they lack murein mucocomplex in their cell walls; as a consequence, penicillin and certain other antibiotics can be used to suppress bacterial growth and in so doing facilitate the isolation of fungi from clinical specimens. Unlike most bacterial pathogens, fungi generally prefer a low pH, and the majority of them will grow readily at room temperature.

D.   General Characteristics of Mycoses

Broadly, the fungi cause diseases of 3 major categories: the superficial mycoses, the intermediate mycoses, and the deep mycoses. Two properties of fungi appear to be of paramount importance in the pathogenesis of the diseases they cause. First, the tissue tropism of the fungus may account for the clinical picture that it evokes. Tissue tropism denotes the predilection of a parasite for a particular tissue or organ of the host. Although many pathogens exhibit tissue tropism (e.g., gonorrheal infection of epithelial cells of genital mucous membranes and shigella infection of the gut epithelium), the basis for such selective localization of fungi has not been established. The tissue tropism of many fungi is marked. Examples are *Histoplasma capsulatum,* which lives within macrophages of the RES; *Cryptococcus neoformans,* which thrives in the central nervous system; *Paracoccidioides brasiliensis,* which lives selectively in mucous membranes and lymph nodes; and *Blastomyces dermatitidis,* which elects skin. The dermatophytes, responsible for superficial mycoses, thrive on keratin; however, some prefer the keratin of hair, some the keratin of nails, and others the keratin of skin.

In addition to tissue tropism, a second property of fungi that is important in the pathogenesis is the ability of many of them to incite sensitivity, especially delayed-type sensitivity, in the host. Often, the sensitivity of the host to fungal antigens accounts in large part for the pathologic effects produced.

Obviously, much remains to be learned about the pathogenesis of the mycoses. Many of the pathogenetic mechanisms of bacteria, e.g., toxin production or capsule formation, are not characteristic of most fungi. Some nonpathogenic fungi produce toxins that, if ingested, in the manner of staphylococcal enterotoxin or botulinum toxin, may be toxic. However, there are no well-established instances in which production of exotoxins or endotoxins by infecting fungi contributes significantly to the disease process, although there is evidence suggesting an endotoxin-like activity for some species. Capsule formation is not characteristic of most fungi, but it is prominent in one pathogenic yeast, *Cryptococcus neoformans.*

Generally, the evidence indicates that fungal diseases are controlled principally by cellular immune mechanisms, although sometimes there is almost certainly an interaction and collaboration between cellular and humoral immunity. It is a common observation that a state of delayed sensitivity to Ag(s) of a particular fungus is associated with immunity to reinfection or with a favorable prognosis if the individual has clinical disease. Specific humoral Abs, on the other hand, often reflect the extent of the infection but are not related to protection. Thus, a marked increase in humoral Ab titer during fungal infections is likely to reflect the amount of fungal Ag being produced and to be correlated with a poor prognosis.

Other compelling evidence that fungal infections are prevented and controlled in large part by cellular immune mechanisms comes from clinical experiences with immunologically deficient patients. It is well established that depression or defects in cellular immunity (CI), either genetic or acquired, predispose to serious fungal infections, whereas depression or defects in humoral immunity usually do not. Often the invading fungi in such instances are normal flora opportunists that are ubiquitous in the environment. Such opportunistic infections with species of *Candida, Aspergillus,* or some of the phycomycetes present a major problem in management of patients whose CI has been suppressed by drugs or other therapy used to prevent rejection of organ transplants or to treat tumors. Cancer patients

TABLE 36-3

Increase in Fungal Infections in a Cancer Hospital during the
Decade 1950 to 1959*

Year	No. of cases	Year	No. of cases
1950	2	1955	13
1951	4	1956	27
1952	9	1957	34
1953	15	1958	22
1954	11	1959	30

* The upward trend has continued since 1959, and a majority of the infections are
caused by *Candida albicans*.

Modified from Hutter, R. V. P., and Collins, H. S.: The occurrence of opportunistic fungus infections in a cancer hospital. Lab Invest. *11*:1035, 1962

are at particular risk of infection because the late general suppression of
CI produced by the malignant disease itself is exaggerated by treatment
with anticancer drugs all of which have immunosuppressive activity. The
magnitude of the problem presented by opportunistic fungal infections is
indicated by the representative data shown in Table 36-3.

A role for immune forces other than those of CI in preventing and controlling fungal infections is indicated by both clinical and experimental
data; however, these forces may contribute less than CI to overall defense
against fungi. Neutrophils have been implicated as playing a part in protection. For example, in candidiasis, the intact neutrophil appears to be
important in preventing systemic spread of the organisms. In addition, it
is well established that diabetics and patients with certain other endocrine
disorders are highly susceptible to certain opportunistic fungi, even though
their CI appears to be essentially normal. It is possible that this increase
in susceptibility is related to neutrophil dysfunction; however, at present
there are few data to explain why these patients are unusually prone to
fungal infections.

Clearly, much remains to be learned about both innate and acquired
immunity to fungi. The current increase in opportunistic fungal infections,
together with the difficulties in treating mycoses, emphasizes the need for
a better understanding of both the pathogenesis of and the immune response to fungal infections.

E. Treatment of Mycoses

The mycoses are often more difficult to treat than bacterial infections
because only a few effective antifungal agents are available (Chapter 6).

Griseofulvin is an antibiotic produced by the mold *Penicillium griseoful-
vum* and certain other species of *Penicillium*. It is fungistatic and is active
against the dermatophytes that cause superficial mycoses of hair, skin, or

nails. This antibiotic is relatively nontoxic to patients, and is customarily given over a period of months. During this time, it accumulates in keratinized tissues and inhibits fungal growth. However, it is essential that the drug be administered until all infected hair, skin, or nails are shed or grow to the point where they can be trimmed to remove the fungi.

Amphotericin B, the most useful of the antifungal polyenes, is produced by various species of the bacterial genus *Streptomyces.* It strongly inhibits the growth of fungi and is effective in treating systemic mycoses and some of the subcutaneous mycoses. Polyene antibiotics act on sterol-containing cytoplasmic membranes; therefore they are not antibacterial (except against mycoplasmas) but they can interact with both fungal and human cytoplasmic membranes, which contain sterol. As a consequence, amphotericin B is not exclusively toxic for fungi and can lead to kidney damage or erythrocyte destruction in the host. It has the added disadvantage of being poorly absorbed from the gastrointestinal tract, consequently, it is injected, usually intravenously. Because of its toxicity, amphotericin B is reserved for use in life-threatening or severe mycoses.

Griseofulvin and amphotericin B are the backbone of antimycotic therapy. Nystatin is another antibiotic that can be used topically. "Preantibiotic" remedies that are still of use include iodide therapy for sporotrichosis and certain other subcutaneous mycoses, and topical applications of various ointments or powders, such as 5% undecylenic acid, 5% benzoic acid, or 3% salicylic acid, for some of the superficial mycoses.

Several new and promising antifungal agents are currently being assessed. These include hamycin, another polyene antibiotic. This agent has an advantage over amphotericin B, in that it can be administered orally; however, it also produces toxic side effects. Although hamycin has been shown to be effective against some of the systemic mycoses in experimental studies, it is not available commercially. Another promising agent is the antimetabolite 5-fluorocytosine. This agent has a few adverse effects which are reported to be comparatively transient. In limited trials, 5-fluorocytosine, given alone or in combination with other agents, has been effective in some systemic mycoses that failed to respond to amphotericin B alone. Also some cases of chromoblastomycosis that had resisted treatment for many years responded dramatically to 5-fluorocytosine. Saramycetin is still another antifungal agent being evaluated. It is a polypeptide antibiotic that has been reported to be highly effective against several of the systemic mycoses, including histoplasmosis, blastomycosis, and sporotrichosis.

References

Emmons, C. W., Binford, C. H., and Utz, J. P.: Medical Mycology, 2nd ed. Philadelphia, Lea & Febiger, 1970.

Fass, R. J., and Perkins, R. L.: 5-Fluorocytosine in the treatment of cryptococcal and candida mycoses. Ann Intern. Med. *74*:535, 1971.

Hutter, R. V. P., and Collins, H. S.: The occurrence of opportunistic fungus infections in a cancer hospital. Lab. Invest. *11*:1035, 1962.

Kirkpatrick, C. H., Rich, R. R., and Bennett, J. E.: Chronic mucocutaneous candidiasis: Model-building in cellular immunity. Ann. Intern. Med. *74*:955, 1971.

Lehrer, R. I., and Cline, M. J.: Leukocyte myeloperoxidase deficiency and disseminated candidiasis: the role of myeloperoxidase in resistance to *Candida* infection. J. Clin. Invest. *48*:1478, 1969.

Lehrer, R. I., and Cline, M. J.: Leukocyte candidacidal activity and resistance to candidiasis in patients with cancer. Cancer *27*:1211, 1971.

Utz, J. P.: Pulmonary infection due to opportunistic fungi. Adv. Intern. Med. *16*:427, 1970.

Vandevelde, A. G., Manceri, A. A., and Johnson, J. E., III: 5-Fluorocytosine in the treatment of mycotic infections. Ann. Intern. Med. *77*:43, 1972.

Wilson, J. W., and Plunkett, O. A.: The Fungous Diseases of Man. Berkeley, University of California Press, 1967.

The Deep-Seated Mycoses

The deep-seated mycoses are often referred to as systemic mycoses. They comprise a group of diseases each of which may range in severity from inapparent to lethal infections, depending on the relative activities of the host and the parasite. The various deep-seated mycoses and their respective etiologic agents will be considered separately.

Coccidioides immitis

A. Medical Perspectives

The etiologic agent of coccidioidomycosis, *C. immitis,* exists in large numbers in the soils of endemic areas of the southwestern USA, of Central America and of South America. A self-limiting form of coccidioidomycosis is seen so often in the San Joaquin Valley area of California that it has gained the common name of "valley fever." The deserts of the southwestern USA offer the unique climate essential for the dissemination of *C. immitis;* a wet, rainy period allows the germination and reproduction of spores, and an ensuing hot, dry period permits air- and dust-borne spread of the highly infectious arthrospores. As high as 90% of the population in endemic areas give positive skin-test reactions to Ags of the fungus, indicating that most people who are regularly exposed to *C. immitis* become infected. However, only about 40% of those who are infected become overtly ill, and fewer than 1% develop severe disease.

B. Physical and Chemical Structure

Being a typical dimorphic fungus, *C. immitis* varies in structure between a hyphal (mycelial or mold) form found in soil and a spherule form found in infected tissues (Fig. 37-1). Since the hyphal form grows most readily *in vitro,* the Ags used for skin testing and other immunologic studies have been obtained exclusively from this form; however, spherule Ags are currently being evaluated. A variety of polysaccharides and proteins are present in coccidioidin, the filtrate of mycelial cultures that is commonly used as an Ag preparation. This mixture elicits a positive delayed-type sensitivity reaction in sensitized individuals, and will also give positive precipitin and complement-fixation (CF) reactions with serum from patients with extensive infections. The chemical components responsible for these various activities are poorly characterized.

As shown in Figure 37-1A, barrel-shaped arthrospores are formed in the mycelium. Within tissues the infecting arthrospore (asexual spore) germinates to give rise to the spherule, which increases in size as the number of contained endospores increases. The original thick wall of each spherule becomes thinner as the diameter increases from approximately 15 μm to about 75 μm. At this point the spherule bursts and releases hundreds of endospores, each of which can form a new spherule (Fig. 37-1B).

C. Extracellular Products

Few data are available concerning extracellular fungal products of possible importance in the pathogenesis of coccidioidomycosis. There is no evidence that either endotoxins or exotoxins are produced.

15

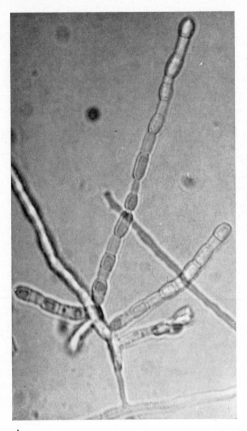

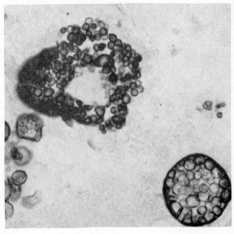

B

Figure 37-1. *Coccidioides immitis.* A, Mold form with arthrospores. B, Tissue form in the lung, showing an intact sporangium with well-defined endospores at the lower right and in the center a ruptured sporangium, releasing small endospores. (From Emmons, C. W., Binford, C. H., and Utz, J. P.: Medical Mycology, 2nd ed. Philadelphia, Lea & Febiger, 1970.)

A

D. Culture

Sabouraud's glucose agar supports the growth of *C. immitis* at room temperature. Contaminated materials from patients, such as sputum, exudate from lesions, and spinal fluid, contain the spherule form of the fungus; however, when this form is plated onto tubes of Sabouraud's medium, growth of the mycelial form occurs. Extreme caution is necessary when dealing with cultures of *C. immitis* because the *arthrospores readily become airborne by the slightest air current and are highly infectious. Special techniques must be used for handling spore-bearing materials to prevent infection.* Petri dishes should not be used for culture work. Many laboratory workers have become infected and some have developed severe disease.

The colonies form a white cottony mycelium at first, which soon turns buff or grayish brown. At this stage of the growth cycle the appearance of the mycelium has been described as "moth-eaten." Sporulation begins within 3 days to 2 weeks, depending on cultural conditions.

The mycelial form of *C. immitis* is readily isolated from contaminated soil. The hyphae are relatively wide, branching and septate.

The spherule form has recently been cultivated *in vitro* on special media.

E. Experimental Models

Mice and guinea pigs can be infected with *C. immitis,* by either inhalation or injection. Guinea pigs have been used extensively in the study of immunologic responses during infection.

F. Infections in Man

The usual route of infection is the respiratory tract; airborne arthrospores are inhaled and some of them reach the lung. About 60% of infected individuals remain asymptomatic but become skin-sensitive to coccidioidin by about 3 weeks after infection.

The acute and most common form of the disease resembles influenza. The initial symptoms consist of cough, fever and malaise. One to 2 weeks later, about 3 to 5% of patients develop sequelae attributable to hypersensitivity reactions, the most frequent being skin lesions (erythema nodosum or erythema multiforme) or joint symptoms ("desert rheumatism").

A chronic, progressive, granulomatous disease occurs in fewer than 1% of those infected; this is often fatal unless intensive treatment is given. Patients with this form of coccidioidomycosis apparently have some defect in their immune response to the fungus that allows continued growth of organisms and widespread dissemination of the infection. The granulomatous lesions resemble the tubercles of tuberculosis. The infection may be disseminated to many parts of the body, including bones, viscera and central nervous system; however, the GI tract is remarkably resistant to infection.

Amphotericin B is the only effective therapeutic agent readily available for treatment of systemic coccidioidomycosis.

G. Mechanisms of Pathogenicity

The fact that primary infections with *C. immitis* usually cause a self-limiting disease or no symptoms at all suggests that the principal mechanisms of pathogenicity of this fungus are related to its ability to induce hypersensitivity. It is probable that the early transient allergic manifestations in the skin and joints of some patients represent immune-complex hypersensitivity reactions, and that the chronic systemic form of the disease results from a defect in the cellular immune response.

H. Mechanisms of Immunity

Cellular immunity normally develops after exposure to *C. immitis,* and its level is probably correlated with the degree of delayed sensitivity in the skin.

It is of interest that the incidence of dissemination varies greatly, depending on genetic influences. Whereas about 1 in 400 Caucasians with diagnosed coccidioidomycosis develops disseminated disease, the incidence is about 14 times as high in Negroes and 100 times as high in Filipinos! The reasons for these differences are unknown, but are obviously related to different capabilities in developing an immunologic response to the fungus.

I. Laboratory Diagnosis

Although the diagnosis of coccidioidomycosis is usually made on the basis of clinical findings, culture is helpful in the chronic, disseminated forms of the disease.

Sputum or other clinical specimens can be examined directly by means of a KOH wet-mount slide preparation, which reveals characteristic spherules. Culture of such material on Sabouraud's glucose agar will yield typical colonies, usually within several days at room temperature or at 37°C.

J. Reservoirs of Infection

The soil is the only reservoir of infection.

K. Control of Disease Transmission

Only under rare circumstances is coccidioidomycosis transmitted by any means except inhalation of airborne spores. Therefore, effective control depends principally on prevention of dust dissemination by such measures as installing lawns or pavement, or oiling or watering soil. The efficacy of this kind of control was proven during World War II; it was observed that a number of workers involved in building Air Force bases in endemic areas became ill with coccidioidomycosis following exposure to contaminated dust. Measures were taken to decrease dust inhalation, with a consequent dramatic decrease in the case rate. An obvious rule is that workers who must be heavily exposed should wear masks.

Histoplasma capsulatum

A. Medical Perspectives

Histoplasmosis, caused by H. capsulatum, shares many characteristics with coccidioidomycosis. Both diseases extend over a spectrum from self-limiting to chronic, granulomatous lung infections, and both are endemic in certain geographic locations. However, histoplasmosis is the more widespread of the 2 diseases and occurs in many parts of the world, notably in the USA along the Mississippi River, along other large rivers draining into the Mississippi, and in many areas along the East Coast.

For many years, only the severe disseminated form of histoplasmosis was recognized. Largely as a result of massive screening tests for tuberculosis in the USA, it was realized that the rate of infection with *H. capsulatum* is high in endemic areas. Roentgenographic examination revealed that many individuals in these regions had healed, calcified lesions resembling those of primary tuberculosis, even though a surprising number failed to give a positive reaction to the tuberculin skin test. Upon skin testing, however, these subjects were found to have delayed sensitivity to histoplasmin, an antigenic extract of *H. capsulatum*. Thus infections with *H. capsulatum,* like those with *C. immitis,* result in clinical disease in a minority of persons infected and severe disseminated disease is a rare event.

B. Physical and Chemical Structure

Histoplasma capsulatum is a dimorphic fungus, occurring in mycelial form in soil and *in vivo* as a typical oval yeast (about 2 to 4 μm in length) within macrophages (Fig. 37-2A). The yeast cells multiply by forming single buds and propagate until the macrophage is packed with organisms. The few extracellular yeast organisms found *in vivo* probably represent organisms released by the disruption of infected macrophages.

The mold form, found in soil, produces microconidia (2 to 5 μm in diameter), which are the infectious forms (Fig. 37-2B). The mold form also produces characteristic macroconidia, which are large (8 to 15 μm in diameter), round or pear-shaped structures with thick walls and many surface projections (Fig. 37-2C). Although these macroconidia are usually erroneously referred to as *tuberculate chlamydospores,* it is more accurate to call them spiny or warty spores.

Antigens have been prepared from both the yeast and mold forms of *H. capsulatum,* and generally a battery of Ags is used for serologic testing.

C. Extracellular Products

Although *H. capsulatum* produces many extracellular products, none of them is known to be directly related to the pathogenesis of histoplasmosis.

D. Culture

Histoplasma capsulatum can be cultured to yield either the yeast or mycelial form. On blood agar at 37°C, the yeast form develops. Grossly, the colonies are small, smooth, moist and white or cream-colored.

On Sabouraud's glucose agar at RT, the mycelial form predominates; colonies are white and cottony, deepening to a buff or brown color with age.

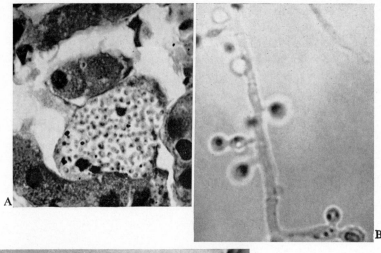

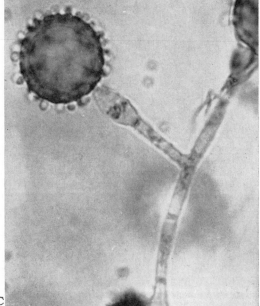

Figure 37-2. *Histoplasma capsulatum.* A, Yeast forms within a Kupffer cell (macrophage) of the liver. B, Mold-form hyphae with microconidia. C, Macroconidia. (From Emmons, C. W., Binford, C. H., and Utz, J. P.: Medical Mycology, 2nd ed. Philadelphia, Lea & Febiger, 1970.)

E. Experimental Models

Many laboratory animals are susceptible to histoplasmosis. Although a single spore or as few as 10 yeast cells may infect a mouse, a dose of 10^6 or more is required to produce a fatal infection.

F. Infections in Man

Being airborne, the spores of *H. capsulatum* most often infect the respiratory tract. The infection may be inapparent, or may occur as a primary acute disease, in a chronic cavitary form, or in the severe disseminated form. When symptoms are present they may include fever, cough and chest pain or more severe manifestations and complications of respiratory infections, such as dyspnea and pleurisy with effusion. Localized pulmonary histoplasmosis resembles tuberculosis in its histopathology.

In the occasional patient who develops severe disseminated histoplasmosis, infection may spread to virtually any portion of the RES. Lesions are often present in the spleen, liver, lungs, lymph nodes and other organs. Amphotericin B is used to treat the patient with the disseminated disease.

G. Mechanisms of Pathogenicity

The propensity of *H. capsulatum* to propagate within nonimmune macrophages accounts in large measure for the pathogenic properties of this fungus. However, little is known about the ways in which the organism causes disease.

The name *H. capsulatum* is a misnomer chosen for the fungus many years ago when staining artifacts were mistaken for capsules.

H. Mechanisms of Immunity

See Chapter 36.

I. Laboratory Diagnosis

Histoplasma capsulatum can be cultured from clinical specimens such as sputum. Biopsies of lymph nodes or other infected organs contain large numbers of the fungi within macrophages. Although the organisms can be seen in tissue sections stained with hematoxylin and eosin, special stains such as methenamine-silver or PAS (periodic-acid-Schiff) improve their visualization.

J. Reservoirs of Infection

Soil is the principal reservoir of H. capsulatum, especially soil that is enriched by the feces of birds or bats. Thus, areas around chicken houses, under starling roosts, and in caves inhabited by bats frequently contain large numbers of the fungal spores. Birds do not become infected, apparently because their high body temperature inhibits the organism. Bats, however, are susceptible to histoplasmosis, and *H. capsulatum* can be recovered from bat guano. Within caves, where bat guano mixes with soil, *H. capsulatum* grows well. A number of cases of histoplasmosis have occurred among cave explorers as the result of inhaling large numbers of infectious conidiospores. For this reason, histoplasmosis has been called "spelunker's disease."

K. Control of Disease Transmission

The control of histoplasmosis depends on eliminating or avoiding highly contaminated soil foci. Prevention of soil contamination would seem to be the best policy, because it is virtually impossible to eliminate *H. capsulatum* from soil once it becomes established there. Soil can be decontaminated to some extent by the use of formaldehyde or other chemicals. Effective control of dissemination of *H. capsulatum* spores has also been achieved by covering contaminated dusty areas with a layer of clay or shale soil several inches thick.

Blastomyces dermatitidis

A. Medical Perspectives

North American blastomycosis is seen most often in Canada and the USA, especially in the northern Mississippi River Valley and the Ohio River Valley. The causative fungus, *B. dermatitidis,* is also known as *Ajellomyces dermatitidis.*

This form of blastomycosis is being recognized with increasing frequency in many parts of Africa.

B. Physical and Chemical Structure

Blastomyces dermatitidis is a dimorphic fungus that grows in tissues or cultures at 37°C as a thick-walled, budding yeast, and in cultures at room temperature as a mycelial form. Lateral, rounded conidia (3 to 5 μm) are borne along the hyphae, and presumably are the infectious form. The yeast forms are spherical, 7 to 20 μm in diameter, with a wall almost 1 μm thick (Fig. 37-3). They produce only one bud at a time, which helps to distinguish the organism from similar species.

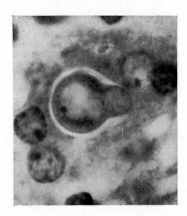

Figure 37-3. *Blastomyces dermatitidis.* (From Emmons, C. W., Binford, C. H., and Utz, J. P.: Medical Mycology, 2nd ed. Philadelphia, Lea & Febiger, 1970.)

C.   Extracellular Products

A culture filtrate containing extracellular products, called blastomycin, analogous to coccidioidin and histoplasmin, is used as an Ag preparation for skin-testing and serologic tests.

D.   Culture

Blastomyces dermatitidis can be cultured on blood agar at 37°C to yield colonies of the yeast form that appear waxy and become wrinkled. On Sabouraud's glucose agar at room temperature, mold-form colonies are produced.

E.   Experimental Models

Guinea pigs and mice have been used for the study of *B. dermatitidis*. Intraperitoneal injection of the organism into mice gives rise to abscesses on the omentum.

F.   Infections in Man

North American blastomycosis occurs in one of two major forms. In one form of the disease the lesions are limited to skin and usually to one part of the body; the lesions may persist for many years in an otherwise healthy person. The other form of the disease is a widespread infection caused by dissemination of *B. dermatitidis* from a primary focus, usually in the lung.

Pulmonary blastomycosis begins as a subacute respiratory infection and gradually increases in severity over a period of weeks to months to eventually resemble tuberculosis or carcinoma. The fungus may become disseminated by way of the blood stream to involve many parts of the body.

Cutaneous blastomycosis begins as a papular lesion of the skin or as a subcutaneous nodule that ulcerates. The skin lesions tend to spread peripherally.

G.   Mechanisms of Pathogenicity

Little is known about the mechanisms of pathogenicity of North American blastomycosis. It is of interest that the cutaneous form is thought to occur subsequent to a primary respiratory tract infection, which is usually inapparent. The skin lesions contain few organisms, but huge numbers of lymphocytes and plasma cells are present, suggesting that a chronic immunologic response is a component of this disease.

H.   Mechanisms of Immunity

See Chapter 36.

I. Laboratory Diagnosis

A direct mount in 10% KOH may reveal the characteristic yeast form in pus or sputum. Cultures and serologic studies are also useful in diagnosis.

J. Reservoirs of Infection

Although there is some question as to the reservoirs of *B. dermatitidis,* it is thought to be principally a soil fungus.

K. Control of Disease Transmission

North American blastomycosis is not transmitted directly. Since the reservoirs have not been found, there are no known effective means to control transmission.

Cryptococcus neoformans

A. Medical Perspectives

Cryptococcosis may be a mild or even inapparent infection of the lung or it may become disseminated, often resulting in a subacute or chronic meningitis. In untreated subjects the meningitis is uniformly fatal after a period ranging from a few months to as long as 20 years. It was formerly called "torula meningitis" because the old name for this fungus was *Torula histolytica.*

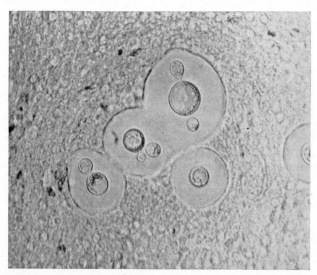

Figure 37-4. *Cryptococcus neoformans.* Note the thin-walled, budding yeasts surrounded by large clear areas of polysaccharide capsules. (From Emmons, C. W., Binford, C. H., and Utz, J. P.: Medical Mycology, 2nd ed. Philadelphia, Lea & Febiger, 1970.)

B. Physical and Chemical Structure

Cryptococcus neoformans occurs in the form of a budding yeast, 4 to 20 μm in diameter, with a polysaccharide capsule (Fig. 37-4). The cell wall is thin, as compared with other yeasts of comparable size, and tends to collapse, resulting in crescent forms.

The capsules of cryptococcus are often very large and may measure 10 to 20 μm in width. The capsular polysaccharides have been classified into 3 antigenic types: A, B and C.

Recently, it has been shown that some strains of *C. neoformans* have a sexual phase that identifies them as *Basidiomycetes*.

C. Extracellular Products

The only product known to be important is the capsular polysaccharide, which can sometimes be demonstrated in the serum of patients with cryptococcosis.

D. Culture

Cryptococcus neoformans is readily cultured on Sabouraud's glucose agar at room temperature. It will also grow at 37°C, which helps to distinguish pathogenic from some nonpathogenic strains. Mucoid colonies are formed; these are cream-colored at first but darken to a brownish shade.

E. Experimental Models

Mice and rabbits are susceptible to cryptococcal infections.

F. Infections in Man

Like many other mycoses, cryptococcosis presents various clinical pictures. The common mode of infection is via inhalation; however, primary infections may be inapparent or mild. On x-ray study, lesions may be found to be large and solitary, or diffuse and widespread. Occasionally, workmen exposed to large numbers of the fungi develop a severe pneumonitis, but more often the lung disease is discovered by chance because the symptoms are so mild. It is of interest that cryptococcal lung lesions do not calcify after healing; consequently, it is possible that many cases of primary pulmonary cryptococcosis go undiagnosed.

From the lung, or possibly from other portals of entry, the fungi may disseminate, usually via the hematogenous route, to involve virtually any organ. *Visceral forms* often mimic tuberculosis or cancer. In about 10% or fewer of those infected, bones and joints are involved (*osseous form*). *Cutaneous* and *mucosal* lesions, also common, can vary from superficial ulcers to nodules or granulomas, or to carcinoma-like lesions.

Cryptococcal meningitis, the most dangerous form of disseminated disease, resembles tuberculous or other chronic forms of meningitis. The onset is commonly insidious, with intermittent headaches. Vertigo or other CNS symptoms may be observed, depending on the location and extent of the lesion. At autopsy, granulomatous lesions of the meninges or mucoid fungal masses are found. In untreated subjects the disease usually progresses, with increasing CNS deterioration, and ends in death after a few months. Alternatively, the course of the disease may extend for years, marked by remissions and exacerbations; however, without treatment the outcome is invariably fatal.

G. Mechanisms of Pathogenicity

The pathogenesis of cryptococcal infections is poorly understood. Clearly, the antigenic polysaccharide of the capsule is an important virulence factor. It is antiphagocytic, and is produced in such large quantities that it may induce a state of immunologic paralysis, thereby allowing the infection to progress.

Cryptococcus neoformans seems to have a predilection for the CNS, but the basis for this is not known. Continued growth of the fungus leads to accumulation of masses of highly mucoid material that have a gelatinous or myxomatous appearance. In the CNS especially, these accumulations can lead to damage from pressure effects, in much the same way that certain tumors do.

H. Mechanisms of Immunity

The study of immune mechanisms in cryptococcosis is hampered by lack of suitable Ag preparations. Although it is suspected that inapparent primary pulmonary infections occur frequently, without subsequent disease (analogous to many other mycoses) proof is lacking because no reliable skin test Ag is available. Serologic tests are also unreliable because there is considerable cross-reaction between the Ags of *C. neoformans* and those of other fungi.

The weakness of the inflammatory response to the organism is a striking characteristic of cryptococcosis. For example, the discharge from skin lesions that grossly resemble abscesses is not pus but, instead, is composed almost entirely of a mass of fungal cells. Similarly, tissue lesions contain few inflammatory cells but huge numbers of fungi.

Paracoccidioides brasiliensis

South American blastomycosis, caused by *P. brasiliensis,* occurs in various parts of South America, with the highest incidence in Brazil. It is a

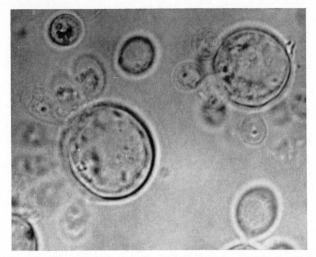

Figure 37-5. *Paracoccidioides brasiliensis.* Note the multiple buds formed by a single cell. (From Emmons, C. W., Binford, C. H., and Utz, J. P.: Medical Mycology, 2nd ed. Philadelphia, Lea & Febiger, 1970.)

chronic, granulomatous disease, but differs from those discussed above, in that the fungus frequently attacks mucous membranes, often in the mouth. Lesions may also occur in the gastrointestinal tract, skin, lungs and lymph nodes.

Paracoccidioides brasiliensis resembles *B. dermatitidis,* but is distinguished by its multiple buds rather than by the single bud characteristic of blastomyces (Fig. 37-5). It is thought that the fungus is introduced into the mouth by vegetation used to clean between the teeth, or for chewing.

References

Emmons, C. W., Binford, C. H., and Utz, J. P.: Medical Mycology, 2nd ed. Philadelphia, Lea & Febiger, 1970.

Lewis, J. L., and Rabinovich, S.: The wide spectrum of cryptococcal infections. Amer. J. Med. *53*:315, 1972.

Negroni, P.: Histoplasmosis. Diagnosis and Treatment. Springfield, Ill., Charles C Thomas, 1965.

Roberts, J. A., Counts, J. M., and Crecelius, H. G.: Production *in vitro* of *Coccidioides immitis* spherules and endospores as a diagnostic aid. Amer. Rev. Resp. Dis. *102*:811, 1970.

Sarosi, G. A., Voth, D. W., Dahl, B. A., Doto, I. L., and Tosh, F. E.: Disseminated histoplasmosis: Results of long-term follow-up. Ann. Intern. Med. *75*:511, 1971.

Seabury, J. H., Buechner, H. A., Busey, J. F., Georg, L. K., and Campbell, C. C.: The diagnosis of pulmonary mycoses. Report of the committee on fungus diseases and subcommittee for clinical diagnosis, American College of Chest Physicians. Chest *60*:82, 1971.

Wilson, J. W., and Plunkett, O. A.: The Fungous Diseases of Man. Berkeley, University of California Press, 1967.

The Intermediate Mycoses

For reasons of convenience, the category of intermediate mycoses is used to encompass those mycoses not caused by either the dermatophytes or the commonly pathogenic fungi of the deep-seated mycoses. The dividing lines between deep-seated and intermediate mycoses are often difficult to distinguish; indeed, the fungi that cause intermediate mycoses can invade systemically if host defenses are sufficiently depressed. However, in a majority of cases, the fungi of the intermediate mycoses cause infections of subcutaneous or mucocutaneous tissues, often with lymphatic involvement but without systemic spread. Included in this category are sporotrichosis, maduromycosis and chromomycosis that principally involve subcutaneous tissues, and infections caused by the so-called opportunistic fungi.

Virtually any species of fungus can cause an opportunistic infection if the host is sufficiently immunosuppressed; however, *Candida albicans* is the most frequent offender. It can infect when host responses are slightly or even imperceptibly out of balance. Consequently, emphasis will be placed on candidiasis as a prime example of the opportunistic mycoses. It should be stressed, however, that many other normally nonpathogenic fungi, such as *Aspergillus* sp., also act as opportunists.

Sporothrix (Sporotrichum) schenckii (Sporotrichosis)

A. Medical Perspectives

Sporothrix schenckii occurs in soil and on vegetation in a widespread distribution over most of the world. It is probable that infections with this fungus occur fairly often; in common with many fungal infections, clinical disease is infrequent. Skin testing for delayed sensitivity is not routinely done; however, in one experimental study of various populations, positive skin-test reactions to Ags of sporothrix were obtained in 10% of hospital patients tested, in 20% of gardeners and nursery workers and in 60% of long-term nursery workers. These results suggest that continued exposure to the organisms eventually leads to subclinical infections and the development of delayed sensitivity.

Because the causative fungi are widespread, and the disease is usually chronic but not fatal, it is likely that sporotrichosis will continue to occur with about the same incidence as it has in the past.

B. Physical and Chemical Structure

Sporothrix schenckii is a dimorphic fungus that occurs in tissues, or in cultures at 37°C, as elongated, banana-shaped or cigar-shaped, budding yeasts about 2 × 6 μm (Fig. 38-1). The mold form possesses slender hyphae, about 1 to 2 μm, in diameter, with flower-like collections of small conidial spores, each approximately 3 × 6 μm, borne on sterigmata (Fig. 38-2). Each hair-like sterigma is so slender as to be barely visible on light

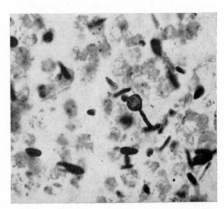

Figure 38-1. *Sporothrix schenckii.* Elongated yeast form in tissues. (From Emmons, C. W., Binford, C. H., and Utz, J. P.: Medical Mycology, 2nd ed. Philadelphia, Lea & Febiger, 1970.)

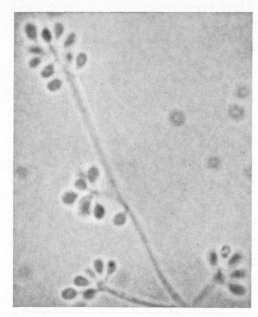

Figure 38-2. *Sporothrix schenckii.* Mold form in culture. Note the slender hyphae with conidia. (From Emmons, C. W., Binford, C. H., and Utz, J. P.: Medical Mycology, 2nd ed. Philadelphia, Lea & Febiger, 1970.)

microscopy. The hair-like appearance of the sterigmata gave rise to the genus name *Sporotrichum* (trichum = hair).

Although the cells contain Ags that may be active in agglutination, precipitation and C-F tests, these Ags have not been well characterized.

C. Extracellular Products

Extracts from culture filtrates have been used as antigenic preparations in testing for cutaneous delayed sensitivity to *S. schenckii*. There are no extracellular products that are known to contribute to pathogenesis.

D. Culture

At room temperature on Sabouraud's agar, *S. schenckii* grows in the mycelial form as brownish, wrinkled mold colonies that appear in about 5 days. On blood agar at 37°C, typical creamy yeast colonies are produced.

E. Experimental Models

Rodents can be infected by intraperitoneal injection.

F. Infections in Man

Human beings are infected most often by *S. schenckii* on thorns, splinters or other objects that penetrate into subcutaneous tissue. The organisms are

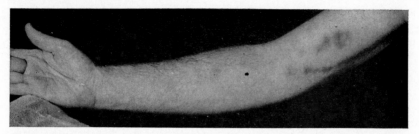

Figure 38-3. Chancriform lesions of primary cutaneous sporotrichosis, extending along lymphatic channels. (From Emmons, C. W., Binford, C. H., and Utz, J. P.: Medical Mycology, 2nd ed. Philadelphia, Lea & Febiger, 1970.)

ubiquitous in dead, decaying organic matter and on many living plants. Sporotrichosis is not limited to man, but occurs frequently in certain domestic animals and can be transmitted directly from them to man. Rarely, transmission can occur by repeated direct contact with an infected human being, or from the environment through hair follicles of normal skin; however, by far the most frequent means of infection is accidental subcutaneous inoculation of organisms from vegetation or dead organic materials.

Although different forms of disease can result, the most common is *primary cutaneous sporotrichosis* (Fig. 38-3). About two weeks after infection, a lesion resembling the chancre of syphilis forms at the site of inoculation (the chancriform lesion). Within 1 to 2 weeks, similar lesions begin to appear along the draining lymphatic vessel, resulting in a characteristic chain of ulcers.

Sometimes the infection is limited to the skin and does not involve the lymphatics, perhaps because of differences between strains of the fungus, or because of altered host responses.

Sporotrichosis is a chronic disease that may remain localized in subcutaneous tissue or lymphatics for many months or even years, during which the patient does not feel ill. As lesions become necrotic, pus is discharged to the exterior.

Disseminated sporotrichosis is rare. During dissemination the lesions occur in various tissues, including the CNS, bones, joints, or lung. They may resemble the ulcers of the primary, cutaneous form, with production of pus, or they may be granulomatous.

G. Mechanisms of Pathogenicity

The means by which *S. schenckii* causes disease are not known.

H. Mechanisms of Immunity

It is assumed that cellular immunity is of primary importance in resistance to sporotrichosis, but this remains to be proven. Experimental studies of small samples of human populations have shown that cutaneous delayed sensitivity develops in parallel with the amount or duration of exposure to the fungus. Normal individuals often possess demonstrable specific Abs without any history of sporotrichosis; however, cross reactions between Ags of *S. schenckii* and other fungi are common.

I. Laboratory Diagnosis

Diagnosis is based on the clinical picture and the results of cultures of pus from lesions (see Section D). The yeast tissue-form of *S. schenckii* is difficult to see and is not often identified in KOH mounts. Special staining techniques, such as PAS, or fluorescent-antibody microscopy is helpful for direct examination.

J. Reservoirs of Infection

The reservoirs of sporothrix are widespread in nature and include both dead organic materials and living plants.

K. Control of Disease Transmission

There are no established methods of control. Protective clothing or gloves can help to prevent inoculation by thorns or splinters.

L. Therapy

Amphotericin B is apparently effective for treating the occasional patient with disseminated sporotrichosis. Localized cutaneous lesions respond well to orally administered potassium iodide.

Maduromycosis (Madura Foot; Mycetoma)

Maduromycosis or mycetoma is a chronic granulomatous disease of subcutaneous tissues that often involves bones. It can be caused by infection with any one of a number of different organisms, including species of the bacterial genera *Nocardia* and *Streptomyces* (Chapter 35), and about 10 to 15 species of fungi. In the occasional case of mycetoma in the USA, the soil fungus *Allescheria boydii* is a frequent etiologic agent; however, mycetoma caused by other organisms is common in tropical and subtropical areas. For example, thousands of persons with mycetoma, caused by a variety of agents, are treated annually in Sudan.

As the name "Madura foot" implies, the foot is the usual site of infection, although hands are also often involved. The disease is chronic, and commonly deforming because of bone involvement. Diagnosis may be made on the basis of clinical observation and by demonstration of organisms in

KOH mounts of pus from lesions. In infections with *Allescheria boydii,* yellowish to white granules are apparent in the pus. The granules, representing fragments of colonies, may be other colors such as brown or black when other organisms are the infecting agents. The KOH preparations also often show masses of hyphae that are wide (5 to 10 μm) and swollen toward the edges of the mass. Culture may be useful for identifying the organism.

Treatment of maduromycosis is frequently not successful, and amputation may be necessary. It is essential that pus be drained from the lesions; however, even with adequate drainage, antibiotic therapy often fails. When bacteria of the actinomycete group are the cause, either penicillin or sulfonamide therapy may be successful, depending on the infecting organism (Chapter 35).

Chromoblastomycosis (Chromomycosis)

Although similar to maduromycosis in some respects, chromoblastomycosis is much more benign. The infection occurs in the skin or subcutaneous tissue and does not involve bones; therefore it is not deforming. The chronic, itching cauliflower-like ulcerations often occur on the legs of laborers whose skin is exposed to contaminated soil or splinters.

The disease occurs worldwide, but is more common in warm climates. It is caused by certain species of several different genera of fungi, notably *Cladosporium* and *Phialophora* (*Fonsecaea*). The latter are readily identified in pus as black or pigmented yeast-like cells that occur in tetrads formed by fission. Unlike most yeasts, Phialophorae multiply by fission rather than by budding. The dark pigment is also apparent in the mycelial colonies that form slowly on Sabouraud's medium at room temperature. Potassium iodide therapy has proven to be the most effective treatment for chromoblastomycosis.

Candida albicans (Candidiasis; Candidosis)

Candida albicans, a member of the normal flora of mucous membranes of man and many other animals, is the species of *Candida* most often responsible for infections. However, other species such as *C. tropicalis* and *C. krusei* also infect man occasionally. *Candida albicans* was formerly known as *Monilia albicans.*

A. Medical Perspectives

Infections with *C. albicans* occur frequently. They are known in the USA as *candidiasis,* or in the British literature by the more logical term *candido-*

sis. Candida infections represent a wide spectrum of clinical states, ranging from acute, self-limiting infections of the mucous membranes to chronic or fatal disease. At present the opportunistic *C. albicans* is responsible for about a fourth of all deaths caused by fungi in the USA. The incidence of candidiasis and the death rate will probably continue to increase, because predisposing circumstances are expected to increase in incidence (Chapter 36). In addition, the nature of the interaction between the host and *C. albicans* is poorly understood. Until more knowledge is gained, the outlook for controlling candidiasis is not promising.

B. Physical and Chemical Structure

Candida albicans occurs principally as an ovoid to spherical budding yeast, approximately 4 to 5 μm in diameter. Although it is a dimorphic fungus with the ability to form true mycelia, it also often forms *pseudomycelia*. The pseudomycelium is a filamentous structure resembling a mycelium but results from elongation of budding cells, rather than from true mycelial growth. Either of these filamentous forms is referred to as mycelial (*M*) forms, and the budding yeast is called the *Y* form (Fig. 38-4).

Groups of blastospores are formed along mycelia under certain growth conditions, and round, thick-walled chlamydospores occur at the ends of hyphae or between hyphal cells (Fig. 38-5). Chlamydospores represent a resting, resistant spore, and consequently are formed in old cultures or on relatively poor media, such as cornmeal agar, at a temperature of about 21°C.

The cell walls of *C. albicans* contain typical fungal constituents, and in addition possess unidentified components that are toxic for mice (Section G).

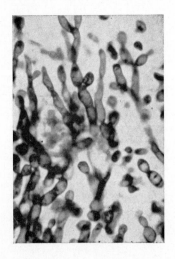

Figure 38-4. *Candida albicans.* A section from the tongue of a patient who died of acute leukemia complicated by candidiasis. Both blastospores and hyphae are frequently seen in tissues during acute candidiasis. (From Emmons, C. W., Binford, C. H., and Utz, J. P.: Medical Mycology, 2nd ed. Philadelphia, Lea & Febiger, 1970.)

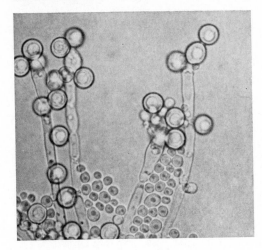

Figure 38-5. *Candida albicans.* Organisms in culture, showing yeast blastospores (smaller spheres) and chlamydospores (larger spheres). (From Emmons, C. W., Binford, C. H., and Utz, J. P.: Medical Mycology, 2nd ed. Philadelphia, Lea & Febiger, 1970.)

C. Extracellular Products

Candida is not known to produce any extracellular products of importance in the pathogenesis of disease. Culture filtrates are used as antigenic preparations in testing for cutaneous delayed-type sensitivity and for *in vitro* immunologic assays.

D. Culture

Growth is rapid on Sabouraud's medium, blood agar, trypticase soy, and many other rich media. Creamy yeast colonies are formed after overnight incubation at 21°C (room temperature) or 37°C; however the optimum growth temperature is around 30°C. After a few days' growth on Sabouraud's agar, colonies contain largely Y forms on the surface, but M forms, both mycelium and pseudomycelium, grow into the agar. The characteristic clusters of blastospores are formed along the hyphae, and chlamydospores are often present (Fig. 38-5.)

E. Experimental Models

Laboratory rodents such as guinea pigs, rabbits and mice can be infected with *C. albicans* and are often used in experimental studies. Like man, the mouse and other rodents are resistant to infection with candida, and large numbers of yeast cells must be injected in order to establish an infection. Most often, the yeast cells are inoculated intravenously or intraperitoneally; in either case, the result is widespread abscesses in many tissues, especially the kidney, and death occurs within a week with most dosages used. Another model involves injection of yeast cells into the mouse thigh to produce a lesion that is self-limiting by about 4 to 6 weeks.

Attempts have been made to produce lesions in the skin and mucous membranes of man and animals. It is usually impossible to infect the intact integuments of normal subjects by inoculating *C. albicans.* If mucous membranes are abraded before inoculation, infection occurs briefly but is soon cleared. Similarly, if skin is abraded and macerated, infection can be initiated, but lasts only as long as the tissue is kept macerated.

It has been possible to colonize, and occasionally to infect, by feeding *C. albicans* to germ-free animals that lack normal bacterial flora, but not to normal animals.

F. Infections in Man

Complex schemes for classifying different forms of human candidiasis have been presented. Perhaps the simplest approach is to consider these infections as a spectrum with a few important protoytpes (Table 38-1).

By far the most common candida infections are the acute lesions of mucous membranes that occur as the result of relatively minor aberrations in the host response. Oral thrush of newborn infants is a good example of this form. The infant's mucous membranes are contaminated during passage through the birth canal, or by contact with attendants soon after birth. Usually, as soon as the normal bacterial flora develops, the yeast infection is controlled; however, premature babies that are immunologically immature may experience severe infections. Other examples of candidiasis of the mucous membranes include infections in the aged, in patients with diabetes or other endocrine abnormalities, and *especially in patients given broad-spectrum antibiotics or steroid therapy. Vulvovaginal and gastrointestinal manifestations are common in these patients.*

Cutaneous infections occur most often as a direct result of mechanical forces that cause abrasion, or of continued excess moisture, or both. For example, *perlèche* is seen in patients who have deep folds around the corners of the mouth; saliva provides a moist environment for fungal growth. *Intertrigo* also occurs in moist folds of skin, such as obese buttocks and groins, and beneath pendulous breasts; this condition is worse during hot weather when excess perspiration keeps the affected areas moist. It may occur between the fingers of workers who keep their hands in water all day and regularly have macerated skin.

Paronychia and other involvement around the nails are not likely to be caused by candida unless there is maceration or some predisposing abnormality of the nailbed.

Certain rare forms of candidiasis occur as a result of serious immunodeficiencies. *Candida granuloma,* fortunately, seldom occurs; it results in horny, disfiguring, granulomatous lesions of the skin. More frequent, but still rare, is *chronic mucocutaneous candidiasis* (CMC), in which the fungi are found only in the superficial layers of skin and mucous membranes, and

TABLE 38-1
Manifestations of Candidiasis in Man

Disease Process	Common Predisposing Factors	Probable Outcome
Lesions of mucous membranes:		
Oral (thrush)	Infancy, old-age, diabetes, antibiotic therapy, steroid therapy	Usually self-limiting; may be chronic over many months
Vulvovaginal	Pregnancy, diabetes	Self-limiting when predisposing condition is cleared
Gastrointestinal, perianal	Antibiotic therapy	Self-limiting after use of antibiotics is discontinued
Perlèche—lesions at corners of the mouth	Wearing dentures	May be self-limiting when dentures are properly fitted
Intertrigo—lesions within folds of tissue such as groin	Obesity, perspiration	Clears with aid of medicated powders to keep affected areas dry
Paronychia—lesions around nails	Maceration	Usually self-limiting
Candida granuloma— production of horny, granulomatous lesions	Immune deficiency	May respond to amphotericin B, at least temporarily
Chronic mucocutaneous candidiasis—fungus grows in superficial layers, does not invade past epithelium	Immune deficiency, usually cellular or combined	Recurs after treatment; few instances of long-term success with immunologic reconstitution have been reported
Disseminated	Malignant disease; other serious diseases	Often fatal. May respond to amphotericin B

never invade. Outstanding features of CMC are its *chronic nature,* with infections often cleared by vigorous treatment only to return soon after cessation of therapy, and its association with *cellular immunodeficiencies* or *severe combined immunodeficiencies.* It has been noted that CMC invariably develops in patients with severe combined immunodeficiencies who survive long enough to be studied, and it is common among patients with a variety of cellular immunodeficiencies; nevertheless, candidiasis does not present a problem in patients with primary deficiencies in humoral Abs.

Disseminated candidiasis is often a terminal event in patients with overwhelming disorders, such as malignant disease. During dissemination the yeast may infect virtually any organ, especially the kidneys.

Use of contaminated equipment by "mainliner" drug addicts has resulted in persistent or fatal candida endocarditis. In addition, certain intravenous catheters and shunts used for medical therapy have allowed entrance of candida and establishment of infection that usually is self-limited when the offending catheter is removed.

Amphotericin B is used to treat disseminated candidiasis; nystatin tablets or ointments are useful for topical treatment of oral or skin lesions, respectively.

G. Mechanisms of Pathogenicity

Despite the fact that candidiasis is the most common opportunistic fungal disease, almost nothing is known about the mechanisms of pathogenesis involved. It has been shown that the cell walls of *C. albicans* contain toxic materials; cell-wall preparations are rapidly fatal for injected mice. However, there is no evidence that this kind of toxicity occurs during the course of infection in man.

H. Mechanisms of Immunity

A vast literature exists concerning the mechanisms of immunity to candida; however, seemingly contradictory observations have been made in different controlled experimental animal models as well as in human studies which, for the most part, have had to be uncontrolled.

There is general agreement that cellular immunity is of primary importance in resistance to candida. Several lines of evidence have led to this general conclusion. Perhaps most compelling is the fact that candidiasis is common in patients with cellular immunodeficiencies, but not in those with humoral immune defects. Other supporting evidence comes from animal studies showing a greater than normal susceptibility to candidiasis in animals immunosuppressed by irradiation, neonatal thymectomy, or other treatment.

Even though cellular immunity is undoubtedly involved in resistance to candida, it remains to be proven that it is of paramount importance. A majority of patients with candidiasis have no evidence of cellular immunodeficiencies and many patients with severe cellular immunodeficiencies do not become infected with the ubiquitous candida. A variety of nonspecific humoral factors have been shown to inhibit or kill candida. Human serum contains a factor that clumps the yeast; transferrin and other iron-binding substances inhibit candida by competing for available iron. The microbicidal peroxidase-H_2O_2-halide ion system found in neutrophils and certain body fluids can kill *C. albicans;* this is the basis for the candidacidal activity of human neutrophils. Experimentally, it has been possible to gain a degree of resistance by immunizing animals with killed candida, and, furthermore, to passively transfer resistance to normal recipients with sera having high humoral Ab titers.

A limited number of patients with CMC have been studied in an attempt to determine the deficiency responsible for their increased susceptibility to candida. The results suggest that any one of a variety of defects may be responsible. Some patients have lymphocytes that do not respond to candida Ags *in vitro,* indicating lack of recognition of Ags. Others produce humoral factors that suppress the response of normal sensitized lymphocytes to candida Ags. Still others have responding lymphocytes that fail to produce MIF.

If cellular immunity is of importance in resistance to candida, and indeed to other extracellular fungi, the principal question is what are the operative mechanisms? Most of the bacterial infections, such as tuberculosis and listeriosis, that serve as models of antimicrobial cellular immunity involve parasites that live within macrophages and that are inhibited by T-cell-initiated changes in the macrophages (Chapter 7). Candida is not an intracellular parasite. During experimentally induced animal infections, the cellular response is principally granulocytic; macrophages appear to play a minor part and to be unable to kill candida to a significant extent. It is possible that certain lymphokines may be antifungal *in vivo,* as they are *in vitro.*

Obviously, much remains to be learned about immunity to candida, and at least some of the tools are now at hand for unraveling the mysterious tangle of interacting host mechanisms.

I. Laboratory Diagnosis

Candida is readily seen in stained pus or secretions. Within tissue sections, special stains such as PAS or methenamine silver make the fungi more readily visible. The organisms are easily cultured, with colonies apparent within a day or two (Section D). The major problem in laboratory diagnosis is in determining whether demonstrable *C. albicans* is the etiologic agent, because it is commonly present in normal flora, and small numbers may rapidly increase, for example, in sputum samples, before the sample reaches the laboratory. Therefore, prompt culture is necessary, and large numbers of candida should be present in fresh specimens if candidiasis exists.

Controversy exists over the relative invasiveness of Y and M forms of *C. albicans.* Many investigators and clinicians claim that only the M form is invasive; therefore, in tissue sections where the Y form is abundant but the M form is lacking it is presumed that there is colonization but not invasion. Conversely, the presence of the M form is taken as evidence of infection. Others claim that infection can occur without invasion by the M form. It has been suggested that lack of certain nutrients leads to the production of M forms, or that they are caused by host responses. *In vitro* studies have defined conditions under which the M form is favored, but whether the same events occur *in vivo* is not known. At present, the controversy cannot be resolved.

A useful test for distinguishing *C. albicans* from similar yeasts is the *germ-tube test*. Organisms in yeast form, inoculated into undiluted human serum, will produce germ tubes within 4 hours, and usually by 1 hour. Other yeasts, and even other species of *Candida,* fail to do so. Sugar fermentations also aid in differentiation of the species.

J.   Reservoirs of Infection

Human beings are the principal reservoir for candida, which is part of the normal flora of most human mucous membranes.

K.   Control of Disease Transmission

Candidiasis will be controlled only when there is a better understanding of host-parasite interactions. At present, control depends on correcting or eliminating predisposing conditions.

References

Catchings, B. M., and Guidry, D. J.: Effects of pH and temperature on the *in vitro* growth of *Sporothrix schenckii.* Sabouraudia *11*:70, 1973.

Emmons, C. W., Binford, C. H., and Utz, J. P.: .Medical Mycology, 2nd ed. Philadelphia, Lea & Febiger, 1970.

Kirkpatrick, C. H., Rich, R. R., and Bennett, J. E.: Chronic mucocutaneous candidiasis: Model-building in cellular immunity. Ann. Intern. Med. *74*:955, 1971.

Pearsall, N. N., Sundsmo, J. S., and Weiser, R. S.: Lymphokine toxicity for yeast cells. J. Immunol. *110*:1444, 1973.

Sethi, K. K.: Experimental sporotrichosis in the normal and modified host. Sabouraudia *10*:66, 1972.

Szaniszlo, P. J., Cooper, B. H., and Voges, H. S.: Chemical composition of the hyphal walls of three chromomycosis agents. Sabouraudia *10*:94, 1972.

Winner, H. I., and Hurley, R.: Candida Albicans. London, J. & A. Churchill, 1964.

Winner, H. I., and Hurley, R.: Symposium on Candida Infections. London, E. & S. Livingstone, 1966.

Young, R. C., Bennett, J. E., Vogel, C. L., Carbone, P. P., and DeVita, V. T.: Aspergillosis. The spectrum of the disease in 98 patients. Medicine *49*:147, 1970.

Chapter 39

The Superficial Mycoses

A group of fungi known as the dermatophytes causes superficial mycoses (dermatophytoses) of keratinized areas of the body, the skin, hair, or nails. A variety of diseases result, the most usual being known by the common names "ringworm" and "athlete's foot." Most dermatophytes are included in 3 genera of *Fungi Imperfecti,* namely, *Microsporum, Epidermophyton* and *Trichophyton.* Approximately 35 species from these genera are known to cause human mycoses.

A. Medical Perspectives

The dermatophytes are found in virtually all parts of the world; however, environmental conditions sometimes favor a higher incidence of some species in certain geographic locations. For example, *Trichophyton schoenleinii* is usually limited to the Mediterranean countries, whereas *T. mentagrophytes* is more widespread, and is common in the USA.

It is probable that every normal person has been infected with at least one of the dermatophytes at some time, often in childhood. Usually the infections are trivial and self-limiting. Part of the population, however, is plagued by long-lasting superficial mycoses that are often resistant to treatment. Even though they are seldom dangerous or life-threatening diseases, the dermatophytoses are responsible for a tremendous amount of discomfort and annoyance for many people.

B. Physical and Chemical Structure

Most of the dermatophytes are molds. They form conidia characteristic of the species; therefore, conidia are important aids in identification of these fungi. Hyphae grow in superficial layers of dead keratinized cells, and form conidia there. The cell-wall material, typical of fungi, covers both the hyphae and conidia. No capsular substances are known to be produced by dermatophytes.

Microsporum. Members of the genus *Microsporum* have macroconidia as their predominant spore form. These are large (20 to 125 μm long), multicellular conidia formed on the ends of hyphae. Figure 39-1 shows the spindle-shaped macroconidia of *M. gypseum* and *M. canis,* two of the common dermatophytes.

Colonies of *Microsporum* sp. are usually tan to brown in color, and become cottony after 2 to 4 weeks. They grow well on Sabouraud's glucose agar at room temperature.

Trichophyton. Microconidia are the prominent spore forms of members of the genus *Trichophyton,* although macroconidia may also be present. The species most common in the USA are *T. rubrum, T. tonsurans* and *T. mentagrophytes;* spores of the latter species are shown in Figure 39-2. Coiled hyphae are formed by *T. mentagrophytes;* the few macroconidia of this species are elongated (8 to 50 μm), and grape-like clusters of spherical microconidia occur along the sides of the hyphae.

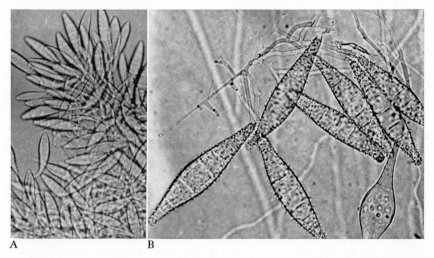

A   B

Figure 39-1. Macroconidia of *Microsporum* sp. A, *M. gypseum.* B, *M. canis.* (From Emmons, C. W., Binford, C. H., and Utz, J. P.: Medical Mycology, 2nd ed. Philadelphia, Lea & Febiger, 1970.)

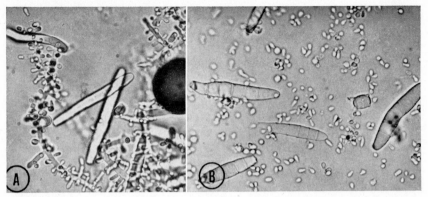

Figure 39-2. *Trichophyton mentagrophytes.* A, Microconidia and B, macroconidia. (From Emmons, C. W., Binford, C. H., and Utz, J. P.: Medical Mycology, 2nd ed. Philadelphia, Lea & Febiger, 1970.)

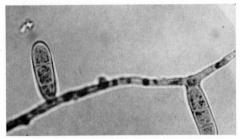

Figure 39-3. Macroconidia of *Epidermophyton floccosum.* (From Emmons, C. W., Binford, C. H., and Utz, J. P.: Medical Mycology, 2nd ed. Philadelphia: Lea & Febiger, 1970.)

The colonial forms of *Trichophyton* sp. vary considerably. Colonies may be smooth or powdery, and may range in color from white, pink, red, or purple to yellow or brown.

Epidermophyton. In the USA, *E. floccosum* is often seen. It bears clusters of oval or club-shaped macroconidia about 8 to 15 μm long (Fig. 39-3), but no microconidia. Its colonies are greenish-yellow and powdery in appearance.

C. Extracellular Products

Little is known about extracellular products of the dermatophytes. All of these fungi utilize keratin and some species are known to produce extracellular keratinases and proteolytic enzymes that allow them to degrade host components used for nutrients.

D. Culture

The dermatophytes are slow-growing, compared with most bacteria. When grown on Sabouraud's glucose agar at room temperature, colonies of some species are apparent after one week, but other species may require several weeks to form visible colonies. Addition of special nutrients, such as vitamins, to the medium enhances the growth of some species. For example, thiamin supplementation stimulates the growth of *T. tonsurans.*

E.   Experimental Models

Host response plays such an important role in the dermatophytoses that it has proven impossible to infect most human volunteers with the dermatophytes. Experimental animal models are also of little value.

F.   Infections in Man

The dermatophytes cause tinea and related diseases. The word *tinea* comes from a Latin root meaning a gnawing worm, and a common name for some forms of tinea is ringworm. However, the name is misleading, for these diseases have no connection with worms. In fact, the fungal infection spreads in an expanding circular form, resulting in ring-shaped, scaly, itching areas on the skin. Other species grow in or on hair or nails. The superficial mycoses are often recognized by such common names as athlete's foot, jockey itch and barber's itch.

Tinea is further classified by the areas in which it is found:

Tinea capitis, a disease of the scalp and hair, is most frequently caused by members of the genus *Microsporum,* but some *Trichophyton* species are often the etiologic agents. In the USA, *M. audouinii* is the most common cause of tinea capitis, but *M. tonsurans* and *M. canis* are also common agents.

Tinea corporis (*tinea circinata*); ringworm of the smooth skin, may be caused by many species of the genera *Microsporum* and *Trichophyton,* but *M. canis* and *T. mentagrophytes* are the most common offenders.

Tinea barbae, or barber's itch, on bearded areas of the face and neck, is usually caused by *T. mentagrophytes,* other species of *Trichophyton,* or *M. canis.*

Tinea pedis, athlete's foot, has been found in well over half of the individuals in populations that have been studied. Its incidence is higher in adults than in children, and higher in men than in women; the disease is exacerbated by hot, moist conditions. The most common etiologic agents of tinea pedis are *T. mentagrophytes* and *Epidermophyton floccosum.*

Tinea cruris, infections of the groin, perineum and perianal regions are most often caused by *E. floccosum.*

Tinea unguium (*onychomycosis*), or tinea of the nails, is caused by the same fungi that cause athlete's foot, but it is especially prone to occur in 40- to 50-year-old women.

Tinea versicolor is a tinea of smooth skin characterized by the changing color of the lesion, hence the name versicolor; the etiologic agent is *Malas-*

sezia furfur. It is of interest that this fungus appears to prefer only keratin of the skin and not of the hair and nails; thus, this infection is limited to the outermost layer of the skin.

Tinea can sometimes result in pustular abscesses of hair follicles, called kerion. The kerion type of infection occurs most often in tinea barbae.

Favus is a severe and chronic type of ringworm, characterized by dermal crusts resembling honeycomb. It can be caused by a number of different dermatophytes, but *T. schoenleinii* is the most frequent agent. Favus is endemic in the Mediterranean area, parts of southern Asia, Africa and the Orient. Patients known to have favus are not admitted to the USA; however, some cases occur in this country, apparently as a result of previous introduction of the fungus by immigrants from endemic areas.

G. Mechanisms of Pathogenicity

All dermatophytes are keratinophilic, but the genera appear to vary as to the kind of keratin they prefer. This preference may determine the site of infection of the various dermatophytes.

Members of the genus *Microsporum* seem to prefer only the keratin of skin and hair, and consequently they rarely invade nails. They grow both inside and outside the hair shaft, forming a sheath of spores on the surface of each hair (ectothrix). Infected hairs tend to break off just above the scalp, leaving a stubble.

Epidermophyton sp. invade skin and nails, but do not attack hair. Thus, they are often implicated as the cause of tinea pedis, tinea cruris, and tinea unguium (onychomycosis), but not tinea capitis.

Trichophyton sp. are not fastidious, but will live on keratin of hair, skin, or nails. Species such as *T. tonsurans* grow principally within hair shafts (endothrix), causing the hair to break off below the scalp surface. This results in bald areas with "black dots" where hairs have been lost. Other species, such as *T. mentagrophytes,* are ectothrix fungi. *Trichophyton mentagrophytes* often causes kerion, probably because of strong inflammatory responses to the fungi within hair follicles.

In general, the symptoms of dermatophytoses are more pronounced when man is the unnatural host than when the fungi are natural parasites of the human host. Thus, *T. mentagrophytes* and *M. canis,* which have animals as natural hosts, tend to incite much more vigorous inflammatory responses in man than *M. audouinii* or other anthropophilic fungi, which have man as their natural hosts. These responses of the host are often a principal factor in the pathogenesis of the disease.

The patterns of growth of the dermatophytes account for the usual clinical picture. The fungi grow in a widening circle or ring that appears brownish to red at the periphery as a result of the inflammatory response there. The center of the ring is scaly; at this site thickened, infected areas of the keratinized layer of the skin tend to scale off. Hypersensitivity to fungal Ags probably leads to the vesicle formation that is often noted.

The sensitivity usually elicited by dermatophytoses can result in *derma-tophytids or "id" reactions.* These resemble contact dermatitis; they occur in regions distant from the site of infection with the fungus. The id reaction is often manifested by vesicular lesions on the hands or elsewhere, which itch and may become secondarily infected or painful.

Common Ags shared by the dermatophytes are capable of inciting a delayed type of sensitivity reaction in the skin of sensitized patients tested with trichophytin, an antigenic preparation made from cultures of various dermatophytes. Apparently the id reaction is analogous to the trichophytin skin test, in that the sensitive patient gives a sensitivity reaction to soluble Ags at a site far removed from the foci of infection. Dermatophytid reactions may be much more severe and troublesome than the actual dermatophytosis.

Thus, the predilection of some of the dermatophytes for certain tissues helps to determine the site of the infection. The pathogenesis of disease may rest principally on allergic or other inflammatory responses of the host to the infecting fungus.

Although dermatophytes often persist in infected superficial tissues for many years, they rarely if ever invade. Either the pathogenic capacities they exhibit on body surfaces are totally ineffective within body tissues or the organisms are unable to persist in the tissues.

H.   Mechanisms of Immunity

The human host is able to limit dermatophyte infections to superficial areas, at least in part, as a result of antifungal factors in plasma. The dermatophytes cannot live in the presence of human plasma or serum.

Delayed sensitivity reactions may be a distinct advantage to the patient in some of the superficial mycoses. When infection is limited to the superficial areas of the skin, an edematous reaction below that area could cause the sloughing and expulsion of infected skin, affording a means of ridding the body of unwanted fungal parasites.

Usually, the dermatophytes establish a workable, long-lasting state of parasitism with their human hosts. They are able to withstand the hypersensitivity responses of the host and, to a large extent, are protected in their exterior environment from both humoral and cellular immune mechanisms. They may often, as in favus, persist in a host for its lifetime.

It has been shown that high concentrations of specific Ab added to media completely inhibit growth of *T. mentagrophytes,* whereas lower concentrations of Ab can cause structural changes in the hyphae and conidia produced. Complement was not present in the media. There is evidence that C plus Ab does not cause lysis of fungi.

Hormonal influences can affect the course of fungal infections profoundly. In tinea capitis caused by *M. audouinii,* for example, children commonly remain infected up until the age of puberty, at which time the infection becomes self-limited. It has been suggested that the increase in long-chain fatty acids in the skin after puberty may be related to clinical improvement. There is experimental evidence that fatty acids and certain oils used on hair inhibit the penetration of some dermatophytes into hairs.

I. Laboratory Diagnosis

The dermatophytes may be recovered from skin scrapings, nails, or hair. Direct examination of KOH mounts (Chapter 36) often reveals hyphae or conidia. Ectothrix or endothrix infections of hairs can be distinguished by direct microscopic examination.

Although the growth of dermatophytes may be optimal at a pH of 6.8 to 7.0, they tolerate a more acid environment and usually grow well on Sabouraud's glucose agar at pH 5.6 to 6.0. Characteristic colonies appear, generally after about 1 to 3 weeks of incubation at room temperature.

Slide cultures (Chapter 36) are especially useful for identifying dermatophytes. Identification is based on the production of characteristic macroconidia or microconidia, as well as on colonial appearance, and occasionally on certain nutritional requirements.

The fluorescence of *M. audouinii* and other *Microsporum* species is helpful in distinguishing infections with these fungi from tinea caused by *Trichophyton*. Hairs that are infected with *Microsporum* usually have a green fluorescence under ultraviolet light, whereas those infected with *Trichophyton* do not fluoresce.

J. Reservoirs of Infection

Depending on the species, dermatophytes that infect man may be normal inhabitants of soil, animal species, or man only. The reservoirs of some of the common dermatophytes are listed in Table 39-1.

TABLE 39-1
Reservoirs of Some Common Dermatophytes

Genus and Species	Reservoir
Microsporum audouinii	Man
M. canis	Dogs, cats
M. gypseum	Soil
M. fulvum	Soil
Trichophyton schoenleinii	Man
T. mentagrophytes	Man, domestic animals, and perhaps soil
T. rubrum	Man
Epidermophyton floccosum	Man

K. Therapy

The dermatophytoses are often self-limiting, although they may persist for many years. Patients with severe or disfiguring lesions may be treated with griseofulvin (Chapter 36). More often, topical treatments are used to alleviate symptoms. Tinea pedis, for example, is made worse by shoes that confine perspiring feet. The warm, moist environment produced favors growth of the fungi. Powders, or other means of keeping feet dry, are sometimes helpful. Antifungal agents such as undecylenic acid are often incorporated into the powders. Ointments containing tolnaftate or fatty acid salts may be effective for treating tinea of the glabrous skin.

L. Control of Disease Transmission

The dermatophytoses are best controlled by avoiding exposure to causative fungi. In infections with *M. audouinii,* the organisms are transmitted from one child to another, especially by contact with caps or other heavily contaminated items. Infections with *M. canis,* on the other hand, are usually contracted from infected animals; owners' pets may be responsible, but stray cats and dogs, fondled by children, are more often the source. Avoidance of such sources of infection helps to control the spread of superficial mycoses.

The efficacy of disinfectant foot baths and similar measures used to prevent the spread of tinea pedis is open to question. Although it is certain that fungi in skin scales may be infectious, experimental attempts to transfer tinea have often failed. Such experiments emphasize the importance of host responses in the establishment of disease. Nevertheless, avoidance of the sources of dermatophytes will protect against infection, regardless of the immunologic status of the host.

Routine sterilization or disinfection of instruments in barber shops and hairdressers' salons has helped prevent the dissemination of certain dermatophytes.

References

Emmons, C. W., Binford, C. H., and Utz, J. P.: Medical Mycology, 2nd ed. Philadelphia, Lea & Febiger, 1970.

Georg, L. K.: Agents of superficial and cutaneous mycoses and of keratomycosis. *In* Manual of Clinical Microbiology, pp. 331-345. Edited by J. E. Blair, E. H. Lennette, and J. P. Truant. American Society for Microbiology, Bethesda, Md., 1970.

Grappel, S. F., Buscavage, C. A., Blank, F., and Bishop, C. T.: Comparative serological reactivities of twenty-seven polysaccharides from nine species of dermatophytes. Sabouraudia 8:116, 1970.

Grappel, S. F., Fethiere, A., and Blank, F.: Effect of antibodies on growth and structure of *Trichophyton mentagrophytes.* Sabouraudia 9:50, 1971.

Hajini, G. H., Kandhari, K. C., Mohapatra, L. N., and Bhutani, L. K.: Effect of hair oils and fatty acids on the growth of dermatophytes and their *in vitro* penetration of human scalp hair. Sabouraudia 8:174, 1970.

Minocha, Y., Pasricha, J. S., Mohapatra, L. N., and Kandhari, K. C.: Proteolytic activity of dermatophytes and its role in the pathogenesis of skin lesions. Sabouraudia 10:79, 1972.

Nozawa, Y., Noguchi, T., Ito, Y., Sudo, N., and Watanabe, S.: Immunochemical studies on *Trichophyton mentagrophytes*. Sabouraudia 9:129, 1971.

Scope Monograph on Human Mycoses. Kalamazoo, Mich., Upjohn Co., 1968.

Wilson, J. W., and Plunkett, O. A.: The Fungous Diseases of Man. Berkeley, University of California Press, 1967.

Glossary

This glossary is limited largely to terms and abbreviations that are not readily found in dictionaries or for which varying definitions may be given. They are for the most part much used terms and in many instances are not included in the index. Special attention has been given to abbreviations.

Abscess: A local collection of pus that represents the liquefied remains of leukocytes (principally neutrophils) and disintegrated tissue.

Accidental host: (see Unnatural host)

Acid-fast: Not decolorized by acid treatment after staining, e.g. the mycobacteria retain certain stains even when treated with acid alcohol.

Acidosis: Abnormal increase in concentration of hydrogen ions in the blood and consequent compensatory mechanisms that alter blood buffers.

Acquired immunity (adaptive immunity): Immunity acquired during the lifetime of the individual; can be acquired either naturally or artificially and can be either active or passive in nature. Usually specific but can be nonspecific; example of nonspecific immunity is the immunity due to interferon.

Active immunity: Immunity acquired as the result of an immune response mounted by the host; may be nonspecific as well as specific.

Adaptive immunity: (see Acquired immunity)

Adenyl cyclase: Enzyme, bound to the cytoplasmic membranes of most animal cells; catalyzes the formation of cyclic adenosine monophosphate from ATP.

Adjuvant: Immunologic; a substance that increases or diversifies the immune response to an Ag. Freund's adjuvants (a) complete = water-in-oil emulsion of mineral oil, plant waxes and killed tubercle bacilli; (b) incomplete = Freund's complete emulsion minus the tubercle bacilli.

Adoptive immunity: Active immunity developed in a recipient as a result of having received immunocompetent donor cells.

Aggressin: A microbial product or component that opposes host defense mechanisms, e.g. capsules that interfere with phagocytosis are aggressins.

Allergen: An Ag or hapten-carrier complex that engenders a state of allergy.

Allergic granuloma: A granuloma developed as the result of an allergic response to the inciting agent.

Allergy: A state of specific hypersensitivity, often employed to designate hypersensitivities due to IgE Ab.

Alloantibody: An Ab produced against a foreign alloantigen.

Alloantigen: An Ag present in some but not all individuals of an animal species.

Anamnestic response (recall or memory phenomenon): An accelerated immune response to an Ag that occurs in an animal previously exposed to the Ag or related Ags; may involve the humoral and/or the cellular immune response.

Angina: Sore throat (there are other uses for this term also).

Anthropophilic: Having a preference for man rather than animals.

Antibiosis: Inhibition exerted by one organism on other organisms.

Antigen mimicry: The circumstance in which a microbe produces an Ag that mimics and is cross reactive with an Ag of the host.

Antiseptic: Disinfectants that are used topically on skin or wounds.

Antiserum: A serum containing Abs; the term is usually employed to designate a serum containing Abs induced by injection of an Ag.

Anuria: A state in which the excretion of urine is severely or totally suppressed.

Apparent infection: Infection associated with clinically evident disease.

Arthropods: Invertebrates with jointed limbs including mites and ticks.

Ascitic fluid: Fluid from the peritoneal cavity.

ASO test: A test for Abs specific for streptolysin O; it is commonly used as an indicator of recent streptococcal infection in the diagnosis of rheumatic fever.

Atelectasis: An airless state of lung tissue with collapsed alveoli; it may be local or general.

ATP: (adenosine triphosphate): A chemical compound that is the major storage form of energy in cells; ATP possesses 2 high-energy phosphate bonds which release energy on hydrolysis.

Attenuated: A derived pathogen that is avirulent or of low virulence. Attenuation may be achieved by genetic selection or by physical or chemical treatment.

Atypical mycobacteria ("unclassified" or "anonymous" mycobacteria): Facultatively pathogenic mycobacteria for man comprising species other than the recognized pathogenic species *M. tuberculosis, M. bovis* and *M. avium.* They are not transmitted from man to man and most species are probably saprophytes.

Bacillus: The name for the genus *Bacillus;* also used loosely to designate rod-shaped bacteria.

Bacteremia: Presence of bacteria in the blood stream; associated with nonseptic as well as septic states.

Bacteriocins: Protein molecules, produced by bacteria, which kill other strains of the same or closely related species.

Bacteriostatic agent: An agent that arrests the growth of bacteria but does not kill them.

Bacteriuria: Presence of bacteria in the urine; may occur in subclinical as well as clinical states.

BCG (bacillus of Calmette and Guerin): An avirulent strain of *Mycobacterium bovis* used as vaccine for tuberculosis.

Beta hemolysis: Complete lysis of RBC's; colonies of beta-hemolytic bacteria on blood agar are surrounded by clear areas of hemolysis.

Biopsy: The procedure of removing tissue from the living animal.

Biotype: A group of organisms all of which have the same genotype but varying physical characteristics.

Blocking antibody: An Ab that can block a specific activity of another Ab or an immune cell. Examples are: the incomplete Ab of brucellosis that blocks agglutination by brucella agglutinins; the incomplete Ab of Rh disease that blocks the "saline agglutinin"; the Ab in the sera of desensitized hay fever patients that blocks the Prausnitz-Kustner skin reaction; the Ab of cancer patients that blocks the action of "killer lymphocytes" on tumor cells.

Blood-brain barrier: A permeability barrier presented by blood vessel walls that restricts the passage of macromolecules, such as immunoglobulins, between the blood and the brain parenchyma. The structural and functional bases of the barrier are not known.

Bubo: A lymph node that has become enlarged as the result of inflammation; often associated with infection.

CAMP (cyclic adenosine monophosphate): Adenosine 3',5' monophosphate; mediates the actions of many hormones; within cells the level of CAMP regulates cellular function.

Capsid: The protein coat of a virus.

Capsular swelling test (Quellung test): Swelling of the bacterial capsule as the result of a specific reaction with Ab; used in serologic identification of encapsulated bacteria; results in opsonization.

Carriage: The act of serving as a carrier of a pathogen.

Carrier: A host who harbors and releases pathogens but shows no apparent disease. A host may shed pathogens during convalescence (convalescent carrier) or for long periods (chronic carrier) or periodically (intermittent carrier).

Caseation necrosis: Necrosis in which the necrotic material is of cheese-like consistency; characteristic of the necrotic lesions of tuberculosis; results primarily from the death of epithelioid cells in the allergic granuloma.

Cellular immunity (cell-mediated immunity): Immunity that can be transferred with cells but not with serum; rests on the specific response of T cells to Ag.

Cervicofacial: Pertaining to both the neck and the face.

CF (complement fixation): Binding the components of C with other substances.

CFU (colony forming unit): One or more cells that replicate and give rise to a single colony.

Chemotaxis: Attraction or repulsion of a cell by a chemical.

Cholecystectomy: Surgical removal of the gallbladder and duct.

CID: "Cellular immune deficiency."

Clean-voided urine specimen: Urine collected midstream after careful cleansing of external urogenital areas to minimize contamination by normal flora.

CMC (chronic mucocutaneous candidiasis): The disease usually occurs in individuals known to be immunodeficient.

CMI (cell-mediated immunity): See Cellular immunity.

CNS: Central nervous system.

Coccoid: Resembling cocci; rounded or spherical cells.

Cold agglutinins: Immunoglobulins in blood plasma or serum that cause the agglutination of RBC's at $0°$ to $4°$ C but not at $37°$ C; occur in primary atypical pneumonia and certain other disease states.

Colicins: Bacteriocins produced by *Escherichia coli*.

Colonization: Growth of organisms on surfaces; may or may not lead to invasion of underlying tissues.

Complement (C): A collective term designating a system of blood proteins, some with enzyme activity, that become triggered to interact either by immunoglobulins aggregated with Ag or with each other or by an alternate pathway.

Compound microscope: A light microscope having two or more lenses.

Consumption coagulopathy: Reduction in one or more of the blood-clotting factors as the result of extensive blood clotting, usually intravascular.

Contact inhibition: Inhibition of growth of normal cells in monolayer cultures that occurs when cells contact each other in the monolayer.

Cord factor: A component of *M. tuberculosis* associated with the capacity of the organism to grow in aggregates resembling skein-like cords.

Corticosteroids: Steroids with certain chemical or biological properties characteristic of the hormones secreted by the adrenal cortex.

Counter-immunoelectrophoresis: Immunoelectrophoresis performed with 2 electrical currents applied sequentially in perpendicular directions to give greater resolution to the precipitin lines formed.

C-reactive protein: An abnormal beta-globulin that appears in the serum of a variety of patients with acute inflammatory diseases. Combines with the C-substance of the pneumococcus to form a precipitate.

CSF: Cerebrospinal fluid.

C-substance: The specific Forssman-like carbohydrate in the cell wall of the pneumococcus.

Cystitis: Inflammation of the urinary bladder, usually as the result of infection.

Cytophilic antibodies: Antibodies which, in the free state, have an affinity for cells that depends on attraction forces independent of those that bind Ag to Ab. Examples are the binding of IgE Abs to mast cells and the binding of certain IgM and IgG Abs to macrophages.

Cytoplasmic membrane (protoplasmic membrane, plasma membrane): The membrane enclosing the cytoplasm of a cell.

Darkfield illumination: A procedure based on the principle of light reflected from the object being observed.

Decubitus ulcers (bedsores): Ulcers of the skin that result from ischemia at local pressure points in dependent parts of the body.

Defervescence: Disappearance of fever.

Delayed hypersensitivity (delayed sensitivity): A specific T-cell dependent sensitive state characterized by a delay of many hours in onset time and course of reaction following challenge with Ag. It can be transferred with cells but not with serum.

Dermatophytes: A group of keratinophilic fungi that invade superficial keratinized areas of the body (hair, skin, nails).

Desensitization (hyposensitization): Abolition or diminution of the sensitive state by administration of Ag, usually in small repeated doses. Applied to the refractory state effected by pollen treatment to prevent hay fever, to suppression of anaphylactic sensitivity to foreign serum with small repeated doses of serum and to the suppression of delayed sensitivity with Ag or hapten.

Differential medium: A medium that permits visual differentiation of colonies of different kinds of organisms.

Dimorphic fungi: Fungi that may exist in either of two forms depending on environmental conditions, e.g. *Histoplasma capsulatum* exists in soil as a mold, but in host tissues as a yeast.

Disinfection: The destruction of any microbe that is capable of producing infection.

DPT triple vaccine: A vaccine containing 3 immunogens: diphtheria toxoid, killed *Bordetella pertussis* and tetanus toxoid.

Dysentery: Inflammation of the intestine, characterized by abdominal pain, tenesmus, and diarrhea in which the feces contain blood and mucus.

Endogenous pyrogens: Substances produced by granulocytes, macrophages, and perhaps other cells that act on the hypothalamus to cause fever.

Endospore: A heat-resistant resting form of bacteria produced within the vegetative cell.

Endotoxin: A toxic moiety of complexed protein, lipid and polysaccharide present in the cell walls of gram-negative bacteria.

ENL (erythema nodosum leprosum): Erythema nodosum lesion that occurs in some patients with leprosy, particularly in drug-treated patients with lepromatous and intermediate forms of leprosy; presumed to represent an Arthus type of reaction and to result from Ag-Ab-C complexes deposited in the vessels of the skin.

Enrichment medium: A medium that favors the growth of one organism over others in a mixture.

Enterobacteria: Bacteria that are commonly associated with the intestine.

Enteropathic E. coli: Strains of *E. coli* that are capable of causing intestinal disease.

Enterotoxin: A toxin that produces pathologic changes in the alimentary tract, e.g. cholera toxin.

Eosinophilic: Having affinity for eosin (a red acid dye).

Epidemic: A disease outbreak affecting an unusually large proportion of a human population; usually subsides within months or a few years at most.

Episome: A fragment of DNA (carrying genetic information) existing either free in the cytoplasm or integrated into the chromosome.

Epithelioid cell: A nonmotile transformed macrophage which characterizes the allergic granuloma; epithelioid cells typically occur in the center of the primary granuloma as closely adherent collections of pale-staining, elongated, epithelial-like cells.

Epithet: The species name or second part of a Latin binomial.

Epizootic: A disease outbreak affecting an unusually large proportion of an animal population.

Erythema multiforme: An acute, inflammatory skin lesion in which red papules, macules or tubercles appear, usually on the head, neck and extremities.

Erythema nodosum: A painful self-limiting lesion in the dermis, particularly over bony prominences of the extremities; it is characterized by an infiltrate rich in lymphocytes and occurs in a number of diseases including rheumatic fever; it probably represents an allergic lesion.

Erythema nodosum leprosum: (see ENL)

Erythematous rash: Red skin eruption occurring in patches of varying size and shape.

Erythrogenic toxin: A toxin produced by group A streptococci that causes erythema of the skin (scarlet fever).

Eschar: A dry mass of necrotic tissue that separates from living tissue, as in certain burn wounds and some infections.

Eumycetes: True eucaryotic fungi.

Exogenous fungal spores: Spores formed on the exterior of hyphae.

FA test: Fluorescent Ab test.

Facultative aerobe: An organism that grows best anaerobically but can adapt to an aerobic environment.

Facultative anaerobe: An organism that grows best aerobically but can adapt to an anaerobic environment.

Facultative parasite: A saprophyte that can assume a parasitic existence.

Facultative pathogen (opportunistic pathogen): A nonpathogenic microbe (parasite or saprophyte) that, under abnormal circumstances, can invade and produce disease. An example is *Candida albicans* infection in immunosuppressed individuals.

Facultative saprophyte: A parasite that can assume a saprophytic existence.

Fermentation: The metabolic process in which the final electron acceptor is an organic compound.

Fluorescent Ab: Antibody coupled with a fluorescent dye.

Formalin: A saturated aqueous solution (about 40%) of gaseous formaldehyde at room temperature.

Forssman Ag: A widely distributed heterophile Ag. For example, when sheep RBC's that contain Forssman Ag are injected into the rabbit (an animal lacking Forssman Ag) so-called "Forssman Ab" is formed.

Frei reaction: Specific skin test reaction to the causative agent of lymphogranuloma venereum.

Freund's adjuvants: (see Adjuvant)

FTA test: Serologic test for syphilis in which a slide preparation of *T. pallidum* is exposed to the patient's serum, washed and finally exposed to a fluorescent labeled anti-globulin serum.

FTA-Abs test (fluorescent treponemal antibody absorption test): A test for syphilis in which the patient's serum is absorbed with Ag of the nonpathogenic Reiter strain treponeme before applying the regular FTA test.

Furuncle: Localized abscess developing from an infected hair follicle.

Genetic transformation: Genetic change(s) induced in recipient bacteria by the uptake and incorporation of short pieces of free DNA from donor bacteria.

Genotype: The genetic constitution of an organism.

Ghon complex: A healed pathologic complex comprising the residium of a solitary lesion (Ghon tubercle) of primary tuberculosis with associated infection of the draining lymph nodes; usually develops in childhood.

Giemsa stain: A stain commonly used for hemopoietic tissue and blood and for visualizing some of the bacteria and protozoa that live in blood cells.

Glabrous skin: Smooth, hairless skin.

Globi: Collections of "foamy macrophages" filled with *M. leprae* and bacterial lipid that characterize the lesions of lepromatous leprosy.

Gram-negative sepsis: A severe toxic, febrile state resulting from infection with enteric gram-negative rods or from parenteral administration of endotoxins of such bacteria.

Granuloma: A lesion comprising a collection of macrophages and macrophage-derived cells (such as epithelioid cells and sometimes giant cells) and often lymphocytes. The epithelioid cell is the hallmark of the granuloma.

Halophilic (salt-loving) bacteria: Bacteria that grow best in high concentrations of salt.

Heat stroke: A heat exposure syndrome characterized by hyperpyrexia, prostration, diminution of sweating, and death; it results from elevated body temperatures of about 106° F and above which are presumed to destroy the thermoregulatory center in the brain.

Hemagglutinin: A substance that agglutinates RBC's; often a specific Ab. Examples are the anti-A and anti-B Abs of the ABO blood group system, and the hemagglutinating enzyme of influenza virus (viral hemagglutinin).

Hematopoietic tissue (hemopoietic tissue): Blood cell-forming tissue.

Herd resistance (herd immunity): The overall resistance possessed by a human or animal population.

Herpes-like lesion: Vesicular lesion resembling the lesions caused by herpes viruses; example, the coldsore of herpes simplex virus infection.

Heterophile Ag: Antigen common to different species.

HSF: "Histamine sensitizing factor"; the factor of *Bordetella pertussis* that renders animals hypersensitive to histamine.

Humoral immunity: Immunity that can be transferred with serum (may also be transferred with cells that synthesize and release Ab); initiated by the specific response of B cells to Ag which in some instances requires the helper activity of T-cells.

Hyperplasia: Increase in tissue mass or size of an organ as the result of an increase in cell numbers.

Hypha (pl. hyphae): One of the branching, usually septate, tubular filaments that make up the growing portion of a fungal mycelium.

Hypovolemic shock: Shock caused by reduced blood volume.

Iatrogenic infection: Infection transmitted to patients by attending physicians.

IC (inclusion conjunctivitis): An eye disease caused by chlamydiae.

Immediate sensitivity (immediate hypersensitivity): A state of specific sensitivity mediated by Abs and characterized by a short onset time and course of reaction after contact with Ag; example, the wheal-flare skin reaction mounted by a hay-fever patient in response to a pollen scratch test.

Immune: In the biological sense the term was first used to designate resistance to injury resulting from infectious agents. Recently its meaning has been extended to include the ability to react specifically with an Ag irrespective of whether or not it is injurious. Thus an animal which, because it possesses Abs, can react specifically with a bland substance such as egg albumin is said to be "immune."

Immune clearance: Clearance of Ag from the circulating blood due to complexing of Ag with Ab; C may also fix to the Ag-Ab complexes and aid in clearance.

Immune complex disease: Disease resulting from the deposition of circulating soluble Ag-Ab complexes in tissues, especially along basement membranes and in vessel walls. The deposited complexes usually contain C. Examples: post-streptococcal glomerulonephritis, systemic lupus erythematosus and vascular lesions of the Arthus reaction.

Immune response(s): Specific response to an Ag involving either B-cells and/or T-cells; comprises the humoral immune response and the cellular immune response.

Immunize: The act or process of rendering an individual resistant or immune to a harmful agent. Often used loosely to designate a specific response to an Ag irrespective of whether or not the response may be protective.

Immunogen: A substance that engenders a specific response, either cellular or humoral, irrespective of whether or not the host is protected. Also used to designate a substance that engenders specific protective immunity.

Immunosuppressive agent: Any agent, physical or chemical, that can suppress specific immune responses. Examples are x-irradiation, azathioprine and antilymphocyte globulin.

Inapparent infection (subclinical infection, latent infection, silent infection): An infection lacking clinical symptoms.

Inclusion bodies: Intracellular masses of abnormal material, often foreign, e.g. viruses or chlamydiae.

Incomplete Abs: Antibodies that can react with specific Ag-determinants but fail to bring about precipitation or agglutination. They are usually IgG Abs and are detected by such tests as the Coombs' antiglobulin test or by adding albumin to the system. So-called nonprecipitating Abs, univalent Abs, nonagglutinating Abs and blocking Abs represent incomplete Abs.

Infection: The presence of microbes in parenteral tissues.

Infection immunity: Immunity that accompanies infection but drops precipitously after infection has ceased; usually, if not always, due to cellular immunity.

INH: Isoniazid hydrochloride; a drug used for the therapy of tuberculosis.

Innate immunity: That immunity which is not acquired but which is inherent to the species; immunity that does not rest on previous experience with a harmful agent or related agents. Innate immunity is in contrast to immunity acquired during the life of the individual as a consequence of experience with the agent or a related agent.

Integration: With reference to DNA it designates the covalent bonding of DNA from a donor organism with the recipient chromosome.

Intercurrent infection: (see Secondary infection)

Intracellular parasite: An organism that normally grows inside a cell; it can be obligately or facultatively intracellular.

K-antigen: An antigenic component present on the surface of certain organisms, particularly gram-negative rods, that serves to protect them against host defenses such as phagocytosis.

Keratinized cells: Cells containing keratins, the water-insoluble proteins that give hair, skin, and nails their horny, tough properties.

Keratinophilic: Having an affinity for keratinized cells, e.g. certain fungi.

Kupffer cells: Fixed macrophages lining the sinusoids of the liver.

L forms of bacteria: Bacteria with deficient cell walls.

Latent infection: (see Inapparent infection)

Latent period (of infection of cells by virus): The interval between penetration of a virus and host cell lysis.

Leukopenia: Abnormally low number of leukocytes in the blood.

Limbs of the immune response: Afferent, central and efferent; the afferent limb relates to recognition, and processing Ag by macrophages, and recognition of Ag by lymphocytes; the central limb relates to the responses of lymphocytes to Ag, including blastogenesis, proliferation, and differentiation leading to the production of Abs and/or "immune cells" (lymphocytes and macrophages); the efferent limb relates to the various activities of Abs and immune cells.

LPF: "Lymphocyte promoting factor"; the factor of *Bordetella pertussis* that causes the lymphocytosis of pertussis.

LPS (lipopolysaccharide):   Example, endotoxin of gram-negative bacteria.

Lumbar puncture: Puncture of the spinal canal in the lumbar region, usually for the removal of cerebrospinal fluid or introduction of medications.

Lymphadenopathy: A disease process affecting lymph nodes.

Lymphokines: Biologically active soluble components or products of lymphocytes that are secreted or liberated as the result of various stimuli, including Ags and mitogens.

Lymphoreticular system: The system comprising lymphoid tissue and associated cells and components, including reticulum cells and reticular fibrils.

Lysogenic conversion of bacteria: A change in the properties of a bacterium that results from carriage of a prophage, e.g. the conversion of a nontoxin-producing bacterium by the action of a prophage.

Lysozyme: an enzyme that degrades murein, a component of the cell walls of many bacteria.

M protein: An acid-resistant, heat-resistant, type specific, surface protein of group A streptococci; it is both the key factor of virulence and the effective immunogen. It is also found in other bacteria including *D. pneumoniae*.

Maceration: Softening or disintegration of tissue resulting from excessive exposure to a liquid or other agents, e.g. the skin of the hands often becomes macerated following long exposure to moist conditions.

Macroconidium (pl. macroconidia): The larger of two types of conidia (spores) produced by fungi that bear both large and small (microconidia) spores.

Menadione: 2-methyl-1, 4-naphthoquinone; water-insoluble substance with vitamin-K activity.

Meningocele: A protrusion of the cerebral or spinal meninges through a defect in the skull or vertebral column, resulting in a cyst filled with cerebrospinal fluid.

Metastatic lesions: Lesions produced by the transfer of the causative agent from a primary focus to a distant location via blood vessels or lymph channels.

Microconidium (pl. microconidia): The smaller of two types of conidia (spores) in fungi that bear both large (macroconidia) and small spores.

MIF (migration inhibition factor): A lymphokine that inhibits the normal migration of macrophages in culture.

Mitsuda reaction: An allergic granulomatous response to the Mitsuda skin test with killed *M. leprae*. The response is positive in the majority of normal adults and in patients with the tuberculoid form of leprosy but not in those with the lepromatous form. A negative response is of value in establishing the diagnosis of lepromatous leprosy.

Morbilliform rash: A skin rash that resembles the fine, rose-red maculopapular rash of measles (morbilli).

Mycelium (pl. mycelia): The mass of hyphae, often cotton-like, that comprises a colony of mold.

Mycetoma (maduromycosis): A chronic infection caused by various fungi, actinomycetes, or streptomycetes.

Myxomatous: Mucinous, mucoid.

NADase: An enzyme that degrades nicotinamide-adenine dinucleotide.

Natural host: A host in which an organism naturally perpetuates itself.

Normal microbial flora (indigenous microbial flora): Microbes that normally perpetuate themselves on the body surface of essentially every individual of a species; they usually cause no harm to the host.

Nosocomial infections: Hospital-related infections.

Ophthalmia neonatorum: Acute purulent gonococcal conjunctivitis in the newborn usually acquired during passage through the birth canal.

Opportunistic pathogen: (see Facultative pathogen)

Opsonins: Substances that combine with particles and in so doing promote phagocytosis; often Abs and C.

Pandemic: A widespread epidemic.

PAP: Primary atypical pneumonia; it is due to *Mycoplasma pneumoniae*.

Parasite: An organism that lives in or on another organism.

Parenteral (outside the intestine): Parenteral tissues are tissues underlying the surface integuments of the body. For example, materials are injected "parenterally," e.g. subcutaneously, intramuscularly, intravenously, etc.

PAS: Periodic-acid-schiff stain which imparts a bright-red color to fungal cell walls and other carbohydrate-rich substances; this abbreviation is sometimes also used for para-aminosalicylic acid.

Passive immunity: Immunity acquired from without through acquisition of either immune serum or immune cells including T-cells, B-cells, plasma cells and macrophages.

Pasteurization: Use of mild heat to kill all vegetative pathogens.

Pathogen: A parasite that is capable of producing illness in a significant number of healthy individuals lacking acquired immunity.

Pathogenesis: The sequence of events that leads to disease including modes of injury and development of lesions.

Periodontal: Surrounding a tooth, as the periodontal membrane; a periodontal abscess involves the side of the tooth root.

Periplasmic enzymes: Enzymes loosely attached to the outer surface of the cytoplasmic membrane.

Perlèche: An inflammatory condition at the angles of the mouth, often caused by infection with *Candida albicans*.

Petechial rash: Small, rounded, hemorrhagic spots on the skin or mucous membranes.

Phagocyte: A cell possessing the specialized function of engulfing particulate material, also called "professional phagocyte" to differentiate it from cells that only rarely phagocytize material.

Phagocytosis: The process by which cells ingest particulate materials and enclose them within vesicles (phagosomes); the particles may be engulfed by the action of pseudopods of the cell or by simple invagination of the cytoplasmic membrane followed by internalization of the phagosome.

Phagolysosome: A vesicle resulting from the fusion of a phagosome with a lysosome(s).

Phagosome: The cytoplasmic ingestion vesicle of phagocytosis bounded by cytoplasmic membrane.

Phenol coefficient: A measure of the disinfectant capacity of a substance compared with that of phenol under standard conditions.

Phenotype: The outward expression of the genotype.

Pinocytosis (cell drinking): The ingestion of fluids by cells; it involves ingestion mechanisms similar to those of phagocytosis.

Pleomorphic microbes: Marked variation in shape and size of microbes of a given species.

Polyvalent antiserum: An antiserum containing Abs specific for more than one Ag or microbe. Often used for prophylaxis or therapy of disease.

Pott's disease: Tuberculosis of the spine.

PPLO: Pleuropneumonia-like organism (mycoplasma).

Prophage: The nucleic acid of a temperate phage following its integration with the bacterial chromosome

Protoplast: A cell that has had its cell wall removed.

Pseudo-membrane: A "false membrane" or membrane-like material consisting of fibrin and necrotic material.

Pseudomycetes: Bacteria that resemble the fungi (eumycetes) in that they usually form hyphae-like filaments and may produce spores.

Psychrophile: A cold-loving organism, e.g. a species of microbe that grows best at temperatures below 20° C.

Pure culture: The progeny of a single organism.

Pyelonephritis: Inflammation of the kidney including the renal pelvis; it usually results from infections of the kidney.

Pyocins: Bacteriocins produced by *Pseudomonas aeruginosa.*

Pyogenic microbe: A microbe that induces the formation of pus.

Pyrexia: Fever.

Pyrogens: Substances that induce fever. Endogenous fever-inducing substances liberated from body cells, including neutrophils and macrophages. Exogenous pyrogens include substances liberated from bacteria that cause fever apparently by injuring cells with resulting liberation of endogenous pyrogen.

Quellung reaction: Swelling of the bacterial capsule as the result of combining with specific Ab (see also Capsular swelling test).

R factors: Plasmids consisting of RTF (resistance transfer factor) responsible for conjugation and R genes that code for resistance to antibiotics; a single R factor can transmit resistance to a number of antibacterial agents simultaneously.

RBC's: Red blood cells (erythrocytes).

Reactivation disease: Disease that reappears due to the renewed activity of residual organisms of preexisting disease; sometimes erroneously termed "endogenous reinfection." An example is reactivation tuberculosis.

Reinfection: An infection that occurs after recovery from a previous infection with the same agent. Reinfection is, of necessity, exogenous and not endogenous.

RES: A functional system derived from mesenchyme comprising macrophages and reticular tissue. The recent tendency is to extend the term to include all elements of the lymphoid system.

Reservoir of infection: A source or storehouse of an infectious agent.

Resolving power (of the microscope): Power to distinguish between two neighboring objects or points.

Reticular cell (reticulum cell): A cell that occurs in lymphoid tissue in association with reticular fibrils. It has a pale-staining nucleus and a fine cytoplasmic membrane that is difficult to visualize; its function is not known.

Reticular tissue: Reticulum cells and associated reticular fibrils found in lymphoid structures, e.g. lymph nodes, bone marrow, and spleen.

RF: Rheumatic fever.

Rheumatic fever (RF): A sequela of group A streptococcal infection.

Rose spots: Small erythematous areas in the skin of typhoid fever patients.

RT: Respiratory tract.

RTF (resistance transfer factor): The plasmid genes responsible for conjugation and subsequent transfer of R factors; RTF together with R (resistance) genes make up an R factor.

Rubelliform rash: Resembling the pale-pink rash of rubella (German measles).

S: Smooth, pertaining to the appearance of bacterial colonies; also used as an abbreviation for Svedberg units, the units of sedimentation (as in 70 S ribosomes).

Saprophyte: An organism that normally exists on dead organic material.

Secondary infection (superinfection, intercurrent infection): Commonly used to designate an infection that is superimposed on an existing infection due to another agent. The term has also been used in rare instances in which the superimposed exogenous infection is caused by the same agent (reinfection).

Selective medium: A medium that restricts the growth of unwanted, but not wanted organisms in a mixture.

Sepsis: Illness due to the presence of pathogenic microbes and their toxins in the body, especially pyogenic microbes.

Septic shock: Shock (often fatal) that results from a state of acute sepsis.

Septicemia: Presence of microbes in the bloodstream with associated sepsis.

Sequela (pl. sequelae): A morbid condition that follows as a consequence of a foregoing disease.

Serotyping: Immunologic procedure employing specific antisera to distinguish between closely related organisms (commonly strains within a species); it is based on antigenic differences.

Shwartzman phenomenon: A local nonimmunologic inflammatory reaction characterized by hemorrhage and necrosis and produced by the injection of sequential doses of endotoxin. It probably occurs naturally under special circumstances and can be generalized as well as localized.

Silent infection: (see Inapparent infection)

Sinus tracts: Pathways through tissues produced by the pressure of accumulated pus; often the pus escapes from the tissues when the tract opens to the outside.

Somatic: Pertaining to the body, except for the germ cells; in bacteria, Ags that are a part of the bacterial cell, rather than secreted, e.g. the lipopolysaccharide Ags that are part of the cell walls of gram-negative bacteria.

Spheroplast: A cell wall-deficient bacterium that retains some of its cell wall material.

Splenomegaly: Enlargement of the spleen.

Sporulation: The act of forming spores.

SR mutation: Mutation of bacteria involving organisms that produce smooth (S) and rough (R) colonies.

Sterigma (pl. sterigmata): A narrow, pointed structure arising from a cell and supporting a spore.

Sterile: Free of all living organisms.

Subclinical infection: (see Inapparent infection)

Superinfection: (see Secondary infection)

Surface phagocytosis: Phagocytosis which demands that the particle be trapped against a surface.

Syndrome: A group of symptoms and signs that, taken together, characterize a disease or lesion.

TAB vaccine: A vaccine formerly used to give partial protection against typhoid fever and other salmonella-induced enteric fevers; the vaccine consists of killed *Salmonella typhi* and paratyphoid A and B organisms.

Temperate phage: A bacteriophage that can either become integrated into the host cell DNA as a prophage or can replicate in the host cell cytoplasm causing cell lysis.

Tenesmus: Painful but unsuccessful efforts to expel feces or urine.

Terminal host: An individual host that cannot pass the organisms on to another host.

Thrombocytopenic purpura: Hemorrhages in the skin, mucous membranes and elsewhere (purpura) resulting from lack of platelets.

Thrombophlebitis: An inflammation of veins leading to the formation of blood clots (thrombi); it is often due to bacterial infection.

Tissue tropism: The property of a parasite that enables it to localize selectively in a tissue, often resulting from a specific affinity of the organism for a certain type of cell in a tissue.

Toxigenic: The ability to engender a toxic state in an animal.

Toxinogenic: The ability to produce a toxin.

Toxoid: A modified exotoxin that has been treated to destroy its toxicity but not its antigenicity.

TPI test (treponema immobilization test): A test for syphilis based on an Ab that acts with C to cause immobilization of *T. pallidum.*

Transcription: The process of transferring genetic information coded in DNA into messenger RNA. The copying of the message of DNA into RNA by a process that involves base pairing of complementary RNA with the DNA and polymerization of the bases so ordered.

Transient microbial flora: Organisms that propagate transiently on body surfaces.

TRIC agents: The chlamydiae that cause trachoma and inclusion conjunctivitis.

Tuberculin test: An intradermal test with tuberculin. The test is useful as a screening measure for detecting tuberculous infection. A positive reaction indicates that the individual is or, in the very recent past, has been infected with *M. tuberculosis.*

Tuberculins: Preparations derived from culture filtrates of tubercle bacilli used in skin tests to detect infection with *M. tuberculosis;* old tuberculin (O.T.), a glycerine-containing heated culture filtrate; purified protein derivative (PPD), a preparation derived from O.T. The active components in tuberculins are proteins and protein fragments having molecular weights of less than 10,000.

Tyndallization (intermittent sterilization): Sterilization of media by heating near the boiling point after several successive intervals of incubation of 12 hours or more to allow spore germination.

Unnatural host (accidental host): A host in which an organism does not naturally perpetuate itself.

URT: Upper respiratory tract.

UT: Urinary tract.

Vaccine: A suspension of organisms (commonly attenuated or killed) used for immunization. Often used loosely to designate any material employed for active immunization.

VDRL test (Venereal Disease Research Laboratory Test): A flocculation (precipitation) test for syphilis.

Vector: A living agent that transmits microbes, e.g. an arthropod that transmits rickettsiae between animal hosts. Conveyance may be mechanical (mechanical vector) or the microbe may multiply, transform, or undergo life cycle changes in the vector (biologic vector).

Vegetative microbe: The growing form of a microbe.

Vincent's disease (Vincent's angina, trench mouth, necrotizing ulcerative gingivitis): Infection of the oral mucosa characterized by ulceration and formation of a gray pseudomembrane; fusiform bacteria and spirochetes are found in abundance in the lesions.

Viridans streptococci: Streptococci that produce colonies in blood agar surrounded by zones of greenish color and associated partial hemolysis; they occur in a number of different systematic groups.

Virulence: The quality of being poisonous or malignant; disease-producing power or pathogenicity of a microbe; sometimes used to designate degrees of pathogenicity of strains of parasites within a species.

Virulence factors: Factors that endow a microbe with the property of virulence. Only certain factors of virulence may be evident (key factors).

Waterhouse-Friderichsen syndrome: A syndrome characterized by bacteremia, especially acute meningococcemia; it is manifested by massive skin hemorrhage, shock, and acute adrenal hemorrhage and insufficiency.

WHO: World Health Organization.

Widal test: A specific agglutination test used in the diagnosis of typhoid fever.

Wild-type strains: Strains of microbes with the genetic constitution of the majority of strains of that microbe found in nature.

Index